Craniosacral Rhythm

AF856828

Publisher: Sarena Wolfaard
Commissioning Editor: Claire Wilson
Project Manager: Christine Johnston
Design Direction: Sarah Russell
Illustrations: Susanne Noller and Michael Hartmann
Photographs: Toni Blättler

Craniosacral Rhythm

A practical guide to a gentle form of bodywork therapy

Daniel Agustoni

Translated by David Beattie and Elaine Richards

Foreword by Ruediger Dahlke

CHURCHILL LIVINGSTONE
ELSEVIER

EDINBURGH LONDON NEW YORK OXFORD PHILADELPHIA ST LOUIS SYDNEY TORONTO 2008

CHURCHILL
LIVINGSTONE
ELSEVIER
An imprint of Elsevier Limited

© 2008. Daniel Agustoni. All rights reserved.

This translation is based upon Craniosacral-Rhythmus © 2006.
The translation was undertaken by the Publisher.

The right of Daniel Agustoni to be identified as author of this work has been asserted by him in accordance with the Copyright, Designs and Patents Act 1988.

No part of this publication may be reproduced, stored in a retrieval system, or transmitted in any form or by any means, electronic, mechanical, photocopying, recording or otherwise, without the prior permission of the Publishers. Permissions may be sought directly from Elsevier's Health Sciences Rights Department, 1600 John F. Kennedy Boulevard, Suite 1800, Philadelphia, PA 19103-2899, USA: phone: (+1) 215 239 3804; fax: (+1) 215 239 3805; or, e-mail: *healthpermissions@elsevier.com*. You may also complete your request on-line via the Elsevier homepage (http://www.elsevier.com), by selecting 'Support and contact' and then 'Copyright and Permission'.

ISBN: 978 0443 067372

British Library Cataloguing in Publication Data
A catalogue record for this book is available from the British Library

Library of Congress Cataloging in Publication Data
A catalog record for this book is available from the Library of Congress

Note
Neither the Publisher nor the Author assume any responsibility for any loss or injury and/or damage to persons or property arising out of or related to any use of the material contained in this book. It is the responsibility of the treating practitioner, relying on independent expertise and knowledge of the patient, to determine the best treatment and method of application for the patient.

The Publisher

ELSEVIER your source for books, journals and multimedia in the health sciences
www.elsevierhealth.com

Printed in China

Working together to grow libraries in developing countries
www.elsevier.com | www.bookaid.org | www.sabre.org
ELSEVIER BOOK AID International Sabre Foundation

The Publisher's policy is to use **paper manufactured from sustainable forests**

Contents

Preface

During a training course in massage in 1989, I experienced a remarkably pleasurable and deep relaxation. The instructor in charge showed us a simple hand position that we were to use to apply touch to the head of our partners as we practiced in pairs; he offered no further explanation. He came to each pair in turn as we worked, likewise applied touch to the person's head, and occasionally remarked, 'the cranium and the body slowly inhale … and exhale …'

Perhaps past experience had prepared me: the various courses I had already attended, the many sessions of biodynamic therapy as devised by Gerda Boyesen and many years of meditation had rendered me familiar with deep relaxation and ready to commit to a profound 'letting go'. After a few minutes of this application of touch to my head, my relaxation deepened. At the same time, I knew precisely where I was at that moment (place, time, position in the room, and who was touching my head).To my surprise, I was at the same time exceptionally relaxed and present. I felt at once safe, securely held and weightless, as in my mother's womb or floating free in space. This happened, deepened, and all without any technique being performed on me.

Days, even weeks after this first 'craniosacral experience' all I needed to do was to close my eyes and attune myself, and immediately the relaxation would intensify and a subtle craniosacral flow would pulse through the whole of my body, into every cell. Fortunately, after my remarkable experience I had asked the instructor in charge of the course what it was that he had shown us. He gave a little smile and said, 'that is craniosacral therapy'.

Impressed by the deep relaxation and the experience of receiving touch in the entirety of my whole self, I knew that this is where my future direction lay. I had a deep desire to discover more about this fascinating method, and explore it in depth. I could never have predicted then the paths (both inward and external) along which this gentle form of bodywork would lead me! There followed an initial course, full-length training courses, assistant placements, and attendance at courses held by many teachers of different branches of craniosacral therapy. After some years of craniosacral practice, I founded the Sphinx Craniosacral Institute in Basel, where I have now been teaching for 10 years. Lectures and courses for various institutions in several countries also followed.

On the basis of my own experience and especially my teaching, I realized how important it is for beginners to have easily-understood explanations on how to carry out a thorough basic treatment, to complement their instruction. So it was, that this practical guide began to take shape, 10 years ago. The first of four editions appeared in 1999.

This work, *Craniosacral Rhythm* [originally *Craniosacral-Rhythmus*, in German], became established as a standard text for beginners and those with an interest in the subject. My second book, its companion volume, 'Craniosacral-Selbstbehandlung', appeared in German in 2004 (published by Kösel-Verlag).

Over the years, I have continually updated the first edition of *Craniosacral-Rhythmus* and expanded it to create the present new edition [now in English, published by Churchill Livingstone]. This practical guide provides information for lay persons and those with medical training about this form of bodywork therapy and how it works, and presents the most important background principles and basic techniques. The original book has also been enlarged with the addition of certain chapters and with the addition of further tips derived from actual practice.

It is an important concern of mine to convey to the reader the sort of basic appreciation that will enable the best possible understanding of the essence of this subtle form of bodywork. The self-palpation, self-treatment techniques and guided journey around the body that this book provides will help build up the practitioner's own experience of the craniosacral rhythm, an expression of the *Breath of Life*. For the benefit of first-time readers and those who want to 'dip into' the book, some particularly important points and essential links have been repeated from time to time.

The time is right to help successful methods of 'gentle medicine' to become more widely accepted and to achieve the position they deserve. Across the world, more and more physicians, physiotherapists, midwives, practitioners of complementary and alternative medicine and therapists – among other reasons because of the limits of allopathic medicine – have shown great interest in craniosacral therapy, because its effects include a harmonizing influence on the central nervous system, resulting in a broad treatment spectrum.

The great demand in some practices underlines the increasing need of many people for the kind of treatment forms offered by complementary medicine, energy medicine and holistic medicine in supporting and assisting healing.

Today, craniosacral therapy is in use on every continent. There are now projects (e.g., in Ukraine, Honduras, and India) in which physicians, healthcare workers, physiotherapists and other professionals are being trained in craniosacral therapy and needy adults and children are receiving treatment.

The holistic form of treatment described in this book helps considerably in preventive health treatment and regeneration from within.

It gives me enormous pleasure that 'Craniosacral Rhythm' is now also available in English.

My wish is that craniosacral treatment will be available in many places and able to contribute to relaxation and healing and to quality of life and joy, both on the personal and the collective level.

Basel, Spring 2007 Daniel Agustoni

Acknowledgments

I should like to express here my heartfelt thanks to all my teachers, in particular to Dr William Martin Allen, from whom and with whom it has been my privilege to learn so much over the past years. I should also like to thank all the craniosacral therapists, teams and study groups with whom I have repeatedly learnt and experienced new things.

I owe a major debt of gratitude to the founder and pioneer of cranial osteopathy, William G. Sutherland, and also to Viola M. Frymann, Rollin E. Becker and John E. Upledger. It was Dr Upledger who simplified this form of therapy and – by including the element of therapeutic dialog – made it accessible to a wider public.

My special thanks are due to James Jealous for his *Biodynamics of Osteopathy*. It is your collective spirit of enquiry and courage that has enabled us today to achieve such magnificent successes with craniosacral therapy and cranial osteopathy.

I am indebted to all those colleagues and friends who have supported me in my work on this book. Special thanks go to Petra Reinmuth, Heini Müller and Joachim Lichtenberg for their detailed review of the manuscript. I am also deeply grateful to Christine Mäder in the administrative office of the Sphinx Craniosacral Institute, to Elli Sexauer and Karin Wenger, and to the models Amélie B. Kim, Garimaa B. Wettengel and the children.

Sincere thanks go to my photographer, Toni Blättler, and to Michael Hartmann and Susanne Noller for the line drawings, and to Tom Schneider for his help in designing the poster.

I am grateful also to Dr Ruediger Dahlke for his foreword to the original German edition of this book, to my two translators (Elaine Richards and David Beattie) for their diligence and expertise, and to Churchill Livingstone for publishing this English edition.

I should like to record my special thanks to the clients attending my practice and to the delegates on my training courses because for me craniosacral therapy is an ongoing process of learning and growing together.

Note from the author

The techniques and treatment approaches mentioned in this book are among other things drawn from the research and practice of W.G. Sutherland, H.I. Magoun, V.M. Frymann, R.E. Becker, E.W. Retzlaff, J.E. Upledger, J.S. Jealous and W.M. Allen.

The use of 'he' or 'she' when referring to individuals such as the practitioner, therapist, client or other person is for ease of reading and relevance to the individual illustrated; it should not be taken to imply masculine or feminine identity generally. In every case, the one should be assumed to include the other.

Note on the legal position

All treatment suggestions, advice and instructions in this book have been carefully scrutinized and tested by the author. Nevertheless no guarantee can be given. The publishers and authors do not assume any responsibility for any injury and/or damage to persons, property or finances.

The methods described in the book are no substitute for treatment by conventional medical or other recognized natural health practitioner when dealing with serious health problems.

The practice of body work is subject to different regulations in different countries and administrations. You should seek advice on the legal position from your legal advisers, professional association or authorities such as the government department of health before offering treatment to patients or sick people or in return for payment.

The responsibility for any treatment carried out is your own.

A word of advice: If you wish to give treatment to healthy individuals (e.g. friends or family as an aid to relaxation), you are advised to attend specialist courses, undergo supervision and receive treatment yourself from a craniosacral practitioner. If you wish to give treatment therapeutically, you are advised to follow a well-established course of further specialist training in craniosacral practice lasting several years.

Foreword

Ruediger Dahlke

Not many new therapeutic approaches have experienced as rapid a spread as craniosacral therapy – and this has happened despite the fact that there has so far been so little detailed popular literature on the subject, apart from the very personal account *Your Inner Physician and You* by John E. Upledger, to inform therapists and interested lay persons about this therapeutic method. Daniel Agustoni's book fills this gap: written by an experienced practitioner, its approach is highly practice-oriented; on the one hand it provides a way for therapists to feel their way into and learn about this treatment approach, and on the other, it offers practical exercises to enable interested lay persons to slowly work toward craniosacral rhythm, a phenomenon that was discovered so late because it oscillates so deep inside the center of the human person.

The idea that 'all life is rhythm' was declared by Rudolf Steiner. The concept that 'all life is dance' was pronounced by the former Harvard academic psychologist Richard Alpert and later teacher Ram Dass. Today, even the quantum physicists tell us that everything in this universe is a matter of waves and wavefunctions, from the innermost parts of the atom to the outermost reaches of the universe. So it is hardly surprising that the nervous system too oscillates in its own intrinsic rhythm, the craniosacral rhythm. Everything suggests that this rhythm is indeed the most fundamental of all; certainly it is the first to appear, it is already present in the fetus and it remains longer than any other at the leaving of our bodies, in the process of dying. It therefore seems no exaggeration to speak here of the pulse of life, with as much justification as we do when speaking of the cardiac rhythm, that of the heart.

If it remains difficult to this day for entrenched adherents of conventional medicine even to acknowledge the existence of the craniosacral rhythm, this difficulty may partly be connected with the fact that it requires much greater sensitivity to sense the craniosacral rhythm than it does for example to perceive the cardiac pulse.

There are on the other hand, many more prejudices to be overcome before it becomes acceptable to believe that it could exist: generations of medical students in our universities have learnt that the cranial bones unite solidly in the course of childhood and from then on for the rest of a person's life form a mechanical unity. It is precisely here, through motions felt at the cranial bones – which have so long been thought immobile – that sensitive hands 'illegally' as it were, detect the craniosacral rhythm.

We also need to remember that even the cardiac pulse that we take so for granted today and can detect and sense so easily had difficulty at first in becoming recognized. More than 100 years after the discovery by William Harvey of the circulation of the blood, the Bavarian surgeon Reisinger at the University of Munich was able to laugh at Harvey and his 'supposed circulation'. To this very day, a streetname in the hospital quarter of Munich recalls the obstinate surgeon; you will search in vain for a street named after Harvey.

To us today, the idea of the circulation of the blood as a coherent, closed system with the heart at its center is a self-evident fact. Perhaps the fact that it took so long to become accepted could also be connected with the fact that Harvey put forward his discovery too much along the lines of an analogy of the world, or at least, he explained it in such images. He saw the circulating blood of the human body as obeying the same laws as the waters of the earth, so that the concept was still based in the macrocosm–microcosm thinking of Paracelsus.

If such an easily comprehensible story had such a hard struggle to overcome the forces of university medicine that were ranged against progress, we might fear that craniosacral rhythm, demanding as it does such sensitivity, would need far longer to achieve recognition and receive attention in the universities.

A constantly growing number of alternative therapists and the many in need of help who put their trust in the power of Nature is not prepared to wait that long. The triumphant march of craniosacral therapy is bypassing the universities, as so many groundbreaking discoveries have done before, and it is in some cases spreading even more quickly and effectively as a result. My own experience in the interpretation of disease symptoms leads me to think that the route outside that of conventional medicine may turn out to be a more successful means of spreading new methods; the advantage here is that they face stern competition, in a system of direct responsibility and usually without reimbursement of costs. The only survivors of such competition will be those methods that can prove themselves. Anything that can gain acceptance despite a (healthy) handicap must be to some extent effective, because no-one would be willing in the long term to have treatment that costs money and achieves nothing. This is of course an argument that also applies to traditional homeopathy, the interpretation of disease symptoms, and many others.

When we consider how much more information is derived from Chinese pulse diagnosis than by taking the pulse in the western manner, we can gain some idea of the subtle detail available in the information we could obtain from the rhythm of the system of fluids bathing the brain and spinal cord, and conducted by their surrounding membranes. Whereas a western physician is mainly able to discover from the pulse that the patient is still alive and how rapidly the patient's heart is beating, a traditional Chinese healer can use the various qualities of the pulse to obtain information about almost every organ system in the body.

In this respect, good craniosacral therapists are more like the masters of Chinese pulse diagnosis.

The extent of the importance of this innermost rhythm of life becomes a little clearer if we remind ourselves that the essential process by which we develop into human beings takes place along the spinal column. We still have to learn in our early years to raise our spinal columns upright to stand up straight as a human being. The feature that made us human millions of years ago continues to do the same today. In India, it is believed that our development toward humanity is a lifelong matter, and one that takes place along the spinal column. Beginning in the sacral region, the Kundalini energy serpent has to make her way from chakra to chakra to reach the head or cranial region. Buddha, the Enlightened One, is often shown with a rearing king cobra behind him, arching over his brow to indicate that his life energy has risen to the crown chakra. The craniosacral stream of energy is in unhindered rhythmic flow.

Even the names used in western medicine recall the sacred, speaking of the 'sacrum' as if this medicine too knew that all development toward health and so to the sacred begins here in this region at the base of the spine. It too realizes the link between health and the fully developed potential of consciousness and that this in turn is associated with the head. In this respect, the discovery of the craniosacral rhythm might also be seen as the rediscovery of an ancient knowledge that has only been forgotten in the west. This might also be the reason for the rapid spread of this method among therapists and its equally speedy acceptance by patients: the ground might already have been there, as it were, ready for this work to occupy it. The reclaiming of previously existing knowledge always takes less time than fresh discovery.

The appearance of this book gives me great pleasure, since Daniel Agustoni was one of the early users of this method in Europe; also because a friend is publishing his book of practical craniosacral work and because I was to some extent able to assist at the birth as regards the production of the first German edition. I hope that the book will further establish this valuable method and help many people to their own experiences of the Breath of Life.

Johanniskirchen, November 1998 Dr Ruediger Dahlke

Section 1

And yet the cranium does move:

Overview, theory, and introduction

1.1 The range and variety of craniosacral treatment – an overview

The where, how, and what of treatment and its results

Craniosacral treatment is a gentle, manual form of bodywork. It is a varied and effective method that can be used alone in its own right, or, with greater and deepening experience, in combination with other methods. The craniosacral rhythm is present even while the person is still an embryo; it is an expression of primary respiration. At the other end of life, when we leave our bodies in the dying process, the ebbing and flowing motions of this rhythm can be felt like a very slow tide for longer than the rhythms of breathing or heartbeat.

The main regions treated are the head (the *cranium*), torso and base of the spine (the *sacrum*). This is where the name *craniosacral* comes from. Treatment can involve listening to the craniosacral rhythm at various points on the body, or at a single point for some time, and the use of various specific techniques to treat and harmonize the craniosacral system.

The practical guidance in this book will mainly show the procedures for *basic structural treatment*. The treatment can be performed in different ways, depending on the practitioner's training and experience and therapeutic approach.

The particular personality of therapist and patient, the relationship of trust between them, and their harmonious therapeutic rapport are a further influence on what happens and how the treatment session proceeds. This means that the course of a craniosacral treatment session can take a great variety of forms as experience and confidence increase.

The client lies on the massage table in normal, everyday clothing, for about 45–60 min. Treatment involves very light touch; on the head this is approximately in the range of 1–3 g.

The craniosacral system consists externally of the bony structures already mentioned, and internally of the membranes surrounding the brain and spinal cord (the *meninges*) and the fluid contained there (*cerebrospinal fluid*, CFS). The free, as far as possible unrestricted flow of the CSF, together with the motion of the membranes of the central nervous system and the bony parts of the craniosacral system, assists a great number of vital functions of the body. Slow rhythms such as the craniosacral rhythm play a decisive role in the development and growth of the brain and spinal cord and their ability to function.

The fluid protects the brain and spinal cord, for example in the case of a blow or injury. It also nourishes the brain and spinal cord and drains away impurities.

Various explanatory models have been suggested to account for the fascinating phenomenon of the craniosacral rhythm. One theory proposes a semi-enclosed, hydraulic fluid pressure system; variations in the volume of the cerebrospinal fluid are assumed to bring about movement of the bones of the cranium; this motion in turn causes the craniosacral rhythm. The rhythm has a frequency of about 6–12 cycles/min, and can be sensed, by means of palpation, over the whole of the body.

The *tide* theory is a model to explain the fluids and potency of the *Breath of Life* principle. It says that the mid-tide is driven by means of the long-tide, and itself drives the craniosacral rhythm. In this way, macrocosmic rhythms and forces affect and bring about the body's rhythms.

The craniosacral treatment described here supports the autonomic and central nervous systems and locomotor system. It intensifies the self-regulation of the body, its self-healing forces and immune resistance, and produces a more balanced craniosacral rhythm. The treatment reduces or resolves restrictions and barriers in the craniosacral system; the subtle support given to the natural motion of the cranial bones and all the body fluids also helps give more room and freedom of motion for the brain as a whole, leading to better functioning and increasing its immense potential. For example, the widening of their entry points benefits the cerebral arteries, and the exit points of the cranial nerves and veins also have more room.

Craniosacral treatment simultaneously assists several different body systems, and relaxes the body *from the outside in*. The more even craniosacral rhythm in its turn, improves homeostasis, by which the body maintains its internal environment. The more harmonious rhythm operating from the center out towards the periphery helps release restrictions *from the inside outward*.

Consequently, this type of bodywork has a wide range of application: it is important for regeneration and maintaining health on the one hand, and on the other it aids healing in the treatment of disorders, syndromes and diseases. Indications and contraindications are given on page 63 and in the Appendix.

Another effect is to train and widen the senses. All our senses are gateways of perception, by which we receive impressions and sensations from what is within and outside ourselves, that is, from our own selves, the world around us, and our social environment. They can even enable religious or spiritual perceptions and experiences.

The craniosacral practitioner:

- accompanies and assists the natural process of self-regulation and self-healing by means of the treatment given
- promotes the client's ability for self-help by providing:
  - — greater self-perception; awareness of the body as a whole entity
  - — understanding of the functioning and the wisdom of the body
  - — confidence and the enabling of the self to change and develop
  - — information on self-treatment.

Craniosacral therapists support their clients on several levels by their presence. It is possible to address and become aware of, these levels of support during the treatment. Agreeable touch has the effect of 'touching' the person, and releasing something in that person.

Evidence of the positive application of touch therapies has been provided by more than 90 studies. The results of these can be found via the homepage of the Touch Research Institute in Florida, at: www.miami.edu/touch-research/home.html

Body, mind, and spirit are a natural unity. Touch can therefore evoke various levels of what it is to be human, individually or in combination at:

- the physical level (physicality and energy)
- the emotional level
- the intellectual/mental level; that of the mind
- the spiritual level; that of the soul.

A number of concepts and interpretations exist to account for these levels. It would be equally possible to speak of the physical, ethereal, astral, mental, spiritual, and cosmic spheres. These are an expression of primary respiration, the indwelling treatment plan and wisdom; it is called by names such as 'the inner healer'. They are also expressed by means of physical signals of the body and lead to sites of health, of restriction, and of release. An area of stillness is created in which healing can take place and the 'body-mind-spirit' unity experienced. Our self-perception is no longer separate and fragmented, but a perception of ourselves as an immediate, united whole, with all its potentials.

The craniosacral rhythm fluctuates in a very subtle, slow way, and so the way in which we detect it is *not by means of thinking and knowing, but mainly by continual sensing and perceiving*. Craniosacral bodywork is therefore a training in the consciousness and perception of the body, both for the client and for the therapist. Craniosacral therapy exercises its harmonizing and self-regulatory effect not only on various physical levels, but can also be felt clearly to affect such things as the emotions, on important insights, or the flow of energies in the person's own body. It enables and establishes a new sense of the body.

Because of the variety of ways in which the therapy works, a number of different complaints may be eased or resolved in the course of several sessions. For example, the successful treatment of back pain may bring with it the additional effects of a reduction in sleep disturbances and hyperactivity. Experience from the practice of craniosacral work shows that this method is often very effective, enabling many everyday complaints that have not yet become chronic to be reduced, or resolved in 6–9 treatment sessions, before they become a serious health problem.

Who should give this treatment, how, and who should receive it?

The basic structural craniosacral treatment shown in this book improves the motion of the cranial bones and the membranes surrounding the brain and spinal cord, and the flow of the CSF. There is an overall harmonization of the craniosacral system and its rhythm.

A trained craniosacral therapist is able to use such means as an extensive ability to assess the whole body, specific methods of structural release, the ability to assist spontaneous motions of unwinding, intraoral work (inside the mouth), and treatment of pivot points known as fulcrums. The knowledge and experience of trained craniosacral therapists enables them to perceive and treat the body as a whole entity.

They will at the same time work with the *free movement*, in accord with the functional and biodynamic approach being used. So no active testing of the motion *restriction* will be performed; instead they will observe and assist the slow, rhythmic motions as an expression of health and the *Breath of Life*. To give the right kind of treatment in this field calls for trust, patience, and a great deal of experience. Presence is the main way to accompany the indwelling force of the slow body rhythms, at the same time as maintaining the therapeutic space for the client.

This basic attitude, together with an understanding of the 'neutral' and extended approaches, assists natural self-regulation. Advanced options for harmonizing the craniosacral system are many and various, both in specific ways and at deeper levels.

Therapists should be trained in how to conduct the dialog and interact with the client during treatment. They should offer presence and empathy, but without identifying themselves with the client; they must be able to establish appropriate boundaries between themselves and their clients. They should offer empathy rather than sympathy, and be aware of their therapeutic responsibility. Craniosacral therapists should accompany events with their focus on the resources, using the sources of strength in the client in the treatment. This helps clients to deal positively with strong feelings, with the insights they discover, and with new bodily sensations. This approach fosters self-confidence and self-reliance. Deep-seated, entrenched traumas and barriers can begin to resolve through trust in an experienced craniosacral practitioner and in the therapeutic process.

The variety of approaches available means that craniosacral bodywork can accompany and assist people before and during birth, during their physical development and the stages of personal growth and change, through to their time of death. Moreover, it can extend our consciousness and strengthen the link with our capacity to love.

Craniosacral treatment usually leads us on from the head to the entirety of bodily sensation. It may sometimes cause us to feel light-as-air, with wide and unbounded horizons; at other times perhaps grounded and centered. We extend our faculty of awareness of touch sensation and feel for ourselves that we are sentient beings and a unity. This awakens and aids healing processes also on the psychical level.

Craniosacral therapy is successfully used throughout the world:

- in the preparation for birth
- during the birth process and postpartum
- in speech therapy and therapy in special education, for speech and learning difficulties and hyperactivity
- in ergotherapy
- in dentistry
- in the treatment of chronic complaints
- before and after operations, to relax the tissue and to hasten wound healing

- following personal shocks and trauma such as falls or accidents; after sudden bad news
- following collective shock and trauma such as natural disasters or war, for victims and their loved ones
- in rehabilitation and care
- in the care and support of sportsmen and women, musicians and professional groups who are constantly performing at maximum level
- for people in general who face major demands in their professional or private lives
- for well-being and spiritual growth
- for relaxation and regeneration, including 'burn-out'
- at the end of life.

Given the great number of fields of application and wide spectrum of effects, it is highly desirable for midwives, masseurs and masseuses, naturopaths and natural health practitioners, physicians, dentists, psychologists, complementary therapists, and other professionals in the health field to engage successfully in the use of this method.

Craniosacral bodywork can also be learned by lay persons to achieve experience of the self, and by family members of the chronically sick and others in need of care. For the best outcome, this calls for a sound foundation in anatomical knowledge, intuition, self-reflection, and the ability to slow down and be ready for stillness. The qualities needed to enter easily into resonance with primary respiration are a fundamentally attentive, open attitude that allows space, and is itself clear and centered. It is important to have sufficient personal experience, that is, of receiving craniosacral treatment oneself, apart from attendance at specialized courses; this makes the person more relaxed and able to understand and realize from experience how varied the effects of treatment can be. This is as essential as regular practice.

General principles and the range of treatment approaches

Principles of craniosacral therapy

The practice of craniosacral therapy is based on the following fundamental principles:

- the body is a unity
- the person is a unity, made up of body, mind and spirit
- there is interaction between structure and function, in which each influences the other
- the body is able to:
  - — regulate itself (self-regulation)
  - — heal itself (self-healing)
  - — maintain its state of health.

Treatment takes equal account of all these basic assumptions.

Our individual personal histories (birth, development, influential experiences, diseases, accidents, falls or operations – both physical and spiritual traumatic events) can cause a reduction, restriction or blockage of our self-regulation or self-healing and our ability to maintain our health. Our bodies have an amazing ability to *compensate* temporarily for major and minor restrictions; this limits the flow of body fluids, the flow of information of the living matrix, and the flow of vital energy in general (Oschman, see p. 119 and Further Reading).

If the imbalance of the individual becomes too great (partly also a consequence of our excessive pace of life and the modern lifestyle), then we find there is a permanently compensated imbalance, which needs to be *decompensated*. If the cause is not removed at this stage, a *continuing* decompensation diminishes the flow of vital strength and body fluids; this in turn can lead to disease processes.

Structure and function influence each other: when we listen carefully with our hands, sensing gently and precisely the way the various tissues of our bodies are made up and the freedom of motion each has, we can perceive the *function/motion* in the *structure* – and in relation to the respiratory rhythm, the craniosacral rhythm, and slower rhythms.

It is possible to sense and to promote both the intrinsic motion (termed *motility*) and the capacity for movement in the entire surrounding environment of the structure (*mobility*) for all the structures of the body (e.g. cranial bones, organs, or body segments).

The guiding principles of the craniosacral model include those set out by W. G. Sutherland for cranial osteopathy:

- the inherent motility of the brain and spinal cord
- the fluctuation of the cerebrospinal fluid
- the motility of the intracranial and spinal membranes
- the mobility of the cranial bones
- the involuntary motion between the two iliac bones.

The range of different treatment approaches in craniosacral therapy

Cranial osteopathy has continued to develop constantly over a period of about 70 years; craniosacral therapy over the last 20. A variety of treatment approaches has emerged. All these approaches in craniosacral therapy encourage slow rhythms of 2–14 cycles/min, and promote a more balanced craniosacral system. As with other methods, different approaches lead to the same goal. Which approach will the client best respond to, and which seems most suitable at that moment?

In my opinion, we do not need to weigh up whether a particular approach is better in principle. Wide training and experience enable the craniosacral practitioner to decide on the basis of clients' differing life histories and immediate needs which treatment approach will be better or more effective, and when. Our guide in this is the slow rhythms and the wisdom of the body, which indicates the way to go.

The biomechanical, structural approach mainly uses various direct and indirect release techniques. Following the cogwheel model established by W.G. Sutherland (see Further Reading), it is based on biomechanics, and thus on the release of restrictions/dysfunctions in the regions of the torso, head and limbs. This occurs extensively in the connective tissue and especially at the level of the bones and membranes of the craniosacral system.

The structural functional approach also employs a structural type of treatment, but there is *no active testing of the motion restriction*, so this approach does *not* confront the system with the motion barrier. Instead, the practitioner's attention focuses mainly on the *free motions and rhythms* which express vitality and health. These indicate the 'direction of ease'; the motion that is possible. The result of allowing space and listening non-invasively to the motions that reveal themselves is often that the cranio-sacral system is helped to balance itself. At the same time as the release occurs, a new balance emerges spontaneously, a balance of the whole body matrix with its pivot points (fulcrums).

The biodynamic approach takes as its guide both the craniosacral rhythm (of approximately 6–12 cycles/min) and, primarily, slower rhythms, which are particularly thought of as an expression of primary respiration, the 'Breath of Life'. Structural treatment, the active search for dysfunctions and their release, is not central to this approach.

If the mid-tide or long-tide manifest themselves, the beginner is advised to remain neutral and present, and at the same time to allow space, rather than using manual, structural techniques. Then, by maintaining this neutral presence, go with the self-correction of the whole body matrix.

In the mid-tide (which has approximately 2–3 cycles/min), there is a change in perception; the ability to distinguish the body structures (skin, connective tissue, bones, dura mater) by sensitive listening all but disappears and is no longer even important. What is perceived instead is the body as a whole, the 'fluid body'. Working at this level, it is possible to provide greater support and assistance to the body in its own self-regulation, down to the level of the body cells. The fluid body is more than the flow of the cerebrospinal and other body fluids. It also includes the 'biosphere' or aura, the entire bioelectrical field in and around the body.

A 'potency' can often also be sensed, manifesting itself in the motions of the mid-tide and long-tide. The midline and the knowledge of our embryological development are drawn into the 'intrinsic treatment plan' that increasingly reveals itself as the 'neutral' deepens.

The long-tide (1 cycle in 100 seconds, 1/100 s) permeates the entire planet. It breathes the *Breath of Life* into all that lives, and can be sensed both within and outside the body as the practitioner gains experience.

Structural treatment is more than simply the treatment of axes of motion and dysfunctions: I believe that the human person as a whole is continuously present in the biological, the energetic and the intellectual–spiritual process. Each system of the body (e.g., the respiratory, cardiovascular, and digestive systems) that plays its part in the organization of the body as a whole has its own function and also influences the other systems. Viewed as a whole, sensations, emotions, creativity, prayer, meditation, and spiritual experience are also functions, which are not static but dynamic processes and help to influence the functions of the body and so also its structure.

It is not usually helpful to mix completely different approaches and their associated techniques. If, however, the practitioner has come to know the individual approaches thoroughly through many years of experience, and can achieve resonance with the client and the capacity of the client's body and being as a whole to express itself, a fluent transition can be made from the structural-functional to the biodynamic approach and the reverse. To do so does, however, require the practitioner not to force the person being treated to conform to a particular schema or concept the practitioner has.

This might mean, for instance, that it is better not to carry out any active, invasive techniques at first, but to begin by familiarizing oneself with the patient's tissues and craniosacral rhythm. The 6–12 cycles/min of the craniosacral rhythm is, in its own right, a rhythm of the tides by which the body expresses itself, and a phenomenon whose qualities of motion I believe it should be possible to palpate in detail. It is only as the practitioner gains experience and becomes more reliably familiar with the body's intrinsic rhythms that it becomes helpful to treat the client at the level of the fluid body.

Important points

Improvement in an individual's health, perhaps through touch that 'tunes in' to the client and presence that allows the client space, does not necessarily mean that you now know craniosacral therapy in all its variety and possess all the basis of knowledge to carry it out; it may however be an indication that you are on the right road to achieving this.

A sound basis of knowledge of the underlying anatomy and physiology is enormously important, as is the ability to distinguish the levels of the body and the motion of the craniosacral rhythm. It is a combination of theoretical understanding *and* highly developed practical skills that help you to understand the associations and processes occurring during treatment. Attendance at specialist craniosacral courses, together with a great deal of practice, exchange and experience are all needed to create the ability to apply craniosacral therapy effectively and lastingly for the well-being of the client.

In the biodynamic field, a practitioner who is not 'neutral' but is instead proceeding too quickly or with too much mental direction, could easily ignore the real inner treatment plan and so bring sensitive regions out of balance.

The client is not fixed or manipulated in a treatment model that solely delivers healing, or by its associated techniques; the client is not forced in any way.

It is helpful to begin in a functional way, that is, to listen first of all to the slow motions of the body such as breathing and the craniosacral rhythm and the balancing of tension in the connective tissue. After listening for a while, a practitioner who is unprejudiced and in 'neutral' will be able to assess which routes and techniques will be helpful, or which the client's system will accept.

The overall situation of the client plays a major part in the decision as to which of the various treatment approaches will be best. All, if correctly used, encourage relaxation, improved balance of the craniosacral system, and self-healing.

The practitioner will also establish whether the client tends to be hypertonous, i.e. sympathetic-system-activated, or hypotonous, i.e. parasympathetic-system-activated. Which part is absent or in need of balance? An experienced practitioner is able to detect this and assist the client in that respect.

Treatment that is 'in tune' and successful therapy is also significantly influenced by other factors. These include the therapeutic rapport – Is the practitioner able to meet a given client where that client actually is? How can the practitioner engage and attune to the client? – and the relationship of trust between practitioner and client, and the resource-oriented dialog that accompanies and assists therapy.

If we orient ourselves by rhythms, motion, and function, our attention is directed towards *health*. Our intention and perception assist the therapeutic process. Directing our resource-oriented focus toward free motion rather than restrictions, we strengthen that which is healthy and positive, instead of concerning ourselves primarily with dysfunctions and the pathological aspect. This is a fundamental factor and should be taken into account in the comprehensive craniosacral treatment that I present in this book.

I believe that we should continually develop our abilities in palpation and train ourselves in distinguishing the different motions of the craniosacral rhythm. The greater the scope of the treating practitioner's knowledge, experience and perception and non-invasive presence, the more the self-regulatory mechanisms will be able to perform their task. In this connection, I should like to recommend Leon Chaitow's book 'Palpation Skills' (see Further Reading).

Palpation and the process of learning to distinguish the qualities of the craniosacral rhythm call for patience and trust. Acquiring comprehensive competence is a challenge for the beginner. It is often easier to begin by familiarizing yourself with the craniosacral rhythm of approximately 6–12 cycles/min; this is more helpful than listening to slower rhythms too early in the belief that you can distinguish them.

This is another reason that this book presents a basic craniosacral treatment that is mainly *structural and functional and designed in relation to the craniosacral rhythm*. The biodynamic approach using slower rhythms has quite deliberately not been addressed in detail in this book.

This has the further advantage that you can discover and practice some of the basic techniques for *the torso* that are explained here, even while you are not yet able to sense the craniosacral rhythm, or sense it only occasionally. The craniosacral rhythm may become clearer to detect once the relaxation in the torso region has occurred.

All the rest depends on practice, including:

- slowing down of the self
- relaxation of the self
- listening, waiting, trusting
- being still
- perceiving slow motions and the indwelling power within them in the stillness
- listening and experiencing amazement.

The theoretical knowledge of structure and function is very important; it is also important to understand the complex interrelationships that exist. However, this can sometimes assume too much importance for the beginner, perhaps because you have such high expectations of yourself and put pressure on yourself, or are unwilling to admit that you have too little patience or still lack experience. However much information we absorb and however many questions we ask and have answered – in the end what matters is the development of our specific palpation abilities, our field of awareness and consciousness of the body.

You can experience all this, and can deepen these capacities by regular 'practice, practice, practice …', also by giving yourself the privilege of receiving craniosacral treatment from experienced practitioners. You can continually develop your own awareness of touch sensation by palpating your own body rhythms and by craniosacral self-treatment.

The aim of treatment is not simply to bring about more balanced qualities in the craniosacral rhythm; it is above all to achieve the following: improved self-regulation of the body as a whole, improvement in the flow and the exchange of all body fluids, greater well-being and deep relaxation. The dialog enables the client to become aware of the changes occurring during the treatment and establishes new perceptions.

The gentle release of tension (in the body) and the more balanced craniosacral rhythm releases the energy that had previously been bound or held fast so that it is once more available as energy for life and so for health.

1.2 Origin and history

As long ago as the seventeenth century, an Italian researcher discovered that the membranes surrounding the brain, the meninges, move with a rhythmic motion, transporting the cerebrospinal fluid (CSF) via the nerve sheaths to peripheral regions of the body.

The origins of craniosacral therapy can be found in cranial osteopathy, a branch of traditional osteopathy. Osteopathy itself, which was founded by Andrew Taylor Still (1828–1917), also includes further manual techniques (applied to muscles and fasciae, bones and joints) and the treatment of organs (visceral osteopathy).

Cranial osteopathy was developed by William Garner Sutherland (1873–1954), who obtained the title DO (Doctor of Osteopathy) in 1900. Although most anatomical textbooks then (as now) taught that the bones of the cranium are firmly united at the sutures that join them, and permit no movement, he was fascinated by the cranial sutures, in particular the scale-like suture between the temporal and parietal bones.

Sutherland knew that every form or structure has a purpose and a function. He drew the conclusion that the various cranial sutures have an articular function; in that way, they would permit movement. Many years of studies followed. One of his discoveries was that different applications of pressure to various parts of the head (applied for example by using a helmet that he designed himself) bring about different physical and emotional changes and effects. WG Sutherland sensed the slow motions like the ebb and flow of the tide and discovered that the cranium 'breathes'. He spoke of the 'primary respiratory mechanism' that precedes pulmonary respiration and is believed to regulate all other functions of the body. Might this cranial breathing be brought about in part by the inner tissue respiration of the central nervous system? He published his ideas under the pseudonym Blunt Bone Bill, but met with little recognition from most of his osteopathic colleagues for some time. It was not until the 1940s that Sutherland was able to convince some of his fellow osteopaths of his research – and the 'cranial concept' was gradually absorbed into osteopathy as an important foundational principle.

William Garner Sutherland made many discoveries and original advances in his 50 years and more of research and practice. One such discovery was that the cranial bones in the midline exhibit particular motions, and he developed the biomechanical *cogwheel model* that is still recognized today. He found himself moving increasingly from the bone to the membrane level: to the function of the meninges as a whole, surrounding both the brain and spinal cord, and, more specifically, the significance of the intracranial membranes, the 'reciprocal tension membrane' inside the cranium. Another topic that interested him was the significance of the pivot points, the 'fulcrums', and the way that ligamentous and membranous tension become balanced, after which harmony is established with all systems of the body. As time went on, the fluctuations of the CSF, the 'fluid level' and the Breath of Life became increasingly important. Sutherland carried out pioneer research into the origin of 'primary respiration' and the indwelling force within it over a period of decades. From 1948 onwards, another treatment approach took shape (the one now known as the 'biodynamic' approach), drawing on the knowledge he had acquired, and diverging more and more from the biomechanical model.

Osteopathy and cranial osteopathy have undergone various developments and have evolved over the past century.

Students of Sutherland taught structural cranial osteopathy in London and Paris, but much time was needed for it to become accepted and to spread there. Osteopathy has become well known not only in the USA, but also in the UK and France, and has become well established over recent decades.

Rollin E. Becker, DO and Ruby Day, DO, both students of Sutherland, worked increasingly at the fluid level and with slower rhythms in carrying out their research and treatment during their later years. As already mentioned in Chapter 1.1, this treatment approach differs from the biomechanical approach to cranial osteopathy both in its general tendency and in its fundamental principles. The most experienced and most important representative of biodynamic cranial osteopathy today is James Jealous, DO, who was personally taught by R. E. Becker and R. Day.

It was John E. Upledger and other osteopaths who made various forms of cranial osteopathy accessible to a wider public, in particular to physiotherapists, massage therapists, body therapists, naturopaths and psychologists. It is, however, largely due to the work of John E. Upledger, DO that craniosacral therapy began to spread so successfully in the 1980s. He included the emotional level and dialog during treatment, and argues in his books for the model of the fluid 'pressurestat' system. He describes 'energy cysts'; I describe these in this book as inertial fulcrums.

Today the craniosacral method is offered in a number of craniosacral schools and by many physical therapists across the world, sometimes under a different name, with modified or quite different approaches; names include: craniosacral therapy, craniosacral treatment and craniosacral-flow®. Just as osteopathy and cranial osteopathy underwent further development over decades, so the craniosacral method has evolved over the last 25 years.

There are important differences between craniosacral therapy and cranial osteopathy; these include the fact that the craniosacral method as performed today is accompanied by therapeutic dialog, interactive process work and a resource and solution-oriented approach (this is important, e.g., in trauma healing). Craniosacral therapy also usually employs far lighter pressure than is usually the case in cranial osteopathy, and may even apply no pressure at all. This means that it is less invasive, or indeed can be completely non-invasive.

Various approaches within the craniosacral method teach and use a modality without invasive methods. They do not prompt any processes, for example to bring about or strengthen emotional release. However, the different treatment approaches and developments of craniosacral therapy each in their own way promote the craniosacral system, the craniosacral rhythm, and the health of the whole person.

The craniosacral system 1.3

The anatomy: an illustrated account

The three levels of the craniosacral system

The craniosacral system consists outwardly of the bony parts of the cranium, spinal column and sacrum.

Internally it consists of the meninges, which form a semi-enclosed, fairly compact membrane system for the brain and spinal cord.

A third level also forms part of the craniosacral system; in addition to the levels of bone and membrane there is that of the cerebrospinal fluid (CSF), which usually flows rhythmically.

These three levels of the craniosacral system will be presented separately here for clarity. It is helpful for the craniosacral practitioner to be able to differentiate and to discover which level is free or restricted, and where. In reality, all three are interlinked and together form a functional unity.

And yet it does move …

Interestingly, the sutures do not necessarily unite with age, but permit minimal motions in the measurable range on a microlevel. Just as the earth has continental plates that move, so the cranium too is not solidly fused; instead it is a living, dynamic structure. The breathing of the cranium, the craniosacral rhythm, is an expression of the vital force. There are some anatomy texts and some training institutions that have taught for centuries that the cranial bones and sutures are capable of motion.

All instruction in anatomy ought to take account of this insight, at the very least since the many demonstrations that this capacity of motion does exist, namely: that the head and brain form a subtly fluctuating system in which the cranial bones move thanks to articular connections between them, for example according to a biomechanical cogwheel model. The meninges also move, especially the intracranial membranes. There are cerebral cavities called ventricles in certain parts of the brain; in these ventricles the CSF, our inner ocean, undergoes slow motions like the ebb and flow of the tide.

The figures in this chapter show some of the many anatomical structures that make-up the three levels of the craniosacral system. You will find more detailed, fascinating illustrations in atlases of anatomy, and further information on the anatomy and functional details in textbooks of anatomy and neuro-anatomy (see Further Reading).

The cranium, cranial sutures and meninges

One of the effects of palpation and gentle structural treatment of the craniosacral rhythm is to expand the cranial sutures, the articulations between the cranial bones, making them better able to follow their natural motion. This encourages both their intrinsic motion (*motility*) and their capacity to move in relation to their surroundings (*mobility*), and consequently that of the entire craniosacral system from head to sacrum (Figs 1.3.1–1.3.4).

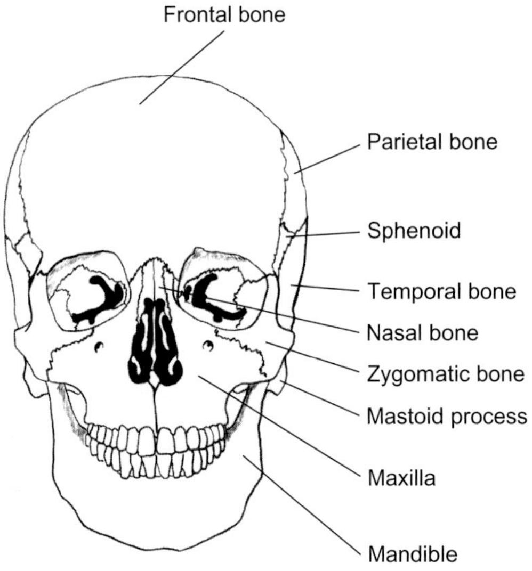

Figure 1.3.1
The cranial bones (anterior).

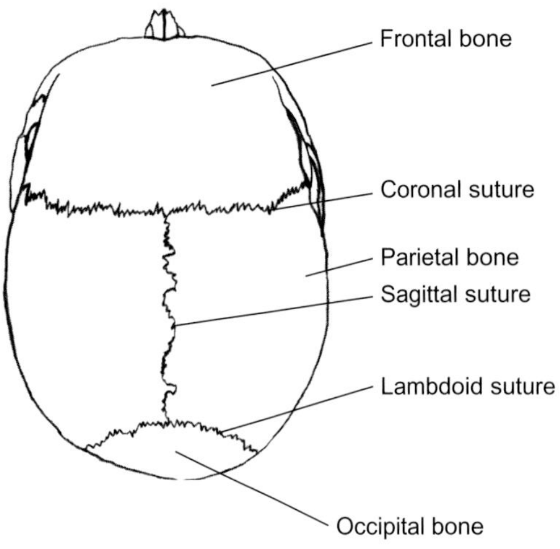

Figure 1.3.2
The cranial bones and sutures (superior view).

This aids the elasticity of the membrane system and improves the fluctuation of the CSF. Improved flexibility and mobility of the meninges benefits the craniosacral system as a whole, the quality of the rhythm and thus all body functions.

As an example, release of the frontal and parietal bones brings about simultaneous stretching of the underlying falx cerebri. The falx cerebri is the inturned arc of dura mater that separates the left and right hemispheres of the brain. Together with the falx cerebelli, which lies centrally inside the occipital bone, this forms the vertical part of the intracranial membrane system in the brain.

Treatment of the temporal bones makes the tentorium cerebelli more flexible. The tentorium forms the horizontal part of the intracranial membrane system.

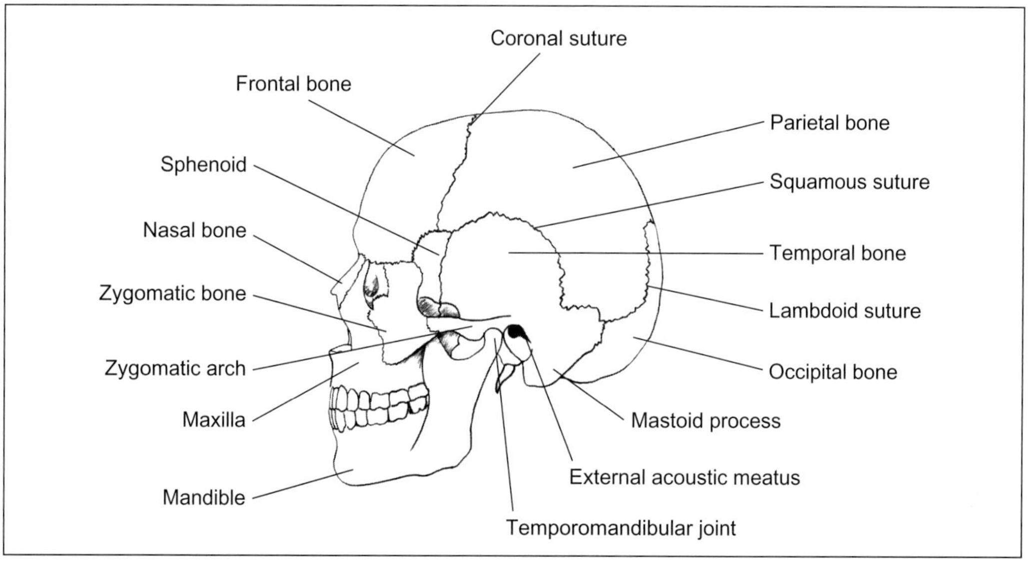

Figure 1.3.3
The cranial bones and sutures (from the side).

Figure 1.3.4
Cranial sutures (the sagittal suture and coronal suture with bregma).

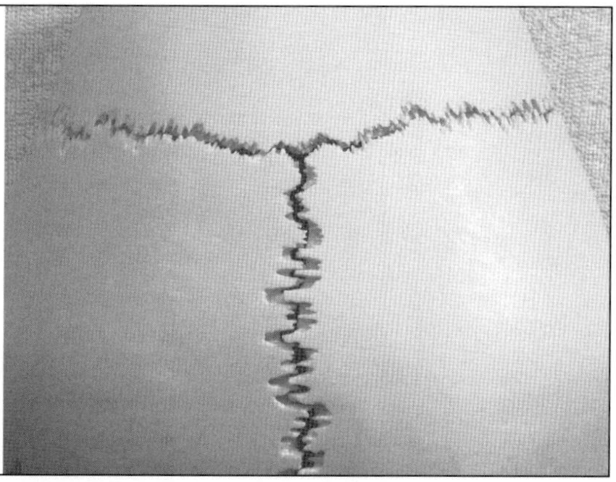

The membrane system consists of three different layers:

- the dura mater
- the arachnoid (arachnoid mater)
- the pia mater.

The cerebral membranes are continuous with the spinal membranes, the one passing into the other at the foramen magnum (Figs 1.3.5–1.3.9).

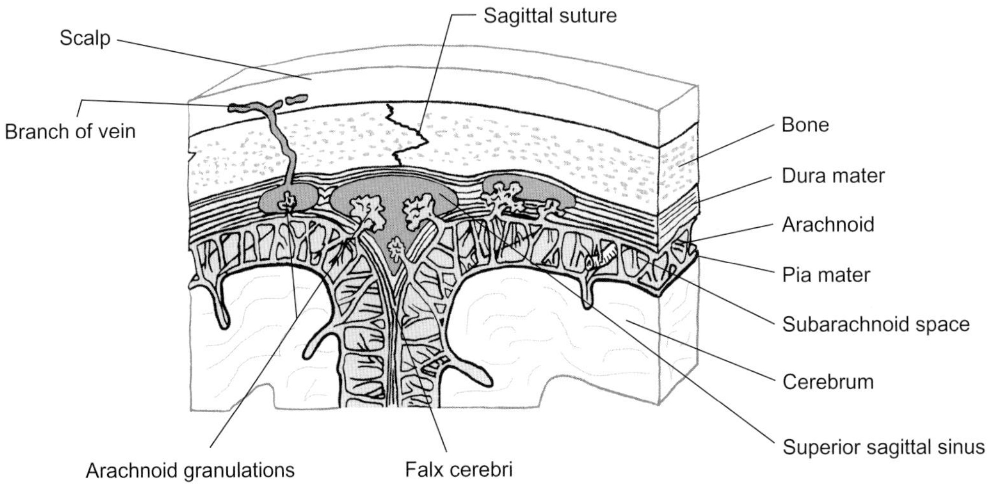

Figure 1.3.5
The meninges in the region of the calvaria (skull cap).

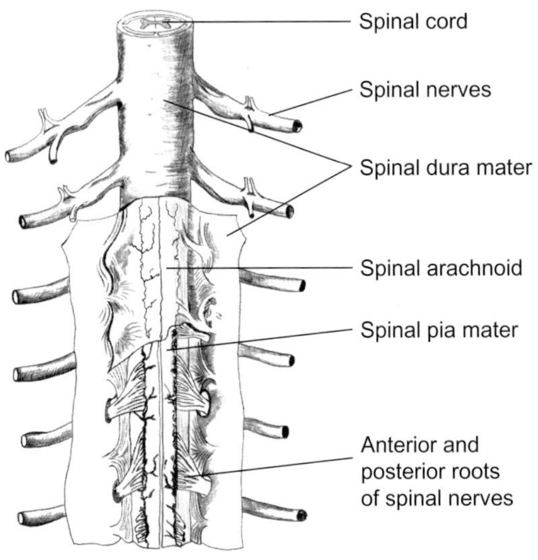

Figure 1.3.6
Spinal meninges.

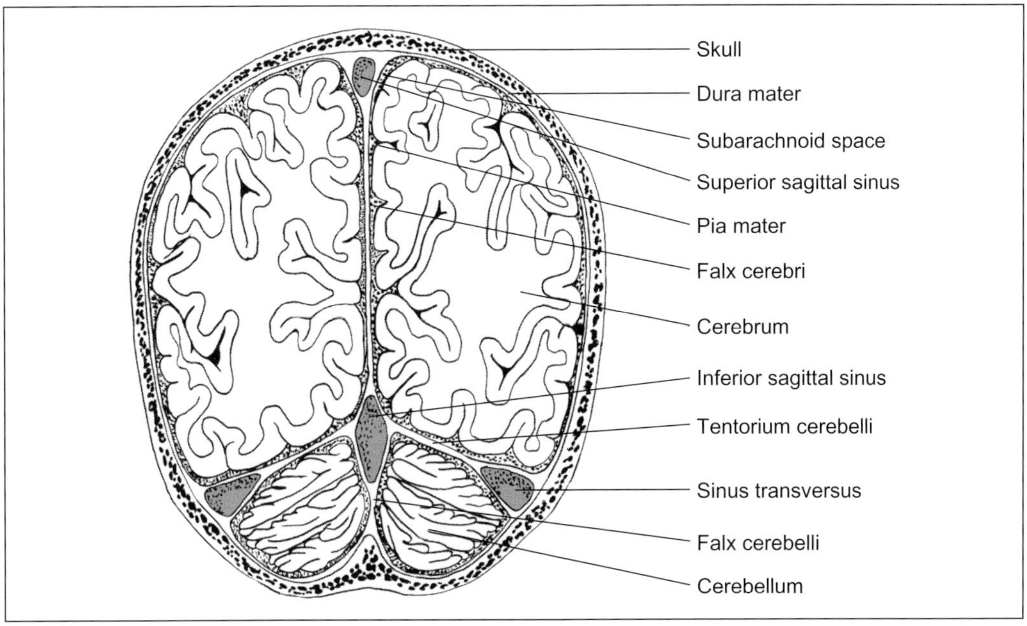

Figure 1.3.7
The falx cerebri, falx cerebelli and tentorium cerebelli. Cranial view.

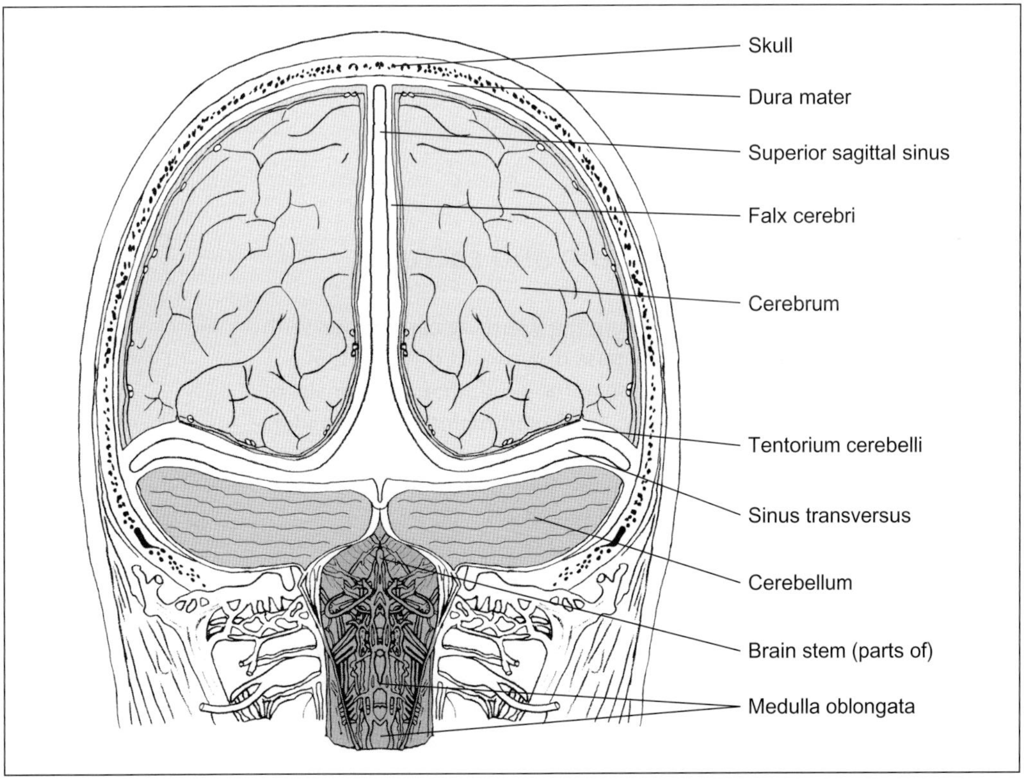

Figure 1.3.8
Posterior view.

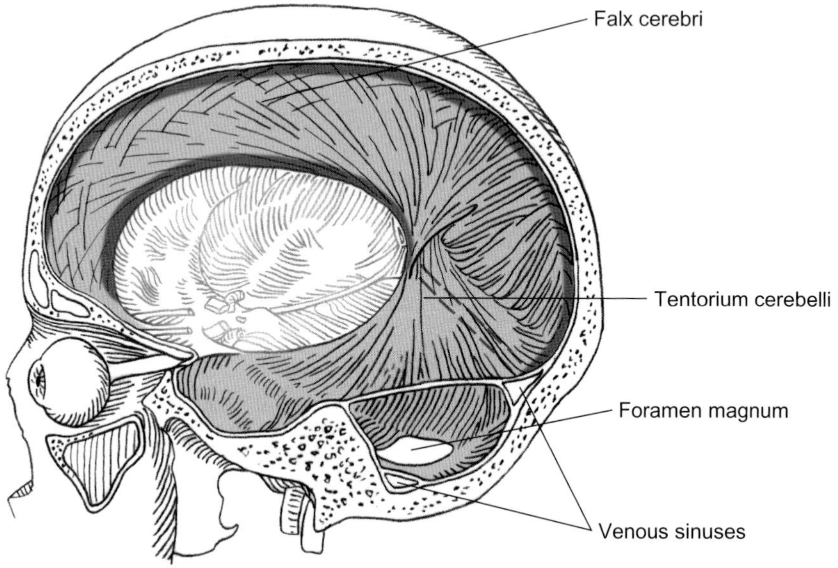

Figure 1.3.9
Lateral view.

The dural tube, spinal column and sacrum

The membranes (or meninges) covering the brain are continuous with those covering the spinal cord. They pass downward through the foramen magnum, and below the base of the skull, they still consist of the same three layers, the dura mater, arachnoid mater and pia mater. The spinal meninges continue down to the sacrum, and protect the spinal cord and spinal nerve roots. The name used for the meninges in the spinal region is the '*dural tube*' (Figs 1.3.10–1.3.15).

The dural tube transmits the craniosacral rhythm onward from the occiput to the sacrum, so that it can also be palpated (i.e., felt) at the sacrum.

The dural tube is attached at the foramen magnum of the occipital bone and also inside the spinal column at the second and third cervical vertebrae and the superior part of the sacral region (S2). It therefore extends beyond the spinal cord and merges with the periosteum (or membrane) covering the coccyx (*os coccygis*).

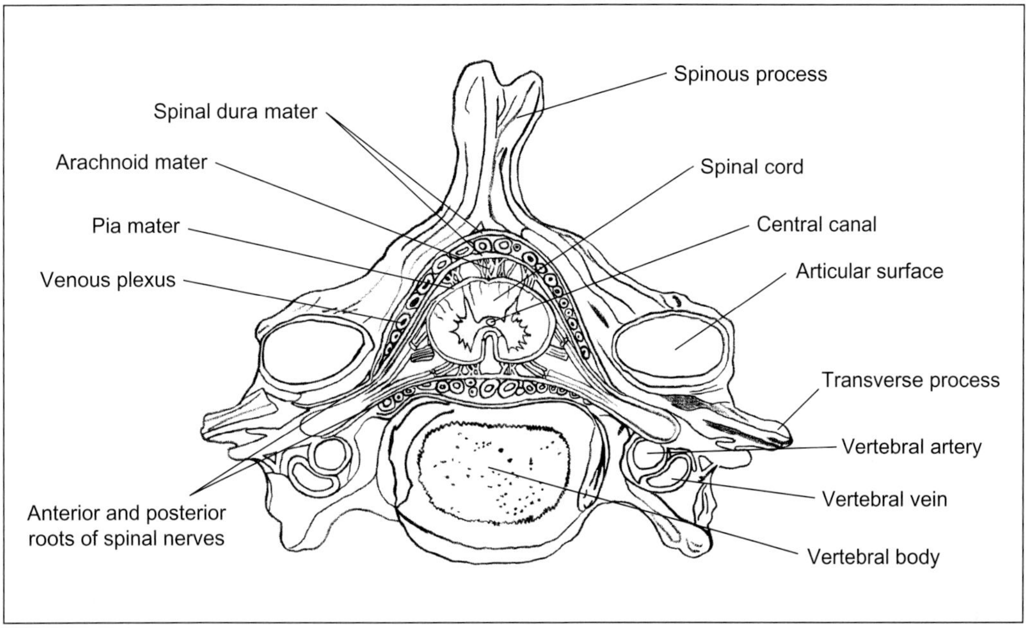

Figure 1.3.10
Spinal column from above.

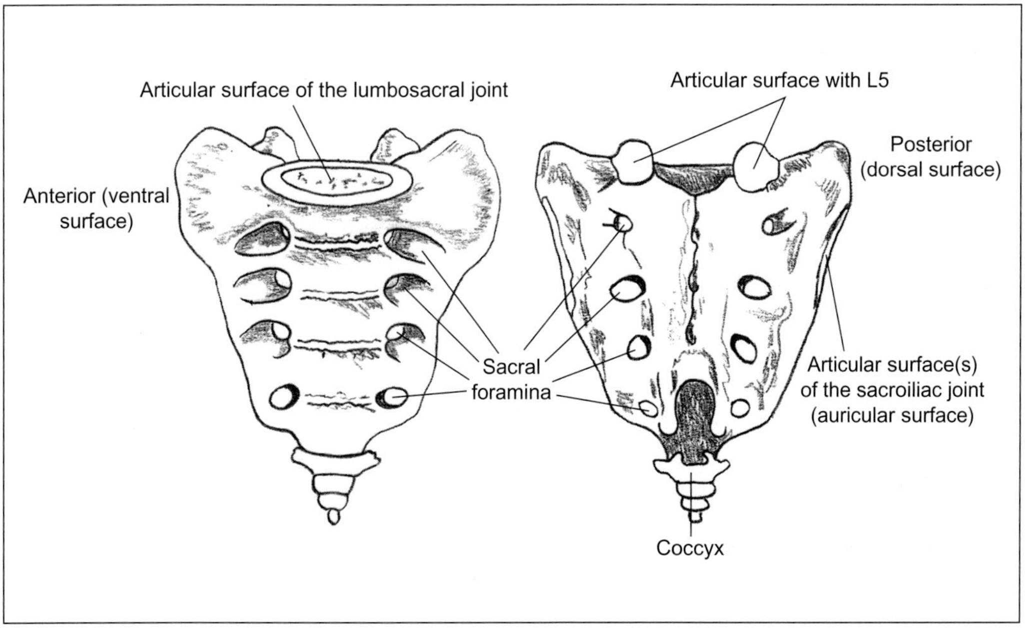

Figure 1.3.11
The sacrum.

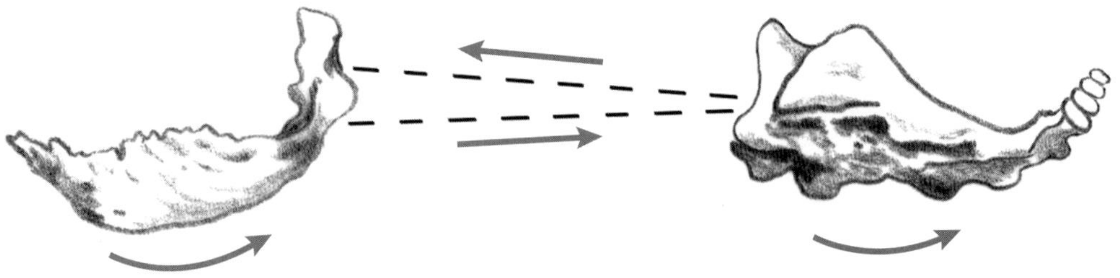

Figure 1.3.12
Direction of motion of the occipital bone and sacrum in flexion (simplified).

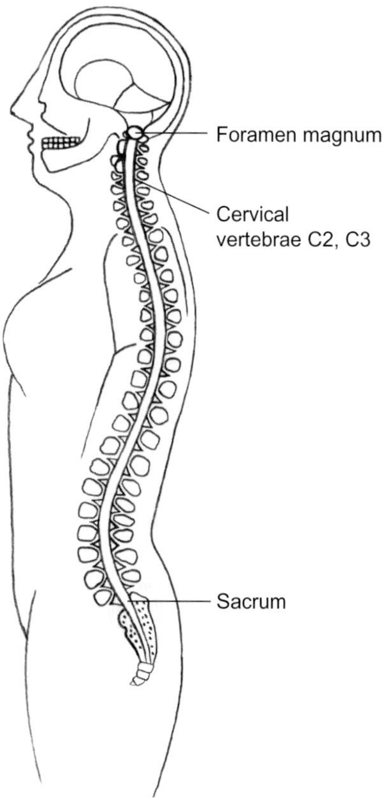

Figure 1.3.13
The dural tube with sites of attachment.

Figure 1.3.14
The central nervous system with nerve exit points.

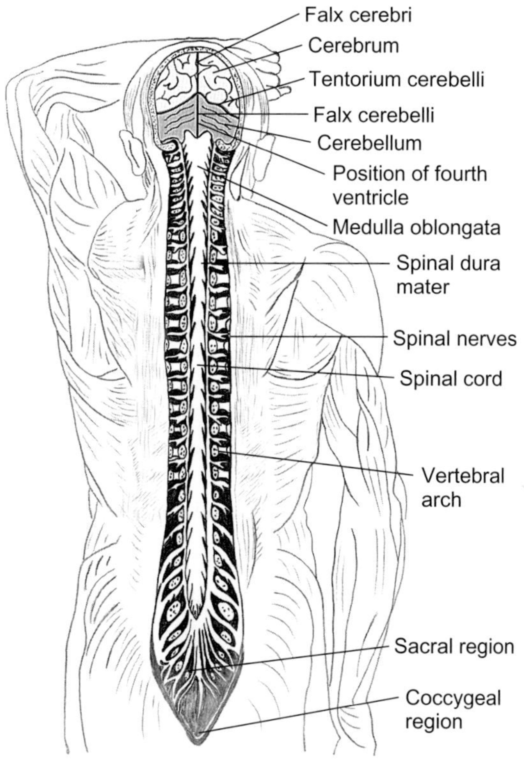

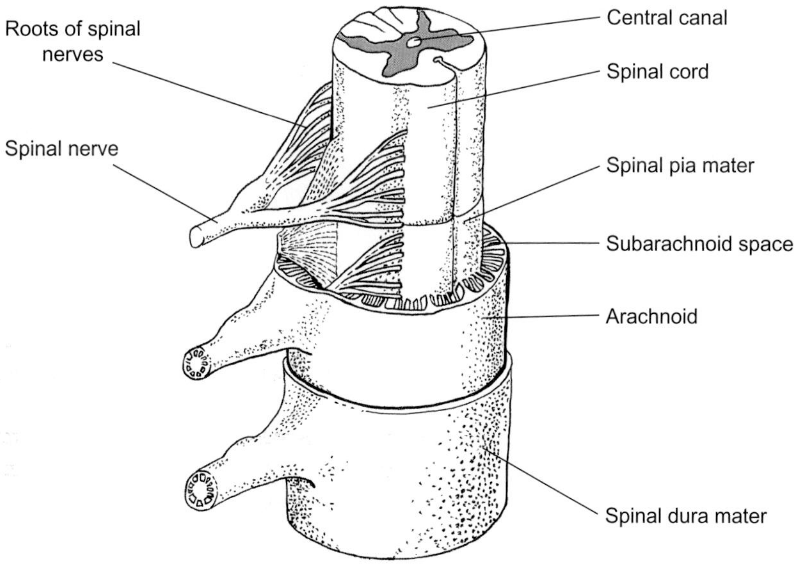

Figure 1.3.15
The nerve exit points with dura mater, arachnoid and pia mater.

The ventricular system

In the interior of the brain there are four chambers called ventricles. They are the cavities containing cerebrospinal fluid (Fig. 1.3.16).

Position of the ventricles: The first and second are lateral ventricles. They lie side-by-side in the region of the cerebrum, in the left and right cerebral hemispheres. The fresh CSF flows downward and anteriorly from these lateral ventricles into another cavity, the third ventricle, which lies almost in the middle of the brain between the left and right thalamus in the region of the diencephalon. From there, a narrow conduit called the cerebral aqueduct (*aquaeductus cerebri*) in the region of the midbrain or mesencephalon leads to the fourth ventricle; this lies between the pons, the medulla oblongata and the cerebellum. All the physiological centers are located in the floor of the fourth ventricle. It is a region that contains many nerve nuclei (Figs 1.3.17, 1.3.18).

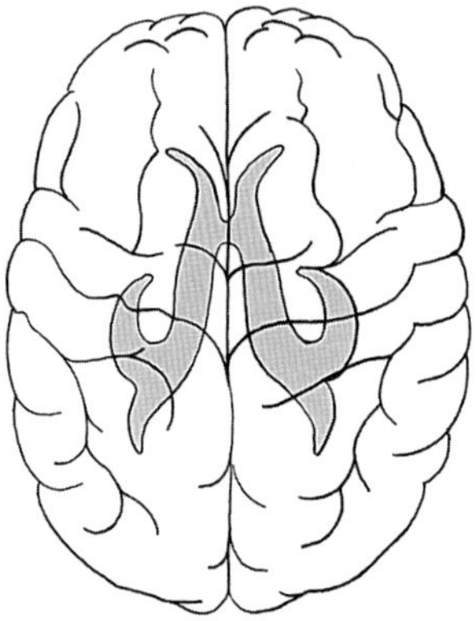

Figure 1.3.16
Position of the lateral ventricles in the brain.

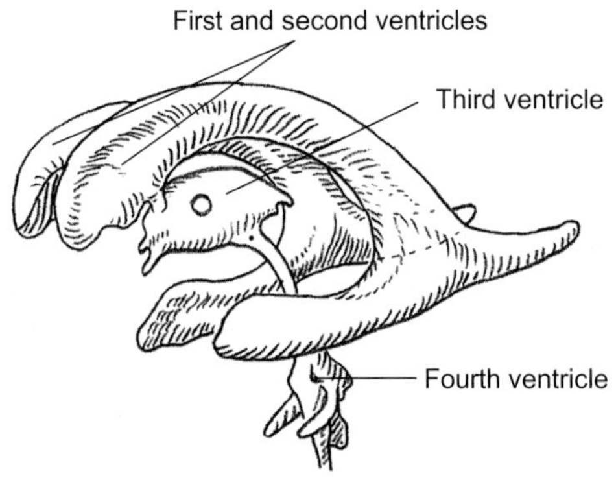

Figure 1.3.17
The ventricles. Lateral view.

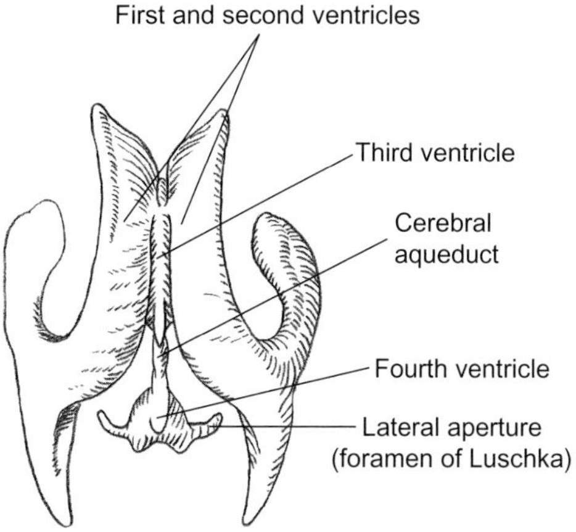

Figure 1.3.18
The ventricles. Cranial view.

The cerebrospinal fluid (CSF)

At certain points on the walls of the cerebral ventricles, there is an extensive vascular fringe, the choroid plexus, which constantly produces vital CSF (*liquor cerebrospinalis*) from the blood.

In healthy individuals, the CSF is clear and colorless. It flows mainly in the subarachnoid space – the space between the skull, which is covered by the dura mater, and the brain – and in its ventricles. In the region of the torso, the CSF flows in the space between the spinal dura mater and the spinal cord.

The CSF in the subarachnoid space bathes the entire brain and spinal cord via the pia mater. It has been proposed that the central canal of the spinal cord may remain partly open in living individuals, so that the CSF can also penetrate there.

The volume of the CSF is fairly slight at around 110–170 mL. This valuable fluid is completely renewed every 5–7 h, depending on the vitality or restrictions of the craniosacral system. This is equivalent to approximately 4–7 times in 24 h. In all, approximately 500–700 mL of cerebrospinal fluid are produced in a period of 24 h.

The CSF and the brain oscillate rhythmically in harmony with one another (Fig. 1.3.19).

Important functions of the CSF

- *Protective:* The specific gravity of the fluid is similar to that of the brain, and together with the dura mater acts as a shock absorber to protect the brain and spinal cord. This is an important function, as it absorbs the vibration that comes from walking, running or from falls and blows. The brain and spinal cord 'float' in the cerebrospinal fluid and are surrounded and protected by it.

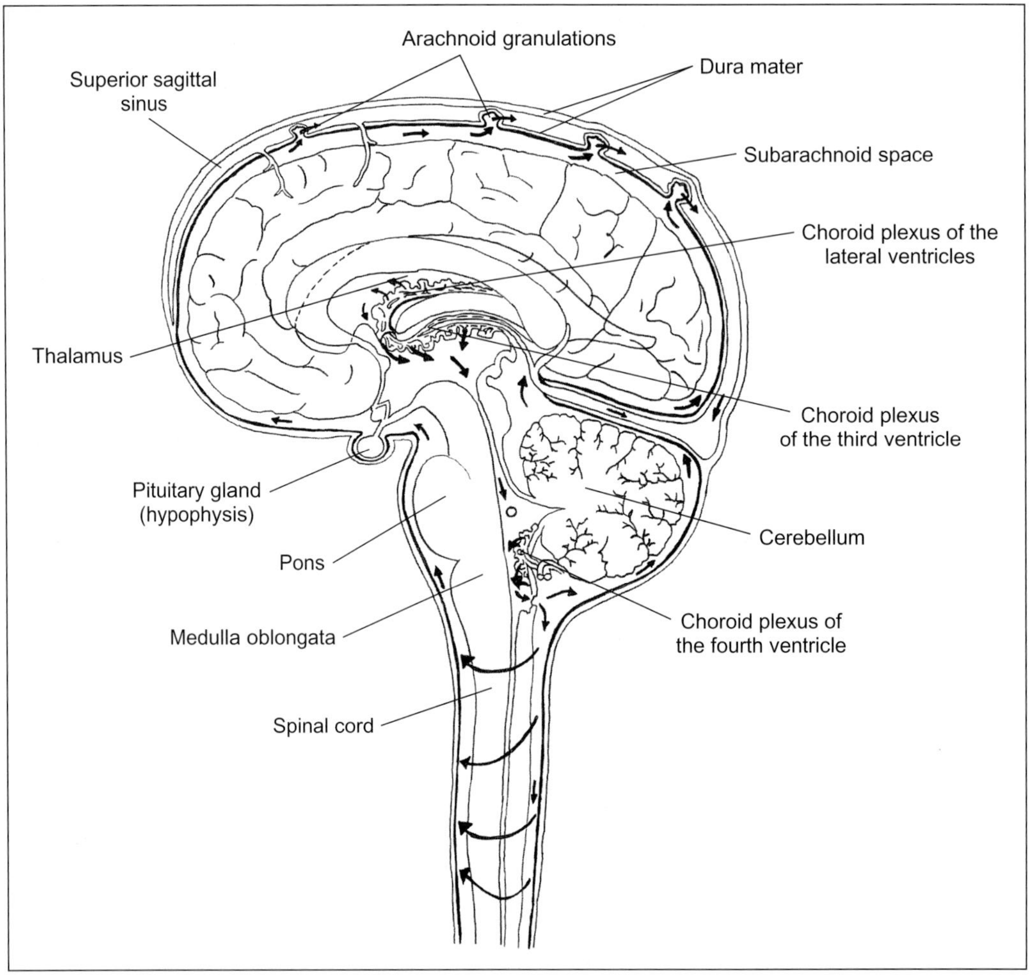

Figure 1.3.19
The production, secretion, distribution and absorption of the CSF in the brain.

- *Nutritive:* The rich composition of the CSF nourishes the brain, the spinal cord and the nerves that emerge from it. Here are some of the substances it contains: glucose, various proteins and dissolved substances in the form of salts, such as sodium, calcium, magnesium, potassium, chloride, phospholipids and phosphates, and cholesterol. Lymphocytes, traces of vitamin C, hormones or neurotransmitters (such as endorphins) have also been found. Metallic ions such as sodium, potassium and calcium are known to be important for transmitting nerve signals or action potentials throughout the central nervous system.
- *Purification and removal of waste products:* An unimpeded, balanced craniosacral system transports the CSF unhindered into many

sites in the brain and along the spinal cord. As this happens, waste substances such as old brain or spinal cord cells or the remnants of past inflammatory processes are washed and transported away.

Medical diagnosis

A diagnostic test can be performed by withdrawing some cerebrospinal fluid, usually from beneath the spinal cord between the third and fourth, or fourth and fifth lumbar vertebrae (lumbar puncture), to test for pathological states of the central nervous system such as meningitis or for bleeding in the ventricles of the brain or subarachnoid space. This method can detect excessive pressure inside the cranium, for instance, which can lead to brain damage, coma or death. Lumbar puncture is generally a rather unpleasant procedure; it often makes the patient feel unwell or produces headaches, because it pierces the dura mater and can cause a sudden change in CSF pressure. In some injuries, inflammations and illnesses, the CSF values are different from normal; one example is the large increase in the leucocyte and erythrocyte (white and red blood cell) count in meningitis.

Reabsorption of cerebrospinal fluid

The CSF is mainly reabsorbed in the vault of the cranium, in the venous sinuses (*sinus durae matris*). There, as the pressure of the CSF builds up, the fluid is drawn out of the system into the arachnoid granulations (*granulationes arachnoideales*) – tiny excrescences that look almost like cauliflower florets. From there, the fluid is reabsorbed into the venous system, in particular via the superior sagittal sinus (*sinus sagittalis superior*), which contains a large number of arachnoid granulations along its course.

In the spinal region, along the spinal nerve exits, some of the CSF is drawn into the extracellular environment and from there, into the lymphatic system. CSF can also filter out of the system at those points where nerves, veins or arteries cross the spinal meninges and subarachnoid space, e.g., via nerve sheaths.

1.4 How the craniosacral system relates to other body systems

The functional improvement of the craniosacral system and the body as a whole

By means of sensitive listening to the slow rhythms of the body, and by administering specific, non-invasive treatments to release tensions in the craniosacral system, the practitioner helps to increase the motility and mobility of the system and so maintain a more balanced craniosacral rhythm.

One of the effects of the basic craniosacral therapy presented here is the release of tension in transverse connective tissue and inertial fulcrums. It treats the cranial bones and sutures, the cranial and spinal meninges and the intracranial membrane system, so releasing the body structures *from the outside in*.

The craniosacral rhythm becomes stronger, more extensive, more symmetrical and more balanced. At the same time, the more balanced craniosacral rhythm moves all the body structures *from the inside out*. These vitalizing, reorganizing motions proceeding outwards from the center to the periphery of the body then help to release the body as a whole from restrictions. The various slow rhythms promote the exchange of all body fluids.

A free craniosacral system and balanced craniosacral rhythm provide considerable support to the functioning of all body systems.

The following body systems are interrelated and influence each other:

- the craniosacral system
- the circulation of the blood (supply of arterial blood and venous drainage)
- the nervous system
- the endocrine system (hormone system)
- the lymphatic system
- the respiratory system
- the locomotive apparatus (muscles, connective tissue, fasciae, ligaments, tendons, joints).

There are close, interactive connections between these body systems. Gentle craniosacral therapy supports these body systems and establishes balance between them.

Craniosacral therapy addresses all these systems, either directly or indirectly, and harmonizes them. The following is an overall summary.

Craniosacral treatment of the head might for instance give the *entrance and exit points of the cranial nerves* more space to perform their function better; this has a positive effect on the processing of all motor, sensory, and sensorimotor stimuli and impulse transmission; it also aids the *balance of the autonomic nervous system*, since it encourages the reduction of stress and assists the process of dealing with external stimuli.

The release of tension in *muscles and connective tissue* benefits the entire body. Some muscles and ligaments are directly connected with bones of the craniosacral system, and so these tissues enfold much of the craniosacral system. Excessive tension in the muscles and connective tissue can adversely affect the craniosacral system; for example, hardening of the muscles of the pectoral girdle affects the upper thoracic vertebrae, the cervical vertebrae, and the transition between these and the cranium. That restricts the motion of the craniosacral rhythm and can also affect body posture, help to cause headaches, and lead to compensatory patterns. Given that the connective tissue runs in both lengthwise and transverse directions in a three-dimensional manner throughout the whole body, the state of tension of the connective tissue is particularly important in determining whether the craniosacral rhythm can be sensed over the entire body, and how evenly it is felt.

Good *arterial and venous perfusion* is also vital; our bodies suffer if the blood circulation is poor, with damage being caused for example to the limbs, the organs and especially the brain. Craniosacral therapy helps improve blood perfusion, and so eases learning difficulties or reduces the likelihood of stroke and heart attacks.

Another important element, besides the circulation of the blood, is the flow of *lymph*, which removes toxins and waste products. When we give craniosacral treatment, our hands also rest on one or more of the body's lymph glands – numbering in all some 700 – and so of course, this encourages the flow of lymph. The subtle motion of an unrestricted, harmonized craniosacral rhythm produces constant lymphatic drainage. To a minor extent, CSF reaches the tissues – the living matrix – in the spinal region and is taken up by the lymph.

Respiration is essential to life and continues throughout our lives, yet little attention is paid to the force of breathing. It is possible to bring about conscious changes in our breathing, although for the most part, it is subconsciously governed by the central nervous system. Craniosacral therapy aids free respiration, helping the elimination of waste substances and leading to greater energy and enjoyment of life.

The significance of the *endocrine system* (hormone system) is highly complex. There is no doubt of its vital function for our life and its effects on us at the physical, mental, and spiritual levels: human development and well-being depend on a well-functioning, well-controlled endocrine system. It contains, for example, the hypothalamus, which is involved in the control of mood reactions and forms the anterior floor of the third ventricle; it lies in the diencephalon. The hypothalamus also governs sleep, hormone secretion, body temperature, water balance, blood pressure and the sensation of hunger. Although it has been the subject

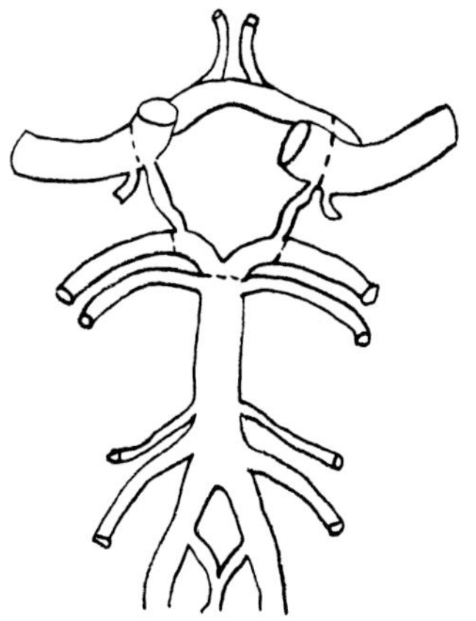

Figure 1.4.1
The cerebral arterial circle around the sella turcica at the sphenoid.

of much research, many of its connections have still not yet been fully clarified.

Below are some more concrete examples of effects of the craniosacral system on individual body systems.

The supply of blood to the brain

The unrestricted provision of blood to the brain is extremely important for the brain's many functions. About 750 mL of oxygen-rich blood are needed every minute for the brain to maintain its functions. The release of the cranial bones has a positive effect on the many entry and exit points: the cerebral arteries and veins, giving them more room in general.

Arterial supply – an example: The most important arteries of the brain are those around the sella turcica, which are interlinked and unite to form a circle of vessels called the cerebral arterial circle or circle of Willis (*circulus arteriosus cerebri*). Release of the frontal bone and of the parietal and temporal bones helps give more room to the sphenoid, which lies in a position surrounded by these other bones. That enables it to resume or improve its natural motion, aiding the motility and mobility of the cranial bones and membranes (the meninges). These motions maintain the flexibility of the cranial base and drain the circle of vessels surrounding the sella turcica, in turn assisting the perfusion of the brain. The increased flexibility of these arteries also helps prevent a blood vessel becoming obstructed or rupturing (and thus it can prevent a stroke) (Figs 1.4.1, 1.4.2).

Venous drainage – an example: The venous blood passes through thousands of vein branches in the brain, until it all collects in the venous sinuses. The most important of these are the superior and inferior sagittal sinuses (*sinus sagittalis superior/inferior*). The used blood passes from here into the transverse sinuses (*sinus transversus*). Finally, the venous blood

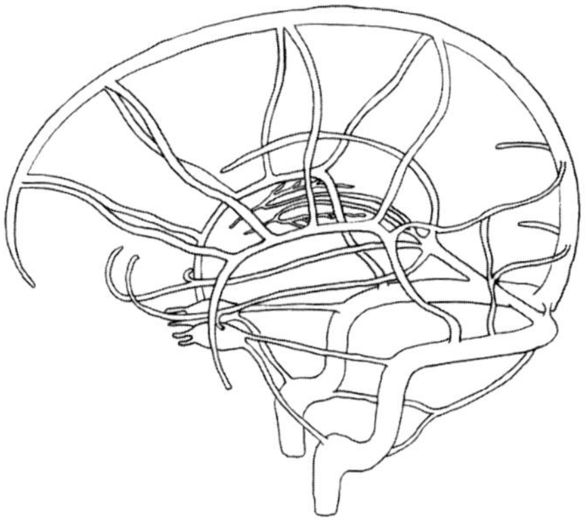

Figure 1.4.2
Venous drainage of the brain.

passes to the cranial base, down to the sigmoid sinus (*sinus sigmoideus*). The blood from many vein branches passes through the internal jugular vein (*vena jugularis interna*) into the superior vena cava and so back to the heart. The superior sagittal sinus runs past the upper border of the falx cerebri and the inferior sagittal sinus past its lower border. There is a particularly large number of arachnoid granulations in the superior sagittal sinus; these reabsorb the CSF back into the blood. The motions of the craniosacral rhythm also assist in preventing a congestion of venous drainage.

The gentle stretching of the falx cerebri that accompanies the lifting of the frontal and parietal bones encourages venous drainage through the sinuses above and below the falx and the straight sinus (*sinus rectus*). Release of the temporal bones and an occipital bone freed of tension and adhesions allow the occipitomastoid suture greater mobility and in particular give more room to the jugular foramen (*foramen jugulare*). About 85% of the venous blood leaving the head passes through the two jugular foramina.

At the same time, release of the cranial bones and membranes allows the cranial nerves and vessels as a whole more room for the optimum performance and control of the vital functions they serve (Fig. 1.4.3).

Balancing the autonomic nervous system

One of the benefits of craniosacral therapy is to strengthen the mechanism that plays such an essential role in self-regulation of the body: the autonomic nervous system. This part of the nervous system stimulates and controls the functioning of important organs, a process that is carried on quite involuntarily and without our being conscious of it. Examples of such processes are the stimulation of the striated muscle of the heart, of most glands, and of the smooth muscle of many organs. Our bodies are able to carry out this control of our vital functions faultlessly over long periods of time. However, if excessive demands are

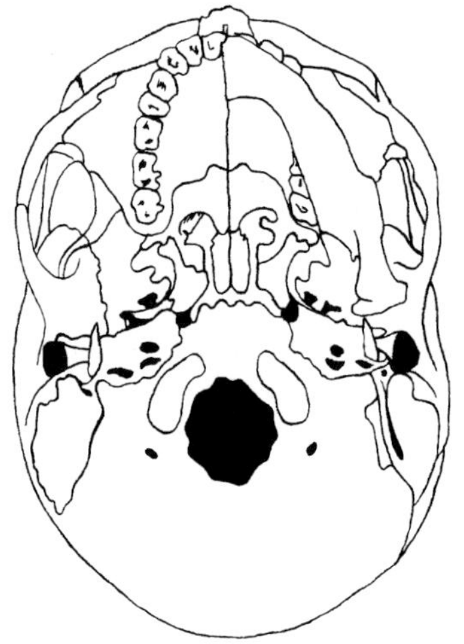

Figure 1.4.3
The exit points of nerves, arteries, and veins at the cranial base (simplified).

made of their self-regulatory powers for any length of time, e.g., through permanent stress, sustained extreme exertion, sleep deprivation, or becoming excessively strained or overburdened, a point can be reached when even the body's self-regulatory mechanism is no longer able to cope and no longer works at its usual capacity.

Craniosacral treatment aids multifaceted self-regulation and strengthens the immune system, so that diseases simply do not arise.

The autonomic nervous system has recently been subdivided into the following categories:

- the sympathetic nervous system
- the parasympathetic nervous system
- the social nervous system.

The traditional model by which it is divided into sympathetic and parasympathetic systems has been established for about 100 years. The research by Dr Stephen Porges and the practical results he obtained in autistic individuals confirm his theory of the social nervous system, which will be briefly outlined later in this chapter. In craniosacral therapy, attention should be paid to the adaptability of the tri-partite nervous system; in other words, to see that all systems are free and able to react appropriately with the external environment.

The sympathetic and parasympathetic systems are continually delivering impulses to exercise control of functions, for example, to the:

- lacrimal glands
- heart
- lungs
- stomach
- parts of the large intestine
- kidneys

- uterus
- genitals
- sweat glands.

The sympathetic and parasympathetic systems balance each other in such a way that there should always be the possibility (according to the situation) for one system to be stimulated without entirely blocking the other. During everyday activities, it is mainly the sympathetic system that predominates, while the parasympathetic system is predominant during stages of rest and relaxation. A balanced autonomic nervous system (ANS) can adapt within a very short time, changing and re-establishing balance without remaining fixed in a one-sided bias.

Permanent stress and the psychosomatic dysbalance that this leads to, are among the main causes of disease in western culture. Millions of people no longer find it easy to relax naturally. Their autonomic nervous system has become accustomed to the necessity for *permanent sympathetic-system stimulation* and is to some extent dependent on it. The natural alternation and balance between the sympathetic and parasympathetic systems are often limited because of excessive sympathetic over-stimulation. If the capacity for balance is lacking, the only option for the ANS, instead of self-regulation (in a broad mid-range region) is often that of descending from high sympathetic stimulation to the opposite extreme of pronounced parasympathetic dominance. This can be expressed as 'shut-down', a breakdown of regulatory capacity in the form of extreme exhaustion or burn-out.

Sadly, it is not only adults who suffer from permanent sympathetic system stimulation; many school pupils also suffer. The combination of this problem, eating the wrong foods and the lack of exercise increasingly leads children to develop learning and concentration problems, ADHD or ADD (attention-deficit disorder, see p. 310). Instead of compensating for the effects of permanent sympathetic system stimulation by administering tranquilizing and stimulating medication and other dependency-creating methods simply shifting the problem, treatment could address the cause and help the ANS to re-learn how to alternate between activity and passivity, and to engage in social participation. Craniosacral therapy, Somatic Experiencing® and other kinds of complementary medicine offer highly suitable methods to achieve this.

The sympathetic nervous system

A major part of the sympathetic nervous system consists of the sympathetic torso, which lies in the spinal cord; it runs down either side, down the spinal column between the first thoracic segment and the third lumbar segment; the alternative name of thoracolumbar segment is sometimes used because of this. The sympathetic nervous system enables us to take action or be capable of action (in the face of stress). This means that the sympathetic nervous system tends to dominate during the day. One of its roles is to transmit signals preparing us for 'fight or flight'.

Consequently, in situations involving activity or great stress for the body, the sympathetic nervous system subconsciously or instinctively:

- increases the respiratory rate
- makes the heart beat faster
- increases blood flow
- increases muscle tonus
- slows digestion
- dilates the pupils of the eye
- makes the liver prepare to release the energy from glycogen so as to meet energy demands quickly
- activates the sweat glands.

The parasympathetic nervous system

The major part of the parasympathetic nervous system lies in the brain stem and in the sacral region of the spinal cord. Some older anatomy books therefore refer to the parasympathetic system as the 'cranio-sacral' system.

This parallel is a very interesting one: craniosacral therapy strengthens the parasympathetic nervous system in particular; it is this that enables the individual suffering from excessive stress and sensory stimulation, to achieve relaxation and regeneration. The parasympathetic system predominates when we are calm and relaxed. Consequently, in situations of calm and relaxation, the parasympathetic nervous system subconsciously or instinctively:

- decreases the respiratory rate
- makes the heart beat more slowly
- promotes digestion and peristalsis
- promotes calm, sleep and recovery.

Along some of their course, the nerves or fibers belonging to some cranial nerve nuclei of the parasympathetic system run in common with cranial nerves CN III, CN VII, CN IX and CN X. There is a resultant effect on the narrowing of the pupils, the sensation of taste, the flow of saliva, the swallowing reflex and – especially in the case of CN X (the vagus nerve) – on the heart, coronary arteries, bronchi, stomach, arteries of the small intestine, and many glands.

The social nervous system and the vagus nerve

Since 1997, the neurobiological understanding of self-regulation has been extended and enriched by the concept of the social nervous system defined by Dr Stephen Porges (in particular his 'polyvagal' theory). The ANS is 'neuroceptive' in that it is constantly monitoring the external influences that surround us. This evaluation of our environment happens not by means of thought but subconsciously and directly by means of the nervous system. It is a process that occurs automatically in all human beings and all mammals, so that we are instantly prepared for fight or flight in dangerous situations. If we cannot do either, the nervous system switches to a self-defensive mechanism and 'freezes' in a reflex reaction of 'playing dead', in effect a dissociation and detachment from the here and now. The neuroception operating in human beings is 'defective,' in that our nervous system reports a threat even when there is no external cause. In a reaction based on previous threatening situations, they feel insecure, and their nervous systems report danger without any obvious cause. Trivial matters lead to confusion, fear, retreat or over-vigorous reactions.

The social nervous system is made up of cranial nerves CN V, CN VII, CN IX, CN X and CN XI, which play an important role in the making of social contacts and sympathetic engagement with others. Emotional ties, relationships, and social engagement are important for human health. These take place by means of facial expression (part of the trigeminal nerve, CN V), all the muscles responsible for facial expression (the facial nerve, CN VII), the intonation of the voice (glossopharyngeal nerve, CN IX and vagus nerve, CN X), the heart and lungs (vagus) and the movements of the head and neck (accessory nerve, CN XI).

The vagus nerve is especially interesting. The control of this nerve derives from a number of different nuclei and nerve origins, and it has many different functions; thus the term 'polyvagal system'. Some parts of the vagus nerve emerge from the medulla oblongata via the posteriorly situated (*dorsal*) nucleus of the solitary tract. In phylogenic terms, this is the older part of the vagus. In situations of danger, it can reduce all the body functions to a minimum, in effect serving to save energy in emergency or danger. In weeks 30–32 of fetal development, another part of the vagus begins to take shape: nerve fibers begin to emerge from the medulla oblongata via the anteriorly situated (*ventral*) nucleus ambiguus. This part of the vagus is myelinated, which means that the reactions occur very quickly. Its functions are most certainly of the social type, since it regulates such things as the facial muscles and the throat, and so controls facial expression and the voice. That extends our capacity to express ourselves, makes us more animated and enables more open, social behavior. This part of the vagus is involved in such matters as expressing love, in making contact with another person and in the search for a partner. If you would like further information, articles by Stephen Porges can be found on his homepage (www.psych.uic.edu/faculty/porges.htm).

Craniosacral therapy need not just be an end in itself, leading the client from tension (sympathetic nervous system) to relaxation (parasympathetic nervous system). It is also effective for the client in the longer term, for example if the client finds the route from tension to relaxation and is able to experience both poles of the situation in an appropriate way, internally, externally *and in social engagement in the here and now*. This also helps the client to encounter others in a freer, more authentic way. Therapeutic dialog during the sessions is also an important aid (see p. 90 and p. 267).

The 'second brain', the enteric nervous system

The vagus nerve has spreading, efferent branches, but also around 31 000 afferent fibers (nerve fibers leading to the brain). A few decades ago, Gerda Boyesen rediscovered the dual biological and psychological function of the gastrointestinal tract (GI tract). The interaction of brain and abdomen on the emotional and neurological level has now become a current topic once more. The neurobiologist Michael Gershon has pointed out some interesting associations in his book 'The Second Brain'. There is an exchange of information between the 'second brain' (which has around as many nerve cells as the brain) and the brain itself, via the vagus nerve. Various areas of the brain and endocrine structures need to receive information about conditions below the diaphragm. In this context, the GI tract, especially the abdominal wall, produces substances manufactured by the body, such as dopamine and serotonin. The enteric nervous system is a large association of peripheral ganglia that function like small organizatory satellite brains and are governed by other autonomic nerves; these operate to switch the enteric nervous system on and off. The vagus nerve can be seen as an intermediary between the 'second brain' and the brain in our heads.

The cranial nerves and their functions

The nervous system receives input from the senses, and integrates the information from these stimuli and the corresponding response. It enables and influences communication between ourselves and our environment. Nerve tissue transmits impulses bioelectrically, by means of minute electrical currents, and passes the message on by means of chemical substances, special messenger substances called neurotransmitters.

Each hemisphere of the brain has 12 cranial nerves. All of these, with the exception of the vagus nerve, are 'only' situated in the head and neck region. Almost all the cranial nerves arise from the brain stem; from there they run in very different directions throughout the head and neck region, depending on their role. Tension release at the cranium gives the cranial nerves more room, especially at their entry and exit points which can become narrowed or overstretched as a result of stress or accidents. Even a tiny reduction in pressure in the cranial nerves helps them to function better.

The individual cranial nerves

Cranial nerve I: Olfactory nerve

The olfactory nerve (*nervus olfactorius*) is a purely sensory nerve that carries the input from the sense of smell. It links the primary sensory cells in the mucous membrane of the nose with the olfactory cortex in the brain.

Cranial nerve II: Optic nerve

The optic nerve (*nervus opticus*) is also a purely sensory nerve, responsible for the transmission of visual information. It begins in the retina of the eyes, and even within the orbit of the eye (*orbita*) it is already surrounded by dura mater and pia mater. Its diameter as it leaves the orbit is around 4–5 mm. The left and right optic nerves meet at the optic chiasm (*chiasma opticum*), passing together over the pituitary gland and diaphragma sellae. The optic tract then passes over the thalamus to the cerebral cortex.

Cranial nerve III: Oculomotor nerve

The oculomotor nerve (*nervus oculomotorius*), together with the IV and VI cranial nerves, control the movements of the eyeball and supply the muscles responsible for raising the eyelids. It passes through the dura mater at the superior orbital fissure (*fissura orbitalis superior*).

Cranial nerve IV: Trochlear nerve

The trochlear nerve (*nervus trochlearis*) is a purely somatomotor nerve, and controls a single muscle of the eye, the superior oblique (*musculus obliquus superior*). It is the thinnest of the 12 cranial nerves.

Cranial nerve V: Trigeminal nerve

The trigeminal nerve (*nervus trigeminus*) is both a sensory and a somatomotor nerve. Its role includes responsibility for the facial and masticatory muscles: its three main branches are the ophthalmic, maxillary, and mandibular nerves. The sensory parts of the trigeminal nerve supply the whole of the face, the mucous membranes of the face and the greater part of the meninges. A motor part of the nerve supplies the mandible or the masticatory muscles. The fifth cranial nerve forms part of the social nervous system, because the face is involved in the expression of feelings.

Cranial nerve VI: Abducent nerve

The abducent nerve (*nervus abducens*) is a purely motor nerve; it is responsible for the outward, i.e. sideways, movement of the eyes.

Cranial nerve VII: Facial nerve

The facial nerve (*nervus facialis*) has motor, parasympathetic, and sensory functions. The somatomotor part supplies all the muscles and nerves of facial expression, and its roles include facial expression, speaking, eating, drinking, and the closing of the eyelids. The parasympathetic fibers run to the various glands (lacrimal, nasal, palatine, and submandibular glands). The sensory part carries taste sensation from the anterior two-thirds of the tongue, where most of the taste receptors are located.

The VII cranial nerve forms part of the social nervous system, because the face is involved in the expression of feelings.

Cranial nerve VIII: Vestibulocochlear nerve

The role of the vestibulocochlear nerve (*nervus vestibulocochlearis*) is purely sensory. It transmits acoustic (hearing) and postural (balance and motion) stimuli via the thalamus to the cerebral cortex and other areas of the brain.

Cranial nerve IX: Glossopharyngeal nerve

The glossopharyngeal nerve (*nervus glossopharyngeus*) has motor, parasympathetic, and sensory functions including the transmission of a special sense – taste. Along with the vagus nerve, it controls the movement of the muscles of the throat. Parasympathetic fibers run to the parotid gland. Sensory branches also transmit sensations of taste from the posterior third of the tongue. This nerve is also responsible for sensation in the mucous membranes of the throat.

The IX cranial nerve forms part of the social nervous system, because the face is involved in the expression of feelings.

Cranial nerve X: Vagus nerve

The vagus nerve (*nervus vagus*) is the longest and most extensive nerve. It has motor, parasympathetic, and sensory functions, including transmission of a special sense, and it extends from the head region down as far as the abdominal region. Its motor role is in controlling the muscles of the throat and vocal cords.

The vagus is the main nerve of the parasympathetic system, and so has a great influence: it has considerable involvement in the parasympathetic innervation of the heart, intestinal motion, bronchi, stomach, intestines, liver, gallbladder, pancreas, and kidneys. One effect of the vagus nerve is to make the heart beat more slowly, and it also transmits sensory impulses for increased secretion of digestive juices. Somatosensory parts run to the meninges of the posterior cranial fossa, the external acoustic meatus and the pharyngeal and laryngeal regions. Special sensory connections transmit information including that from the taste receptors in the throat and stretch receptors of the heart and lungs (respiratory reflex).

The parts of the vagus (the social parts) that emerge from the ventral region of the medulla oblongata supply the organs above the diaphragm; those that emerge from its dorsal region mainly supply the organs below the diaphragm.

The X cranial nerve forms part of the social nervous system, because facial expression, uttered sounds, speech, and voice are involved in non-verbal communication, especially the expression of feelings.

Cranial nerve XI: Accessory nerve

The accessory nerve (*nervus accessorius*) has a purely motor function. Its branches supply mainly the sternocleidomastoid and trapezius muscles (*musculus sternocleidomastoideus; musculus trapezius*).

The XI cranial nerve forms part of the social nervous system, because movements of the head are involved in non-verbal communication, especially the expression of feelings (e.g., turning toward or away from someone; nodding of the head).

Cranial nerve XII: Hypoglossal nerve

The hypoglossal nerve (*nervus hypoglossus*) is a purely motor nerve and supplies the muscles of the tongue. It is therefore important for speaking, eating, and drinking.

The vagus and trigeminal nerves supply the choroid plexus on the walls of the cerebral ventricles. These are where fresh CSF is formed out of the blood.

Brain activity

Increased blood flow to the brain enables improved functioning of the cerebrum and cerebellum. The cerebrum is the largest part of the brain, and the knowledge gained over a lifetime is stored in its cerebral cortex. The cerebrum is divided into two hemispheres, each of which has four parts called lobes. These are named according to the cranial bone that defines their position: frontal lobe, parietal lobe, temporal lobe, and occipital lobe. The cerebellum is involved in the coordination and performance of movement sequences.

An increase in craniosacral motion brings about drainage of the brain stem and reticular formation (*formatio reticularis*), which are very primitive brain structures in evolutionary terms, and bathes them in 'fresh' CSF.

Nerve nuclei in the brain stem coordinate body processes that are important for survival, such as breathing and heartbeat. One of the effects of the stronger, more balanced craniosacral rhythm at the occipital bone is to stimulate function in the cerebellum and brain stem region, something that should be borne in mind when treating individuals with heart or breathing problems or undifferentiated fine motor function.

An interesting additional point is that regulation of *brain frequencies* probably occurs in the two masses of the thalamus. Most people have a direct connection between the two thalamic masses via the interthalamic adhesion (*adhesio interthalamica*) across the third ventricle. Deep relaxation can be consciousness-expanding and has an effect on brain activity, the thalamus and especially the CSF in the third ventricle; parts through which healing processes and spontaneous healing are believed to be especially assisted and brain frequencies positively influenced.

Endocrine organs and the hormone system

The motions of the cranial bones and brain also stimulate the hormone system. Hormones are messenger substances that influence important body functions, human behavior and emotions. The hormones are released into the bloodstream and travel through it to reach their target cells; this is the route by which control and regulation of the hormone system continually takes place.

Release of tension of the cranial bones and meninges gives the cranial base more room; this applies especially to the centrally-located sphenoid. The effect of this is that the craniosacral rhythm is freer to move into flexion and extension/ER–IR. The diaphragma sellae and tentorium cerebelli form two horizontal diaphragms, transverse structures in the brain. The attachments of both include the bony prominences of the anterior and posterior clinoid processes of the sphenoid. The motions of the craniosacral rhythm also help give these diaphragms and all intracranial membranes more motility and mobility. This in turn gives more freedom of motion to the cranial bones and all the other structures. One effect of these subtle motions, for example, is to stimulate the pituitary gland, epiphysis and hypothalamus and so to promote a well-balanced and vital hormone system.

The pituitary gland (hypophysis)

The sella turcica (the 'Turkish saddle') lies in the middle of the sphenoid, within the cranial base. The middle of this 'saddle' forms an open depression, the hypophysial fossa (*fossa hypophysialis*), in which sits the pituitary gland (*hypophysis*). The gland is about the size of a hazelnut; it lies beneath the diencephalon and above it stretches the diaphragma sellae. Above that is the optic chiasm. The pituitary gland consists of the larger, anterior lobe and the smaller posterior lobe. The blood–brain barrier is minimally developed at the posterior lobe, and the substances circulating in the blood can influence the neurons here.

The pituitary gland is a kind of hormonal 'executive organ' for the hypothalamus. The pituitary gland influences other endocrine glands, which in turn influence peripheral organs. For example, the end result of hormone stimulation of the kidney is increased production of red blood cells in the bone marrow; the kidney and the pancreas are responsible for the regulation of blood sugar levels.

The pituitary gland regulates the stimulation of hormone secretion by the adrenal glands, and its hormones also stimulate body growth, protein synthesis, the rise in blood sugar, lactation, and the onset of labor, by releasing the relevant hormones into the blood and CSF as and when required.

The pituitary gland has its own intrinsic motion brought about by its activity and stimulation by the hypothalamus, and also motion caused by the craniosacral rhythm of the sphenoid, on which it is moved to and fro. This has significance for its function.

The epiphysis (pineal gland, pineal body)

The epiphysis lies in the posterior part of the third ventricle in the posterior region of the diencephalon.

The significance that has been accorded to the pineal gland in the past has been more than almost any other structure in the brain. The evolutionary and biological development of this organ is also impressive: it is light-sensitive, and was more pronounced in the past as a 'parietal eye' in certain animals; even, it is thought, in humans. The development of the epiphysis has regressed considerably during the evolutionary process – perhaps because of the increasing development of optical vision by means of the eyes. Among ancient fish and quadrupeds, the 'median eye' was widespread, but few animals today have a superiorly positioned parietal eye; it exists for example in some lizards and frogs.

In many families of fish, the epiphyseal-diencephalon region is receptive to light stimuli. The skin over the pineal organ is translucent.

On the subject of the epiphysis and light, one of the functions of the epiphysis is the production of melatonin, which is involved in regulating the sleep–wake rhythm. It is produced in greater or lesser quantities irrespective of the season of the year or the external light conditions. Melatonin is sometimes taken medicinally to counteract jet lag, and was reputed for a time to have rejuvenating properties and to reduce the risk of cancer. Current research into diseases of the brain and nervous system (such as Parkinson's and Alzheimer's) assumes that melatonin plays a significant role in the removal of unwanted substances from the brain, for example heavy metals such as mercury, which we absorb from our environment and our food.

In the distant past, the seventeenth century, the last century and still more recently, scholars, seers, poets and philosophers have told of the remarkable qualities of the epiphysis. It is also involved in transformation processes relating to immaterial substances. Certainly balanced slow rhythms help to initiate and deepen the intricate task of self-regulation. In ER/flexion, the third ventricle rises in a 'V' shape, and in IR/extension it is lowered, taking the epiphysis with it in its motion.

Neurological wellsprings of consciousness

There are also other structures belonging to the nervous system and endocrine system located in the region of the diencephalon and mesencephalon, which have a profound influence on our humanity (Fig. 1.4.4). Some of these structures are presented here; nevertheless, the reason that our perceptions occur is not because of individual structures and regions of the brain, but because of cooperative events in complex, interactive circuits and feedback control systems, working together as a whole, as a unity, permeated by the spirit, inspired.

Figure 1.4.4
The pituitary gland (hypophysis), epiphysis, thalamus, and hypothalamus.

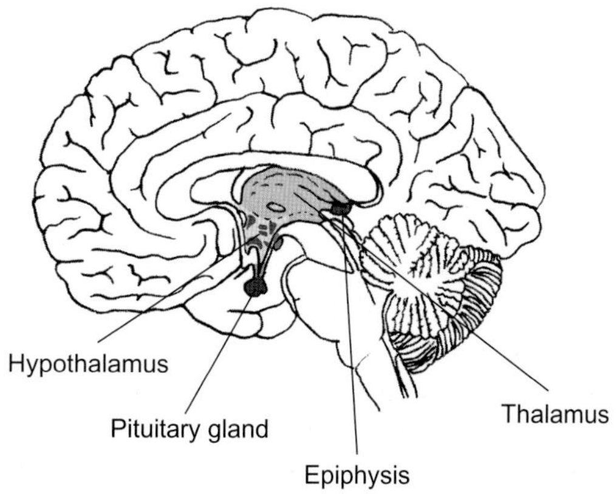

It is interesting to mention, at this point, the most recent results of brain research using the most modern imaging equipment, and also the oriental understanding of the system of energy in the human body, such as the chakras. The brow chakra, also called the third eye, lies at approximately the same horizontal level as the frontonasal suture, third ventricle, hypothalamus, thalamus and epiphysis. These are all regions where the portals of our inner and external perception open and where a natural expansion of consciousness occurs. Medical drugs such as tranquilizers, antidepressants or even anesthetics inhibit consciousness. Sedatives and stimulants mainly operate on or from these wellsprings of consciousness – these centers around the third ventricle and brainstem (including the reticular formation, *formatio reticularis*). If these regions are repeatedly stimulated by the more balanced craniosacral rhythm, it has the effect of increasing self-regulation, and a waking deep relaxation and an expansion of all the senses can spontaneously arise.

The thalamus

The thalamus is a bean-shaped structure about 3×1.5 cm in size and forms the center of the diencephalon. In an adult human, its volume accounts for about 1.4% of total brain volume. The thalamus is the primary collection point receiving all the sensory tracts, including those from all the senses except the sense of smell; from here, the information is relayed to the cerebral cortex. It therefore serves to integrate sensory and motor impulses. As the 'gateway to the consciousness', the thalamus is involved in ensuring that the perceptions of our senses reach our consciousness: it is here, for example, that information on movement is received and passed on. Acoustic information is filtered in the thalamus and relayed to the hearing cortex.

All kinds of information converge here; both our assessment of the external situation and that of our own bodily condition.

The walls of the left and right thalamus form the lateral limits of the third ventricle, in which fresh CSF is produced. Many of the substances contained in the CSF are important carriers of information in the communication of the nerve and hormone systems. Many structures influence and potentiate the CSF here, in the center of the brain.

The fluctuation of the CSF and various slow rhythms stimulate the left and right thalamus, the hypothalamus, and the epiphysis across the midline of the third ventricle. What amazing organization and interplay of Nature …

The hypothalamus

The hypothalamus is situated roughly in the middle of the brain, beneath the thalamus, and is the center of all the body's autonomic processes. It forms the anterior floor of the third ventricle. Under the hypothalamus, the pars tuberalis of the pituitary leads to the pituitary gland. The hypothalamus contains autonomic regulation centers and is in turn connected with centers of the central nervous system. Despite the tiny space it occupies in the brain, no other region apart from the brain stem has as many different and vital control functions as the hypothalamus: it regulates sleep, temperature, water balance, the sensations of hunger and satiety, blood pressure, sexual behavior, learning processes and hormone secretion. It is also responsible for the balance of the sympathetic and parasympathetic nervous system and has an influence on emotions and their physical effects. It consists of multiple circuits that are interconnected and also relate to the limbic system.

Control hormones are also produced in the hypothalamus; these are secretory and inhibitory hormones that pass from the hypothalamus to the pituitary gland and govern hormone production there.

It is also interesting to discover that the hypothalamus plays a part in the reduction and intensification of stimuli. So there is such a thing as all-embracing consciousness, but it is held in check and controlled by our reason and instinct for various reasons, including the important one of protection from being overwhelmed by stimuli. For instance, if the external or internal changes result in the hypothalamus receiving a message to switch from stimulus reduction to greater or more differentiated intensification of stimuli, this brings about a natural extension of consciousness. It then becomes possible, for example, either to listen to the orchestra as a whole or to distinguish various individual instruments.

Some 40 000 nerve fibers run from the hypothalamus to the pituitary gland, and the entire region is stimulated by the more balanced motion of the craniosacral rhythm.

The limbic system and the amygdaloid body (corpus amygdaloideum)

The limbic system includes parts of the cerebrum, hypothalamus and hippocampus and can be understood in functional terms as the *center of emotional behavior and of memory*. Limbic fibers link many nerve nuclei in the diencephalon and mesencephalon. The hippocampus is responsible for the arousal of aggression, emotional behavior and drives. Moods and emotions are located in the limbic system beneath the threshold of our consciousness, and affect motivation.

The amygdaloid body (*corpus amygdaloideum*) is part of the limbic system. It can store and retain a memory of states of excitement and fear. In every harmoniously performed craniosacral treatment that provides the experience of trust and release, the amygdaloid body can let go of part of the memory of trauma from its cell memory. At this moment, in a safe therapeutic context, the client can find the relaxed and anxiety-free experience of new sensations such as the unity of body, mind and spirit, inner freedom or joy. The direct experiencing of the new sensations in the here and now causes these too to be neurologically stored – the earlier traumatic experience is put into perspective, enabling healing.

The immune system and psychoimmunology

Psychological events influence autonomic functions via the limbic system, directly affecting such functions as breathing and the circulation. A harmonious emotional state, calmness, and trust enhance the body's powers of resistance. Worry, anxiety, doubt, and mistrust reduce these powers. The improved regulation of the body as a whole and the harmonization of the sympathetic and parasympathetic systems, the autonomic nervous system, strengthen the immune system.

'Good stress' (Eustress), by which is meant the active, healthy surmounting of the demands of everyday life, has a motivating and strengthening effect, while 'bad stress' (Dystress) such as constant stress, weakens the immune system. Physical stress (wounds, burns, infections, operations) is to be distinguished in this respect from psychological stress (fear, annoyance, performance pressure), although in everyday experience, the two are linked.

The body reacts to both types of stress by one stress reaction

- In response to stress, certain stress hormones are released into the CSF within seconds.
- The hypothalamus is activated, causing a hormone message to be sent via the pituitary gland to the cortex of the suprarenal gland (adrenal cortex), which is stimulated to release glucocorticoids – stress hormones that bring about a rise in blood sugar level and influence carbohydrate metabolism.
- The medulla of the suprarenal gland (adrenal medulla) produces epinephrine (adrenalin) and norepinephrine (noradrenalin). Both these substances stimulate the sympathetic nervous system. This speeds up the activity of the heart and increases blood pressure and blood sugar levels. Epinephrine is also produced by psychological excitement.

Possible consequences of constant stress

- more frequent infections as a result of weakening of the immune system
- less resistance to infections and slower recovery from illnesses
- lack of sleep or an unrefreshing sleep
- reduced ability to learn and concentrate
- tension headaches
- digestive problems
- risk of burn-out
- listlessness
- irregular and unbalanced craniosacral rhythm.

The field of psychoimmunology is receiving increasing attention, even in allopathic medicine – and the hypothalamus influences the immune system. This in turn is closely connected with the limbic system, which has close functional connections with what is happening psychologically. Research has shown that positive thoughts, meditation and prayer strengthen the immune system. The nervous system, hormone system and immune system are ultimately a single network, something that has been pointed out by, among others, Professor Candace B. Pert in her book 'Molecules of emotion. Why you feel the way you feel' (see Further Reading).

In industrialized countries, most people are already under severe and permanent pressure. This 'dystress' increasingly leads to psychosomatic disorders of all kinds, especially back pain and sleep disturbances. Unhealthy stress also places a burden on the cardiovascular system and predisposes to strokes and heart attacks.

Permanent overstimulation of the sympathetic nervous system can produce adverse consequences

- Individuals, along with their nervous system, become so accustomed to permanent stress that they need the stress and become addicted to excitement, including the 'adrenalin kick'.
- The autonomic nervous system ceases to be capable of moderation, and only knows or can only maintain the highest level of sympathetic activity, or at the other extreme parasympathetic depression. In extreme cases, this can lead to 'vagus shut-down' or nervous breakdown, together with long-term autonomic problems.

1.5 The craniosacral rhythm: An expression of primary respiration

The phenomenon of the craniosacral rhythm

The craniosacral rhythm, which has a frequency of approximately 6–12 cycles/min, and also the slower mid-tide and long-tide, are an expression of a phenomenon known in the craniosacral model as *primary respiration* or the *Breath of Life*. Primary respiration, with its various rhythms, is in principle always an expression of health, always striving for the 'perfect blueprint of existence', for originality and for wholeness. The expression of primary respiration always focuses on optimum harmonization of the body as a whole, down to the cellular level.

There are various theories and indicators as to what factors and structures are involved in giving rise to these slow-motion oscillations. No conclusive explanation for the motions of the craniosacral rhythm has yet been found: what causes it, or where or how it is regulated; a number of different influences probably contribute. For me as a practitioner, the question of how far the craniosacral rhythm can be demonstrated scientifically tends to fade into the background. I have encountered many practical instances of therapeutic success, and research has been carried out into how a craniosacral system operates when freely functioning or restricted. For me, it remains an actual phenomenological event as well as an everyday, palpable fact. Over recent decades, other body rhythms have been measured, both slower and faster, in addition to the rhythm of 6–12 cycles/min, in studies using a variety of methods.

In this book, as mentioned above, basic craniosacral treatment involving the craniosacral rhythm of around 6–12 cycles/min is described. Slower rhythms can also be palpated during treatment in addition to the craniosacral rhythm, so a brief account of these will also be given.

My own understanding of the various rhythms was greatly helped in particular by regularly and frequently palpating my own body rhythms and those of other people. Nature all around us also constantly presents us with wonderful displays: a soft wind moving the gently swaying fields and woods; the rolling waves of the ocean, now faster, now slower, and (like the wind) at any single moment, presenting us with the expression of individuality, vitality, dynamism, and power – like the craniosacral rhythm and slower rhythms.

Theories and scientific research achieve recognition and survive until the next discoveries take their place. The answer I give today to the question, 'Where does the craniosacral rhythm come from?' is that I know a number of models to explain it, but that I cannot answer with absolute certainty; nor do I wish to; however I believe it is jointly caused by several different macrocosmic and microcosmic systems and factors.

Where do the ocean waves come from? Why is the swell of the sea sometimes heavy, sometimes light? What precisely lies behind the ebb and flow of the tide? Is it mainly affected by the wind, or currents and undercurrents, differences in temperature or the circulation of water flowing into the seas and evaporating? In what proportions do the sun and moon, the polarity of the earth, the displacement of the earth's axis or the cosmos have an influence; how, for instance, do these affect the polarity of the body itself and body rhythms? The rise and fall of the water at high and low tide are tangible and evident to the senses; something we can feel, see, and hear. So it is with the slow rhythms of the body, which we can learn, with practice, to palpate. If our attitude is too analytical or skeptical, it can lessen our enjoyment of the subject, in the relaxed perception of natural rhythms and the wisdom of the body.

… and all is in motion

As described in Chapter 1, the continual production of CSF, its rhythmic expulsion and drainage into the blood and peripherally into the lymph – probably combined with the force and expression of the mid-tide, a slower expression of primary respiration – gives rise to a slow rhythmic motion of approximately 6–12 cycles/min in the body. This motion is called the craniosacral rhythm (CSR) or cranial rhythmic impulse (CRI). It can be palpated on the head and on the sacrum, and also over the entire body via bones and muscles and especially via the connective tissue.

Explanatory models to account for the craniosacral rhythm

As we have said, various concepts are held among schools, instructors, and practitioners of craniosacral therapy to account for the cause of the craniosacral rhythm and slower rhythms.

One model, which looks to the pressure of the CSF to explain the origin and regulation of the craniosacral rhythm, is that set out by John E. Upledger. This takes as its starting point stretch receptors at the cranial sutures, especially at the sagittal suture between the paired parietal bones: the constant production of CSF increases the fluid pressure and causes the cranium to stretch to varying degrees. Increased fluid pressure in the lateral ventricles causes the parietal bones to move slowly into external rotation (ER), so that the comb-like interlocking digits of the sagittal suture become angled downwards. This activates the stretch receptors lying beneath the suture, which is thought to lead to a reduction in CSF production. That in turn produces a change in motion, initiating internal rotation (IR) – at the same time, CSF is forced into the external CSF spaces. At the end of IR, when the stretch receptors are deactivated, CSF pressure rises again and the parietal bones move into ER once again. This process of pressure adjustment finds expression as the craniosacral rhythm.

The assumption according to this theory is that a connection exists, running from certain receptors beneath the sagittal suture to the third ventricle or laterally to this, to the thalamus, from where the impulses are relayed onward.

Another explanatory model assigns great importance to the exchange process by which blood is turned into CSF.

The following factors probably also contribute to the motion of the craniosacral rhythm

- the brain and spinal cord, which have a degree of motility
- the blood circulation, because the pumping and pulsating activity to some extent also moves other tissue
- the combined firing of groups of neurons, and all local and general activities of the brain.

The craniosacral rhythm, the mid-tide and the long-tide are (as already stated) *different forms of expression of primary respiration*, the 'Breath of Life' – they are *not* the Breath of Life itself. Primary respiration is that same primeval force that breathes life into everything on this planet through all sorts of natural rhythms, that plays its part in giving form by its rhythmic ordering through these rhythms and that perfuses each and every form.

According to the biodynamic model, it is the mid-tide that 'generates' the craniosacral rhythm of approximately 6–12 cycles/min.

The *mid-tide* fluctuates relatively slowly in and around the body with a frequency of 2–3 cycles/min, about 2–4 times slower than the craniosacral rhythm. Usually the mid-tide can be detected after several spontaneous still points. Signs of the mid-tide are when, as we listen, we find that the sense of the structure that we had previously clearly perceived is now fading away, and the rhythm is now becoming distinctly slower. This sensation can seem as if:

- we are distinctly sensing the person's energy field/aura/biosphere
- we are sensitively touching a fluid body in its entirety
- the person's body is fluid/liquid
- we can sense the body as a whole slowly breathing
- we can sense the cells moving
- touch contact has been made with the person's energy body and the individual's bioelectric field is reorganizing itself.

The *long-tide* is the slowest of the three expressions of the Breath of Life, with one cycle per 100 seconds. The long tide is a macrocosmic rhythm operating in the whole of nature right down to the microcosmic realm and can be sensed both outside and within the body.

The long-tide 'generates' the mid-tide.

It is a highly interesting fact that our protoplasm moves in the same rhythm. I do not doubt the rhythm of 1/100 seconds (s) (50 s inhalation; 50 s exhalation), although there are also models, hierarchies, and evaluations created in the biodynamic field that may be imagined or brought about by the practitioner as a result of mental intention or projection rather than by giving adequate respect to the indwelling treatment plan or the needs and capacities of the client.

In the functional and biodynamic approach in particular, the practitioner provides a protected space, and also fulfils the function of a neutral, grounded, centered fulcrum. *If the mid-tide appears, structural techniques like those described in this book, which has a structural-functional focus, are seldom used.* For example, the client's self-regulation and the self-healing processes are promoted and strengthened using the three-step healing process (see p. 246).

At the level of the mid-tide, you should remain in the midst of it, quietly listening and staying with the slow movements and spontaneous still points. You may be amazed at the self-correction that is revealed, manifesting itself in the entire surrounding energy of the patient's body and in the various body structures. These self-corrections can be local, or can take place in the client's body as a whole. Your space-giving, neutral presence and stillness enable and encourage the self-healing processes.

In the biodynamic model of craniosacral therapy, there are some different terms, interpretations, and concepts in existence, and these continue to change and develop.

For example, William Garner Sutherland never referred to rhythms in terms of cycles/min and never spoke of the 'mid-tide' or 'long-tide'. These are more recent concepts, based on certain assumptions. A rhythm of 2–3 cycles/min does not necessarily indicate that this is the mid-tide; it is more a matter of levels of consciousness that are changing, expanding and deepening.

Fortunately, we cannot yet determine and standardize the slow rhythms down to the last detail, because by nature primary respiration is at once free, wild, and timid. The slow rhythms manifest themselves through motion and dynamism – always of the moment and unique – as the expression of a vital, flowing life force. Primary respiration, along with its rhythms, is essentially always an expression of healing force, of health, striving for balance and wholeness.

The craniosacral rhythm and the slow motions it engenders in the body

There are various theories and models to explain how the craniosacral rhythm of approximately 6–12 cycles/min comes about. It has been demonstrated that CSF is constantly being produced in the choroid plexus of the four interlinked cerebral ventricles. The CSF flows out through the three openings of the fourth ventricle into the CSF spaces.

The two lateral openings are called the lateral apertures (*aperturae laterales*) or foramina of Luschka, and the central one is the median aperture (*apertura mediana*) or foramen of Magendie. Here, the CSF passes from the inner CSF spaces into the outer ones, fluctuating in the brain region and along the spinal cord, even being present in small quantities in the central canal of the spinal cord. The center of our bodies is therefore constantly bathed in fresh, nourishing fluid.

The formation of the CSF causes a rise in pressure of the fluid. This together with other factors stretches and widens the subarachnoid space and, via the meninges, moves the cranial bones that are directly linked to it by means of these membranes. This occurs particularly at the sutures, in the craniosacral rhythm. Contrary to the view of many anatomists, the cranial sutures do not become firmly united with age, but function as joints that enable the subtle motions of the craniosacral rhythm. These minute motions of the cranial sutures are on a microlevel. *Experienced craniosacral therapists can palpate beyond this range. They achieve resonance with the motions of the craniosacral rhythm, its force and the various qualities of motion it can express, and with the dynamics of the entire craniosacral system as a functional unity, a whole.*

The fact that the craniosacral system runs from the head via the dural tube down to the sacrum and coccyx, and the CSF is distributed along the spinal cord, means that these subtle, slow motions of the craniosacral rhythm can also be sensed on the sacrum and over the entire body via the connective tissue.

The effect of the CSF is like a wind blowing into the sails (the meninges and intracranial membranes), so that it is able to move the whole system including the cranial bones and to free it from restrictions – in a manner that is at once subtle and dynamic.

Terminology: external and internal rotation (ER/IR), flexion and extension (fl./ex.)

The motions of the craniosacral rhythm can be felt on *paired regions of the body and cranial bones* as *external rotation (ER)* (that is, expanding laterally and becoming fuller and larger) and its opposite, *internal rotation/IR* (reduction in volume; becoming smaller).

For the bones of the midline (the sacrum, occipital bone, sphenoid, ethmoid and vomer), there is an equivalent motion to that which occurs on paired parts of the body: the equivalent to external rotation is *flexion* (fl.), and the equivalent to internal rotation is *extension* (ex.). Other terms met with in instruction and in specialist literature are 'inhalation' (or 'inspiration' (for ER/fl.) and 'exhalation' (or 'expiration') (for IR/ex.) (Fig. 1.5.1).

The terminology that is used to describe the motion is different from that used in physiotherapy. The craniosacral concept is concerned with motion occurring in the head, whereas physiotherapy deals with motion *of* the head. Craniosacral motion is defined in terms of the external,

Figure 1.5.1
The occipital bone and sphenoid and their direction of motion in flexion (simplified).

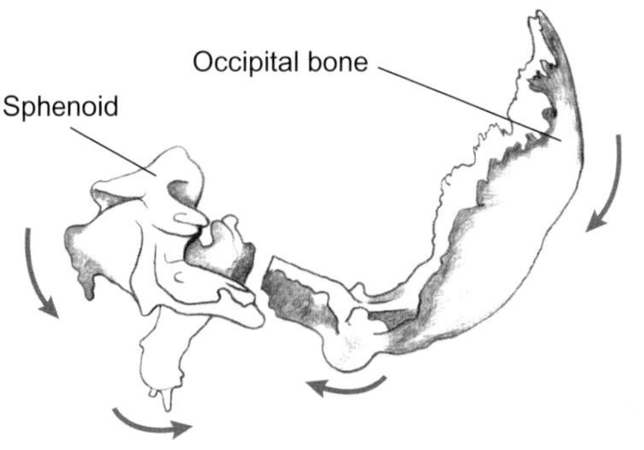

i.e. inferior, cranial base, which is mainly made up of the sphenoid, occipital and temporal bones. If the CSF pressure in the cerebral ventricles increases, the sphenoid and occiput widen upward and outward. The cranial base moves slightly in the cranial direction, so that the pterygoid processes (*proc. pterygoidei*) and occipital condyles (*condyli occipitales*) bend toward each other as observed *at the cranial base from below*, in the direction described as *flexion*. The opposite motion is one of *extension*, in which the pterygoid processes of the sphenoid and the occipital condyles extend away from each other.

The craniosacral rhythm as an indicator of vitality

Indications of the quality of the craniosacral rhythm

The motions of the craniosacral rhythm can be distinguished in terms of:

- strength
- amplitude/range
- right-left symmetry/evenness
- frequency/cycles per min/rate.

Strength: The craniosacral rhythm can be hesitant and scarcely detectable, as contrasted with the clearly detectable, very strong motion that sensitive palpating hands can sense, e.g., leading them inward and outward. Strength is not to be confused with amplitude or frequency.

Amplitude/range: The craniosacral rhythm can display a broad range of flexion and extension motion or external/internal rotation (ER/IR), or it may in contrast exhibit a narrow, limited range. With a little practice, it also becomes possible to palpate whether the range exhibited by the rhythm is greater in ER or in IR (or, whether it exhibits greater flexion or extension). Some individuals and some regions of the body do have a craniosacral system that displays markedly greater flexion or greater extension.

Symmetry: The craniosacral rhythm can be equal on both sides of the body, or it can be more restricted on one side. We palpate the evenness of the motion to the left and right of the midline.

Frequency/cycles per min/rate: The craniosacral rhythm displays a motion measuring approximately 6–12 cycles/min. This is slower than the cardiac and respiratory rhythms and can therefore be distinguished from them. The frequency of around 6–12 cycles/min (1 cycle = one flexion motion plus one extension motion, or ER/IR) is the normal rhythm if the craniosacral system is fairly free of restrictive or traumatic influences or is well able to compensate for these.

If a change in level occurs, as might happen after spontaneous still points, you may also palpate another rhythm: instead of the 6–12 cycles/min, you can detect the mid-tide of 2–3 cycles/min.

Differentiated palpation of the craniosacral rhythm

When palpating the craniosacral rhythm, the aspects that the practitioner focuses on include these four indicators of quality. The craniosacral therapist senses these, observes and evaluates how they change in the subsequent course of treatment and at the end of the session, in the following way:

- Is there an overall harmonization, a balancing of the craniosacral rhythm in terms of greater symmetry and regularity?
- Does the craniosacral rhythm – and with it the person's nervous system or consciousness – have the capacity to change? Is further treatment necessary before the rhythm is detectable at all and becomes more balanced?
- Is the motion greater in flexion or extension (or in external or internal rotation); in other words, is it more in one phase than in the other?
- Is the rhythm more distinct, stronger, and able to be detected at several places on the body? Can a certain strength or dynamism be felt?
- Are external and internal rotations more even, more balanced, on different paired cranial bones or different places on the body?

When we distinguish and differentiate the qualities of the craniosacral rhythm at various places on the body and on the head, our palpation provides us with indications as to where a body structure is either free or restricted. We can identify any possible interrelationships operating across the body as a whole, e.g. where there is evidence of considerable and strong craniosacral motion, indicating vital force and health. We can also recognize the way in which this particular body can best demonstrate and compensate for a dysfunction or avoidance pattern. The craniosacral rhythm always strives for the greatest possible balance and can quickly adapt. We encourage this by our presence, by listening, and by specific, gentle manual techniques.

In order to distinguish external/internal rotation (ER/IR) at individual bones of the craniosacral system (this is also called flexion and extension when it applies to the midline), we need to follow the motion of the rhythm for several cycles.

Example

The following directions of motion can be detected at paired locations, for example on the parietal bones, shoulders, pelvis or feet.

As you palpate, the craniosacral rhythm, a kind of slow whole-body respiration, draws your hands slowly outward and to the side (laterally); this is external rotation (ER).

At its furthermost point the rhythm may pause briefly; then it draws your palpating hands slowly inward (medially); this is internal rotation (IR), and you should follow it to its innermost point.

Here, the motion of this rhythm may turn outward (laterally) again either immediately or after a few seconds' pause, into ER. During ER, it may sometimes stop briefly before continuing in ER, or it may suddenly change direction and move straight back into IR, sooner than it did in the previous cycle.

At the same time as ER/IR, the craniosacral rhythm can be expressed in the longitudinal direction. Longitudinally the body seems to lengthen and then shorten slightly, breathing in the craniosacral rhythm and suffused by it. At the occipital bone, for example, the flexion is sensed *at the same time* as a lateral widening and a downward motion toward the nape of the neck. Extension is sensed here as a narrowing from side to side and at the same time as an upward gliding motion.

How strongly is the craniosacral rhythm expressed? How far does it move, or, how long does the motion of flexion and that of extension last? Do both extend over the same range? Is one side freer than the other? Is the frequency (approx. 12–14/min) just slightly slower than the respiratory rhythm, or very slow (approx. 6–8/min) or even slower?

At this point, I would like to mention the different axes of motion that are used to define the possible directions of motion of each individual bone from the biomechanical point of view. *Since this book is designed for beginners in this method, it will not go into detail by naming the axes of motion of all the bones of the craniosacral system.* These can be found in the publications listed in the 'Further reading' section.

Listen to the motion at various locations on the body and various cranial bones for at least 14 cycles, analyzing the qualities of the rhythm described above.

The craniosacral rhythm can change direction at any time (this change in direction is sometimes but not always associated with a short pause), because by its very nature it tends – like the ocean – always to flow freely and spontaneously.

Sometimes it can also feel as if two flexion (or ER) movements occur one after the other before the extension motion (IR) takes over, or as if the craniosacral rhythm has a staccato character instead of gliding fluently.

Evaluate the craniosacral rhythm by the quality of motion; it is the rhythm you evaluate and not the client. Listen for any changes in the rhythm. Follow it with a fundamentally passive, attentive and open attitude. With this attitude of mind, engage utterly and trustingly with the slow, subtle movements and spontaneous pauses, short or long. The craniosacral rhythm itself knows no right or wrong and can reveal itself differently at any interval – like the ebb and flow of the waves on the beach, never precisely the same …

Which movements appear to be fuller, broader, stronger, more balanced, clearer? As you palpate, note any tendencies, any recurrent imbalance appearing in the motion sequence, especially in relation to the four qualities of the craniosacral rhythm that were listed above.

Account can be taken of the craniosacral rhythm as an indicator of vitality in your overall assessment: *Where the craniosacral rhythm appears reduced, this indicates a restriction in the physical structure of the body.*

Another interesting point is that in coma patients, for instance, a craniosacral rhythm of around 3–4 cycles/min can be palpated, often more pronounced in extension. It is unhelpful, however, to draw over-hasty conclusions or make generalizations. Practitioners would do well to take account of all the sensory and intuitive impressions received during the course of treatment, without allowing themselves or their clients to be bound by them.

The aim of treatment is among other things to harmonize the craniosacral system and alleviate or even completely release restrictions or asymmetries of motion by the end of the session.

Bear in mind: Craniosacral flow happens very subtly and slowly. Even as a beginner you should be able to perceive the craniosacral rhythm clearly if you approach it with inner stillness and centeredness – similar to a state of meditation – and if you apply sufficient relaxation and patience. Remind yourself occasionally: you do not need to do anything actively or want to bring about an effect. All that is necessary is a clear, gentle touch and connection with the place on the body that you are palpating, together with receptive perception. You yourself can relax as you wait for the rhythm to reveal itself to you. This helps you to sense the craniosacral rhythm and its qualities.

Tips

If you cannot yet feel the craniosacral rhythm, or seldom sense it, you may be demanding too much of yourself or are concentrating too much – or it may be that the rhythm is very weak or hard to palpate in the client. You might find it helpful as practice sometimes, to palpate the *respiratory rhythm* at various places on the body, instead of the craniosacral rhythm. This practice should be done both with your eyes closed and – during more advanced practice, for example – with your eyes open and with unfocused, distant gaze.

Strengthening the self-healing forces and increasing well-being

Craniosacral therapy is one of the most comprehensive and at the same time gentlest methods of enabling us to experience ourselves in a relaxed way as a unity. Many disorders come about as a result of disharmony or imbalance, or when important physical, mental or spiritual needs are suppressed over long periods. Such psychosomatic causes can develop into diseases.

Ultimately it is not only a matter of achieving a balanced craniosacral rhythm, but also for the *change* in rhythm to one with greater evenness, strength and range to become evident to the therapist over several cycles. This will assist the craniosacral system – and thus the body and person as a whole – in its self-regulation.

If the craniosacral rhythm on the head, torso and sacrum – and so in the entire craniosacral system – is more balanced than before the treatment, often the freer expression of primary respiration will continue to strengthen self-regulation even days or weeks after the treatment.

If the craniosacral system is freed of restrictions, this has many positive effects besides the free flow of CSF. As previously described, it assists the functioning of many important control centers in the body. When we experience our own actual unity of body, mind, and spirit, this helps us to achieve inner balance, an important process in terms of healing and becoming whole and one that should be considered in every holistic treatment, especially that of disease.

1.6 The still point

Some *still points* arise of themselves: from time to time, the craniosacral rhythm stands still, and this is what we term a still point. It is also possible to externally invite or induce one or more still points.

Spontaneous still points can arise for various reasons. Sometimes it happens entirely by itself, e.g.

- *shortly before* the release of tension in body structures and the body as a whole begins, or when body structures *begin* the release of tension
- *while* the body is carrying out its self-correction
- as a sign that the craniosacral system and all the connective tissue *has now carried out* the self-correction
- so as to be best able to *integrate* changes
- *after* an integration phase on the part of individual structures or of the body and being as a whole.

When the individual is completely relaxed and feels safe and secure and able to trust, the still point often occurs itself, following a period of self-regulation. The still point can last 20 s or some 3–4 min. It is therefore significantly longer than the brief pause in the craniosacral rhythm (previously described) when, for example, there is a change in direction of ER or IR. The still point is a gateway to deeper relaxation.

Still points are very beneficial to the craniosacral system and the regeneration of the whole body, which rests for several minutes in the stillness of its center. During a still point, the entire craniosacral system and other structures associated with it have a chance to reorganize and harmonize themselves.

If a still point occurs, a change in the person's respiratory rhythm is often observed. The individual's breathing may become slower and deeper and the person slips into a pleasant state of deeper relaxation. It is especially during a still point that immaterial transmutation processes of all kinds occur. The cellular level and the energy levels take in the *prana*, the potency of the Breath of Life. Every still point stabilizes and deepens the experience of unity and relaxation in the fact of existence.

After a still point, the craniosacral rhythm re-emerges, usually more strongly than before. This cleanses and nourishes the brain and spinal cord with fresh, invigorated CSF. The qualities of the craniosacral rhythm are often more balanced after a still point, or a slower rhythm, the mid-tide of 2–3 cycles/min, may be palpated. The exchange of all body fluids is stimulated during and after the still point.

Still points help the person to 'let go'. In that relaxation, new experiences can be made on the physical, emotional and intellectual/ spiritual level.

It is also possible for individuals to induce a still point in themselves (p. 167).

You can discover later (p. 155) what the purpose of externally induced still points is and where and how they can be induced.

1.7 Self-palpation of body rhythms on the head, pelvis and thighs

When undertaking the following self-palpation and other self-treatment techniques to increase sensory awareness and help attune to other levels of experience, it is best to seek out a place that is as quiet and as undisturbed as possible. Before we apply touch to perceive the craniosacral rhythm when treating another person, is helpful to learn to palpate and perceive it in ourselves. It is valuable for us as practitioners to become still and collect ourselves (see p. 102 for Golden rules before you begin).

The self-palpation described below is also an aid to relaxation, promoting and expanding perception through your own hands and enabling you to sense a number of structures and motions, rhythms, and interrelationships in the body.

Introduction and preparation

This self-palpation and journey through your own body – a kind of guided meditation – can be performed by laying your hands either on your thighs, on both sides of your pelvis, or on your head. If you are carrying out the self-palpation on your thighs, simply sit down comfortably on a chair and place your hands gently on both thighs. For the self-palpation on the sides of your pelvis, it is better to adopt a position lying down. Self-palpation on your head (which you perform seated) is most easily and comfortably done if you place both elbows on a support arranged in front of you so that the lower part of your arms will be supported by your elbows as you gently touch your frontal or parietal bones, for instance. Make sure that the support is not too high or too low; you could use a blanket folded to the right thickness.

The important point is that you should be able to spend the next 10–15 min sitting comfortably, relaxed, and undisturbed, 'listening' with your hands. You should also make sure that the seat on which you are sitting does not in any way obstruct the blood flow to your thighs. If it does, simply slide forward a little towards the edge of the chair. Do not rest your head on your hands; just let your hands touch your head gently, with a broad contact.

In order to sense your own craniosacral rhythm and that of others, you need personal well-being, centeredness and a comfortable, relaxed position. Make sure that these conditions are all in place before you begin (see p. 102).

Self-palpation

- *Place your hands gently* on both of your thighs, or sides of your pelvis, or on your head.
- *Consciously relax* your hands and wrists, the muscles of your lower arm, your whole arm, shoulders, and entire body including your pelvis and legs. Let go of all tension.
- *If you are seated*, place your feet so that they are as far as possible parallel. Rest the sole of your foot fully on the ground in a grounded, relaxed way. *If you are lying down*, let all your weight rest on the support.
- *Close your eyes*: For the next few minutes, there is nothing to do. Transfer the whole of your attention to your two hands and what you perceive through them.
- *No pressure*: Your touch should not exert any pressure. Instead, you should consciously establish contact with what you feel; on your thighs or on the sides of your pelvis – this will probably be the clothes you are wearing; on your head, your hair or scalp.
- *Gentleness and clarity of touch*: Let your touch become noticeably gentler and quite passive, but without losing the clear contact with the tissue.
- *Spine erect, airway free*: Make sure that your spine is not too bent and that your breath can flow freely. It is helpful to relax your lower jaw slightly so that you are breathing through your slightly opened mouth. Your whole body should remain relaxed.
- *Hand contact*: Now direct your attention more to your hands and sense the whole contact surface. Let your touch become a little gentler still. Now, *using your sensory awareness*, begin to blend with the surface you are touching and the depths of its tissue. The receptors in your hands and fingers can slowly take up the contact with the depths of your thigh, the sides of your pelvis, or your head, and 'dock' there. Allow yourself time, enough for the surface with which you are touching and the body part you are palpating to spontaneously become one.
- *Alternatively*: Touch the level of the skin with a broad contact and clear intention. The receptors do not have to make the connection with the depths of the tissue; you wait *until the tissue begins to expand to meet your hands*.
- *Reduce the intensity of the touch*: If there is any pressure of touch, draw back the pressure; in the fully connected state, it is no longer needed. The touch becomes still gentler, but you can still sense it and you remain in tangible, clear contact.
- *Respiratory rhythm*: Direct your attention to your breath, streaming in and out of your body of itself, so creating the respiratory rhythm. Do not try to alter your breath or breathing rhythm, but remain attentive, observing how it is breathing. Now sense the movement of your respiratory rhythm in your body: do your shoulders or upper body rise gently as you breathe in and lower again as you breathe out?

Perhaps you sense the breath curling around your nostril, or feel the movement of your abdomen or abdominal muscles reaching right down to your pelvis? Perhaps you feel almost nothing, but simply enjoy the experience of being passive for a while and take a few minutes to collect yourself and to be still. Perhaps you sense the flow of your breath in and out as a rhythm that you can detect at various places on your body – including the place where your hands are in gentle contact. Follow the motion of your respiratory rhythm in your body attentively for a while.

- *Perceptual training*: Maybe you do not feel any respiratory rhythm with your hands, but instead sensations such as heat or cold, twitching, hardening or softening of tissues, beating or pulsation, heaviness or lightness. Or perhaps you sense a flow of energy in your body, see images or colors, detect a particular perfume or find some pleasant memory arising within you. Simply receive these perceptions and keep your attention primarily focused on the place where your hands are resting, without altering anything.
- *Which location or region of your body feels good?* What is it that makes you recognize this? What makes you feel this?
- *Heartbeat*: Now turn your attention to your heartbeat. Where do you feel this? In your chest? Under your arms, at your wrists or fingertips? In the region of your neck? Or do you feel your heartbeat at many locations over the whole of your body, including the place where your hands are in contact? Maybe you only sense it occasionally and simply enjoy the experience of being passive for a while and take a few minutes to collect yourself and to be still. There is nothing to do, you can continue to relax and listen attentively with your hands as they rest in gentle but clear contact.
- *Breathing and heartbeat*: Perhaps you can sense the movement of your breathing and heartbeat? As you do so, you can practice consciously shifting your attention slowly, alternately from one to the other, or sensing both together, simultaneously.
- *Craniosacral rhythm*: Now direct your attention to another, more subtle rhythm in your body. On the head, this motion feels like a widening, rather like the slight inflation of a balloon. Then the motion changes to a slight deflation, as if a little air is escaping from the balloon. On the sides of your pelvis and your thighs, you may feel a slow external or internal rotation: this is probably the craniosacral rhythm and its slow, subtle motion resembling ebb and flow. Perhaps you sense this slow fluctuation and flowing for a few seconds and simply enjoy the relaxation. There is nothing to do; you remain grounded, centered, and relaxed. You can let part of your attention rest in the softness of your hands.
- *Respiratory, cardiac and craniosacral rhythm*: Can you sense the motion of your breathing, that of your heartbeat, and your craniosacral rhythm 'side by side'? As you progress, experience makes it easier to transfer your attention consciously between the various motions and rhythms of the body.

- **Before-and-after comparison**
  - — With which tissue level are your hands communicating now?
  - — Are you also in communication with other body structures through this tissue?
  - — How does this tissue feel?
  - — Are there any differences between left and right? If so, what are they?
  - — Has the tissue changed from how it was at the beginning? If so, how?
  - — How does your body feel as a whole – and compared with how it felt at the beginning?

At the end of this palpation exercise, take conscious leave of the place where your hands are resting. Take time to slowly release the hand contact at the deep level. It may be that you value the experiences you have had of bodily sensations and emotions. Take a few deep breaths, open your eyes, and then slowly withdraw your hands from your body. As you draw a few more breaths, stretch your body within the area of well-being and give a pleasurable yawn. Consciously return to the everyday external world.

- How do you now perceive yourself and your environment?
- Has anything changed?
- If so, what?
- What exactly makes you feel this?

The craniosacral rhythm is very subtle and you may not detect it clearly straight away on the very first occasion. You should therefore take time to train your hands, and the many receptors in them, in perception. Often the craniosacral rhythm only becomes evident when you are completely relaxed and are listening with your hands in a way that is quite free of intent.

You can perform this exercise every day or every week as a training in craniosacral perception and the ability to sense. With regular practice, it will noticeably increase your awareness of the body and your palpation skills, and will make you more alert to the wisdom of your body.

All craniosacral self-palpation exercises can also be carried out lying down. In that case, you should find a position in which your body is fully relaxed and in which you do not need to hold on to support yourself. A cushion under your knees/legs takes the stress away from the torso. You can take up hand contact anywhere on your body, because the various body rhythms are transmitted by the muscles and connective tissue to all parts – as long as there is no excessive lack of movement in your body and you are not placing yourself under pressure. Paired, more externally located body structures such as the pelvis and the hip region or various locations on the head are particularly suitable for this 'listening'. Simply take in what you feel with your hands:

- Do you feel greater warmth or cold?
- Do you sense a tingling or pulsation?
- Does the tissue become soft?
- Can you feel the respiratory rhythm or the slower craniosacral rhythm?

- What are the qualities of the craniosacral rhythm?
- Does the craniosacral system enter a spontaneous still point?
- What is the craniosacral rhythm like after the still point?

Sense through your hands, relaxed and without intent, without wanting to change anything. As your experience increases, the sensations you receive of the various types of motion brought about by the various rhythms of the body will become more and more clear.

Body rhythms:

Heartbeat: ≈ 70/min

Respiratory rate: ≈ 16/min

Craniosacral rhythm: ≈ 6–12/min

The more often you practice this self-palpation, the more you will sharpen your perceptions to sense the subtle craniosacral rhythm – an important prerequisite skill for performing craniosacral treatment on other people. There is another benefit: your clear, non-invasive intent and gentle touch usually assist the balance of the craniosacral rhythm, whether or not you are currently able to sense it.

A number of exercises for 'craniosacral self-treatment' and designed to bring about well-being and relaxation can be found in my book 'Harmonizing your Craniosacral System – An Easy and Effective Self-Treatment' (see Further Reading). It has already appeared in German under the title of 'Craniosacral-Selbstbehandlung' (2004). A CD with craniosacral treatments and music is also available; see Appendix 'Music (a selection)' on page 345.

Tips

You may find that you expect or want to achieve too much when you perform this exercise. This is enough to create a slight degree of tension that makes palpation of the craniosacral rhythm more difficult. It is often when the active part of us has given up, when we are left with nothing but the open, receptive attitude and touch, that it becomes possible to sense the craniosacral rhythm.

It is like switching to an inner scale, a blending of your hands with the particular location on the body. This is followed by an act of still, alert, sensitive listening. Remain relaxed, centered and in the flow of your breathing. Being easy and relaxed, and listening without intent, you will often find that this body location will spontaneously begin to harmonize. Let the various slow body rhythms take you with them, and 'stop and stare' in amazement.

Indications and contraindications

1.8

Basic principles

Given the complexity of the anatomical and neurological structures described above and the way that craniosacral therapy works, it is hardly surprising that this method of body work can be helpful in a great many areas. One aspect of this is in the maintenance of health and well-being; but it can also be used to treat various forms of disease, the widespread 'diseases of civilization' or psychosomatic disturbances. Many chronic complaints can also often be eased or resolved by treatment from experienced craniosacral practitioners.

It naturally helps to be able to assess when craniosacral therapy will or will not be advisable. Since each person and each body is different, it is hard to predict the effect and wise to avoid predictions. This would create an additional pressure of expectation, and anything involving pressure and compulsion has little or nothing in common with the craniosacral method.

It is very important to know when it would be wrong to give treatment. It is just as important to keep to these rules, for the protection of both patient and practitioner. We have a duty of care to our clients/patients – and that responsibility also extends to the craniosacral method and its duty-conscious practitioners and natural health therapy as a whole.

Conventional medical advice must be sought without fail where there is a clear disease or disorder and if the patient is unwell for any length of time; treatment of disease must always be left to trained medical experts.

When applying a method that is comprehensive in its effects and can achieve a great deal in terms of effects and responses, it is very important to maintain a self-critical assessment of one's own craniosacral experience and one's own limits. There is a vast difference between individuals who have had no training or have attended a few courses, who have simply received treatment from practitioners, and now wish to treat other people, and individuals who have completed many years of ongoing specialist training and built up a rich fund of experience in their own right. Attendance at specialist craniosacral courses and a post-qualification supervision are strongly recommended before carrying out any of the techniques and basic treatments shown in this book – even if the intending practitioner is already experienced in allopathic medicine or in other natural health methods. Even for such people, courses and comprehensive further specialist craniosacral training improve their store of experience.

If the above advice is conscientiously observed and the contraindications heeded, the possibility of physical harm does not arise on the grounds that craniosacral therapy is very gentle, permitting of space, and is carried out with very slight touch.

The most important indications

- Allergies
- Chronic complaints
- Birth preparation
- Relaxation
- States of exhaustion
- Aid to recovery
- Hyperactivity
- Concentration difficulties
- Headaches
- Learning difficulties
- Painful menstruation
- Excessive muscle tension (hypertonus)
- Back problems
- Sleep disturbances
- Pain symptoms not associated with pathological findings
- Stress
- Stuttering
- Following falls, impacts and accidents
- Syndromes, trauma
- Digestive problems
- Rapid growth spurts
- Grinding of teeth
- Twitching

(A detailed list giving over 100 indications can be found in the Appendix).

The contraindications: basic principles

The contraindications (i.e. instances when a treatment should not be given) distinguish between:

- absolute contraindications
- relative contraindications (as a precaution).

Additional points to consider when assessing contraindications

- The treatment approach.
- The way in which a given treatment is structured, performed and concluded.
- Whether a technique should be performed at all; and, if so, which technique is to be applied and with what intensity.

- The time factor: How long ago was (e.g.) the accident or operation?
- The severity or intensity of (e.g.) an accident or syndrome.
- The amount of experience a practitioner has with the particular method; amount of prior knowledge.
- The practitioner's experience with the particular clinical state, the professional environment in which the treatment is being given (e.g. rehabilitation, neonatal ward, hospital, care home, geriatric care, psychiatric clinic) and the facilities available, e.g., team case discussion or imaging facilities.
- Whether/extent to which the practitioner is familiar with interactive support of the patient's process and trauma healing.
- Clients' ability to deal with the health problem in daily life and to cope with changes during treatment.
- How well clients are connected with their inner personal resources and can relax in the experience of the totality of the body.

All these points are essential in a careful assessment of whether craniosacral treatment is appropriate for an individual, and if so, which method it is best to use. If in doubt, it is better not to give treatment, but to refer the individual to a more experienced craniosacral practitioner.

Absolute and relative contraindications

The following are absolute contraindications:

- acute inflammation (e.g., meningitis)
- severe or open head wounds
- skull fractures
- heart attack (in the acute phase)
- stroke (in the acute phase)
- infection whose course is unclarified (e.g., as a result of tick-bites)

Also absolutely contraindicated: brain tumor, cerebral edema, hematoma (collection of blood occurring as a result of trauma), cerebral hemorrhage, cerebral aneurysms (dilation of an artery as a result of changes in the vessel wall, usually of an artery inside the cranium), often in the territory of the internal carotid artery, and especially the cerebral arterial circle (circle of Willis) – certain parts of this ring of arteries in the brain pass around the body of the sphenoid. These cerebral aneurysms pose the risk of rupture, subarachnoid bleeding or mass intracerebral bleeding. Always confirm in every case that the CSF is 100% free of blood.

These clinical states are not externally recognizable, and may often be unknown to both client and practitioner. It is therefore helpful to clarify any features over the last few months that come to your attention when you take the patient's medical history for the first time, and to see a doctor's prescription; the residual risk is small, but this precaution will help minimize the risk further. Following severe falls, accidents and operations, it is also essential to consult the patient's doctor, both for health and for legal reasons. Patients must bring a doctor's prescription to their first consultation with you.

The treatment approach, the choice of techniques for the particular patient, how intensively and with what aim these are performed, and the spacious presence of the practitioner, are all factors that will determine the nature and intensity of the craniosacral session. They play a part in the decision as to whether to treat in the case of conditions listed under the relative contraindications.

Relative contraindications (precautionary)

- Acute, severe pain.
- Concussion.
- Fresh injuries to the head, spine or sacrum.
- Whiplash injury (this calls for many years of craniosacral experience and best possible knowledge of trauma healing and resource-oriented support as a companion of the client's process).
- Epilepsy (*risk of an attack*).
- Multiple sclerosis (MS) (*risk of an episode*).
- Other diseases mainly affecting the nervous system.
- Schizophrenia, severe psychological illness, borderline syndrome (*Note*: special care is required – these patients need a therapist/ psychotherapist of strong character).
- Osteoporosis is only a contraindication if pressure is applied in giving treatment; otherwise it is an indication.
- During pregnancy: do not use pressure to induce a still point (because this can involve the minute risk of premature delivery) – at most a still point can be invited from the third month, until the seventh month (from then on it can encourage the early onset of labor and so premature birth). In principle, craniosacral treatment is a good preparation for birth. Viola Frymann, who studied under Sutherland, believes that still points in the body always promote homeostasis, in other words the tendency of the body to establish a balance between all body functions.

- As stated above, the relative contraindications are dependent on the degree of experience of the practitioner and on the time since the event.

The efficiency of the craniosacral treatment

1.9

How many sessions at what time intervals?

How many sessions?

Craniosacral therapy is on the whole seldom used as a long-term treatment, because it has a broad range of effects on many functions of the body, strengthens the body's self-healing forces, and at the same time has an integrating effect. The therapy and course of treatment are individual to each person, even when the conditions treated are identical or similar.

Between 6 and 10 1-hour sessions are usually to be recommended for the treatment of many indications. I know many people for whom 4–7 craniosacral treatment sessions were enough to ease the condition, a sign that craniosacral therapy should be continued, since the body as a whole responds well to it. If the progress of therapy is positive, it should not be discontinued too soon – if, for example the client experiences a reduction in pain, even no pain at all, over a short period – so as to avoid a 'relapse' into the old pattern. Continuing treatment can also establish the emerging 'new' and 'healthy' pattern at all levels. The result is not only an improvement in the capacity for compensation of the body as a whole, but also a *fundamental change in body structures at a deeper level.* Thus, during this period, body consciousness begins to expand and become more subtle. Even healthy individuals like to give themselves the benefit of a craniosacral treatment session several times a year – as an aid to general well-being and provision for future health.

Of course, no general prognoses can be made as to the number of sessions that will be helpful, or how many will be needed for the body's self-regulatory mechanism to be strengthened again or for the problems to be successfully treated. Each person is unique, responding quite individually to the craniosacral treatments they receive. There are several different reasons for this, including for example, the experience of the practitioner or the patient's collaboration during the sessions. We should not forget that healing is never a 'linear' process but a constant one of continual balancing until greater homeostasis and wholeness are achieved. Patients may also need to change certain things in the realm of their everyday lives and behavior for the sake of their health, so that the underlying improvements brought about by the craniosacral therapy can achieve long-lasting positive changes for them.

Consider how much time it has taken overall for the body to show evidence of postural defects, herniated (slipped) disks, exhaustion or migraine, for example. Sudden events, too, such as trauma resulting from accidents, leave their traces *in the nervous system*. We know from trauma healing and craniosacral therapy that the amount of time needed for the effects of trauma to resolve themselves and give way to a relaxed and whole sense of the body in the here and now is an entirely individual matter. That also means that orienting and resistance mechanisms also have to be restored, and in this respect it matters to allow the body and being of patients as a whole, enough time in their social learning environment to integrate the changes. This is a more helpful approach than working with excessively high expectations on either side (practitioner or client) and evoking something that might induce more trauma, for example if we hasten the process by provoking response when the resources are inadequate to sustain it.

In the case of chronic complaints that may have been treated unsuccessfully for years or even decades by allopathic medicine and other methods, even an experienced craniosacral practitioner – as well as the client – needs sufficient time, patience and trust. Careful, cautious working in cooperation with the 'inner healer' and the Breath of Life strengthens the client's self-healing forces from one session to the next. In the case of serious accidents or diseases, even partial success often brings an improvement in quality of life. The therapeutic approach to treating whiplash injury, for example, demands a great deal of empathy, patience, experience on the part of the practitioner and mutual trust.

What time intervals between sessions are most helpful?

Practitioner and client should decide together how regularly to arrange the sessions and how much time to allow between them. Various factors should be taken into account in making this decision:

- What is the aim of treatment, the task to be fulfilled?
- Is the wish 'just' to achieve relaxation and release of tension or is it to reduce or release stubborn, chronic pain that has been present for years?
- Does the client already have experience of body work, and how did the client react to it?
- How much mobility does the client have? How does the client deal with the challenge of too much or too little being demanded, or deal with barriers?
- How does the particular level of the body respond to treatment? How does the person as a whole respond?
- Does self-regulation (and, with this, signs such as bowel sounds) begin to operate more vigorously in the first third of the treatment session, in the last third, or in the fourth session?
- How free, inhibited or restricted are the various body structures?
- How great is the body's capacity for integrating changes during and after the session?
- Can the craniosacral rhythm be palpated at all 'listening stations'?

- Is the craniosacral rhythm on the sacrum, occipital bone and sphenoid relatively strong and balanced for several cycles?
- Does the client have a sufficiently good connection with personal inner resources?
- Does the client take time, or create the right environment, to grant the body what it signals it needs?
- What body-awareness does the client have? How much care does the client show in dealing with body and self?

From the great range of points to be considered, it is clear that a prior, standardized treatment plan would be unable to do justice to the individuality of the practitioner and the client.

To begin with, the basic structural-functional treatment and the further elements of treatment shown in this book should be practiced on a number of healthy people; this will help give you a sense of what a relatively vital craniosacral system and rhythm feel like, and how tensions become balanced. When working with the individuality, health and wholeness of a person, the main determining factor is *what the body reveals to us before, during and after the session*, and also what the client tells us through the dialog before, during and after the session.

There is a variety of opinion as to the number of sessions recommended and the time that should be allowed between them. The decision can also be influenced by the personality of the practitioner, by the view held at the school that provided the original training, and – ideally – by experience gained in actual practice. Some practitioners prefer not to arrange several appointments before the first session has taken place, but to begin with just one appointment for the initial session. Once that session has taken place, the practitioner will be in a better position to refer to the factors listed above and to discuss and agree together with the client about possible follow-up sessions and the interval between them. It can sometimes be helpful if the client allows a few days for the treatment to take effect and makes contact again at that stage to arrange the next appointment.

Reactions can vary enormously. The important fact to remember is that often changes are taking place, for example in the sense of greater self-regulation, tension release and health and that these processes very often continue after the treatment session ('Treatment continues to take effect after the session', see p. 269 and Intensification of symptoms due to re-organization, p. 270).

If the *intervals between treatment sessions are too short*, this can be too intensive for the individual (depending on that person's situation) and can evoke greater reaction than is wanted or than is agreeable.

If the intervals between sessions are too long, the positive changes brought about during treatment may not last long enough and the body may quite quickly return to its old pattern.

A further factor determining changes and the integration of these changes is the length of treatment (30 min, 45 min, 60 min or longer) and the treatment approach that the craniosacral practitioner is using. When treating a body that retains a great deal of tension and has a massive cladding of muscle mass, it would be better to plan the first six sessions, say, at shorter intervals of 1–2 weeks. After that, treatment every 3 or 4 weeks might be sufficient. If clients have become accustomed to the craniosacral treatment after a couple of sessions, their bodies often respond to it better and more quickly. The more a body is free and the more its tension is released, the less its energy is retained and reabsorbed in inertial fulcrums. Vital energy is therefore more available for self-regulation and the enjoyment of life.

Thus it is important to both practitioner and client to recognize the individual way in which treatment works and to agree together on suitable time intervals between treatment sessions.

Basic points before beginning treatment 1.10

Certain basic matters need to be clear in the practitioner's mind at the outset, before beginning to administer craniosacral treatment. The following points should be of assistance in ensuring that the treatment takes the best possible course, both for you and for the person receiving treatment. These points are given both as suggestions and as guidelines.

As a beginner in craniosacral therapy, you ought to have received treatment yourself from craniosacral practitioners at least 10 times before giving the first practice sessions. Even if you are already an experienced practitioner of another method, this will help you gain experience of the gentle craniosacral touch and other aspects of a treatment session. This and attendance at specialist courses in craniosacral therapy are essential for the careful practice of craniosacral treatment on other people.

The state of mind and health of the practitioner

It is extremely important that you give treatment only when you are well enough yourself – physically, mentally, spiritually, and emotionally. How can it be possible to aid well-being when the practitioner is personally suffering from extreme physical pain or a depressive mood, or is ill at ease or out of balance?

You yourself are responsible for your own state of mind and health – and it influences the course and quality of the session. To ensure the well-being of your own self as the practitioner, you should take care of your health and of the balance you yourself have. Give yourself the benefit of a periodic craniosacral treatment session with an experienced practitioner. Give yourself enough exercise and relaxation, perhaps by taking your bicycle and cycling through the countryside, surrounded by Nature, by swimming regularly or visiting the sauna, listening to beautiful music, using craniosacral self-treatment methods or remaining in silence and meditating.

Balance, quiet and self-reflection by the practitioner are important in order to achieve the best possible treatment. Without these, the client is likely to derive less benefit from the session and may even, though rarely, experience adverse after-effects. The practitioner should also have a sufficiently high level of energy, and be alert, attentive, centered, 'grounded' and relaxed, before beginning the treatment (see Neutral and stillness, p. 244).

The conscious connection with the 'universal creative force,' caring, alert and spacious presence and regulation of distance all help the practitioner to conserve personal energy rather than expending it, so as not to end a session with a feeling of exhaustion.

Who should treat, and what should be treated?

Craniosacral treatment calls for precise anatomical knowledge on the part of the practitioner, as well as centeredness, intuition, care, and responsibility. One such consideration is that untrained individuals should not treat the sick. Trained practitioners may only treat people with health problems, diseases or disorders when this has been prescribed by a physician or – depending on the regulations in their particular country – when practicing as a recognized natural health practitioner. Regulations governing such treatment vary from one country to another and the legal situation should be fully clarified in advance, for example by making enquiries with professional organizations or public bodies such as the health authorities.

Craniosacral treatment should be available to all for tension release and relaxation and to strengthen self-regulation. There is another point here: we suffer from a general lack of supportive, health-giving touch and caring attention – so we should be kind to ourselves from time to time by doing something agreeable and healthy. For example, parents can support their children in important stages of their growth, and those with handicapped elderly relatives can do something positive for their relations' well-being.

Of course, it almost goes without saying that treatment should be a matter of free will and something the person being treated genuinely wants. It also removes a burden from the parents and relatives of those in need of care if they can hand over treatment to an experienced practitioner outside the family circle and if they too can give themselves the benefit of some craniosacral treatment. In this way, the family members are released from the need to take on the additional role of therapist, and they themselves emerge strengthened from the treatment sessions and with greater patience and strength for their everyday tasks. If you are treating people who are close to you, this personal level of relationship of course makes for a different situation from that in which you are treating someone outside your family and close circle. It helps you and all concerned for you to take care, for example for you to be aware of the dynamics of identification or transference and counter-transference.

General guidelines

An essential question to ask yourself when you are trying to promote a person's well-being is, what is your motive for giving the treatment? You also need to be clear about your basic ethical standpoint. The following points should be sufficient to convey what is involved in your duty of care.

Important considerations
- Treat information concerning the client confidentially! You have a duty of professional confidentiality and must not reveal a client's information.
- Conscientiously examine the indications and contraindications, if necessary seeking conventional medical opinion.
- Therapeutic, energetic and emotional presence during treatment is an essential prerequisite for delivering treatment.
- As the practitioner you should continually regulate the distance between you and your client, on the physical, emotional, mental and spiritual levels.
- You should permit clients their personal space and carefully accompany this.
- Respect your clients' physical, personal, ritual, religious and cultural boundaries and political attitudes.
- Be honest as regards your training, abilities, and experience, and also as regards the limits of treatment.
- Recognize and acknowledge your own limits during treatment, particularly your capacity to cope with stress, especially when dealing with powerful processes and a high level of trauma activation.
- Encourage the growth and autonomy of your client. Be aware of your therapeutic position/function and act exclusively for the good of your client.
- Respect other professional colleagues and other forms of treatment.
- Do not set your treatment charges inappropriately high or low; these vary, among other things according to previous knowledge and training and any additional specialist training that the practitioner may have, and according to the general price level in that region.
- Only call yourself a craniosacral practitioner or craniosacral therapist once you have successfully completed a comprehensive course of specialist craniosacral training at a recognized institution and so acquired the necessary competence.

Guidelines for the practitioner

The general guidelines also apply to the practitioner. The moment two or more people come into contact (which, in craniosacral treatment, is by means of physical contact), it makes sense for practitioners to have as clear an idea as possible about themselves before starting to administer treatment.

Important matters that practitioners and clients may encounter in the course of a series of treatment sessions include:
- basic emotions such as love, fear, anger, pain and joy
- nearness and distance
- intimacy
- sexuality
- reflection by the client during the treatment of issues that involve or matter personally to the practitioner and clarity in dealing with these

- transference – countertransference
- demand and reality
- provocation or avoidance of issues
- the definition of a 'good session'
- practitioner's pressure or urge to succeed
- ability to deal with the 'inner critic' or 'inner doubter'
- empathic involvement
- establishing clear boundaries.

Preparing for a treatment session

For the craniosacral treatment to be a pleasant experience for both practitioner and client, and in order to achieve the best possible outcome, it is helpful to make the best possible preparation; that applies not only to your own inner state, but also to the way you arrange the room in which treatment is to take place. Create a harmonious environment that promotes trust. Here are some tips and ideas.

Surroundings and treatment room

Ensure a quiet environment where you can be undisturbed and where no-one else is allowed to enter while the treatment is being given. If you are working in the family environment or among friends, tell the others in the house that you do not want to be disturbed.

For craniosacral sessions, *a safe, protected, and undisturbed* context is important, a place where you can work undisturbed and your clients can relax. A suitable room is one that is bright but where no-one can see in. Avoid disturbing background noise such as telephones ringing, fax machines, or answering machines on a loud setting. Another way to deal with external noise, if it is not too intrusive, is to treat it as a reason to remain centered and not to allow yourself to be too easily distracted by external influences.

Air the room well before and after each session. The room temperature should be pleasant; you could even increase the room temperature for a while, as the body's sensation of temperature can change, both as a result of lying down (e.g. lowering of blood pressure through relaxation) and as a consequence of events on the physical or mental–spiritual level.

Equipment and aids

You will need the following in order to work comfortably and easily:

- A treatment table. This should be fairly soft and sufficiently broad and long (e.g. 75–85 cm (2 ft 3 in – 2 ft 9 in) wide and about 2 m (6 ft 6 in) long) and adjustable in height. There are massage tables available that contribute enormously to the comfort of treatment for both practitioner and client and are durable enough to last for decades. You should also ask the specialist supplier to show you accessories such as a stool on castors (with hydraulic height adjustment), knee roll bolsters and table extensions. If you are not yet ready to buy a treatment table, there are alternatives:

— A sturdy table with the same dimensions as above. There needs to be enough leg room at the top and bottom ends of the table, so that your legs and knees are not restricted. On top of the table you should place an underlayer of material that is as soft as possible, such as foam or a soft beach mat or camping mattress with a thick, soft blanket, to provide a padded surface. Put a clean sheet on top for reasons of hygiene.

— Another method is to place a robust tabletop on three stable trestles that you can fold away when not in use. The tabletop can be stored behind a cupboard when not needed, and the folded trestles will not take up too much room. Pad the tabletop in the same way as described above for the table; otherwise, two isomats and a soft, thick blanket would suffice as an underlayer. Inflatable mattresses are not very suitable, however, as they do not provide sufficient stability. The materials listed can be obtained quite cheaply from DIY stores.

- A freshly-laundered sheet made of linen, cotton, or other material (you may wish to choose a fabric with as low a synthetic content as possible).
- A stool on castors with hydraulic height adjustment or two stable chairs.

Tips

If the client happens to be very tall, the treatment table too short, or no extension is immediately available for the massage table, you can sit with one or two rolled-up blankets on your knees to provide an area of support for your forearms. That will give you enough space for your arms and hands, which will rest stably and serve as a fulcrum to enable you to give the treatment in a relaxed way.

It helps to have two or three chairs for yourself and your client to use during the arrival stage, for the dialog before the session begins, and as a place to leave such items as spectacles, watch, jewelry or belt. It is useful to have mineral water and drinking beakers, for refreshment and for washing out impurities; tissues are also useful to have available. If there are jewels in the room, it helps to cleanse them from time to time – rinse them for a few minutes in flowing water and then leave them to dry in the sun for at least 1 h to recharge.

For intraoral treatment (only for advanced students and practitioners) you will also of course need finger cots and disposable gloves.

- Cushions or blankets to provide the correct working height that will be comfortable for you when sitting at the treatment table: upright, with arms resting on the table to the maximum extent possible.
- A blanket, in case the client feels cold.
- A pillow (and two towels) to support the client's head and cervical spine as necessary.
- Knee roll bolsters, additional blankets or large towels: when someone is lying down for some time, especially if they have backache, lumbago or a herniated disk, it is advisable to take the weight off the lumbar region and abdominal muscles; rolled-up blankets under the knees can be adjusted to provide the right height, and they relieve the weight on the torso.

The power of aromas

It is easier to relax in a well-aired, pleasant-smelling treatment room: the scent of essential oils passes straight from our noses to the brain. Aroma lamps can be bought in many places. When selecting the aroma, I do recommend taking care to choose 100% pure essential oils and room sprays. Use a subtle quantity, and do always ask clients if they are allergic – some people are. If you are setting up and using a practice room, you will find the occasional use of incense and myrrh, for example, helpful for energetic cleansing and disinfecting.

Music as an aid or distraction

It is best to let the client decide whether the room should be filled with relaxing music during the session. Music can assist the client's inward journey, stimulate the senses, bring relaxation and so assist treatment; but it can also be a distraction and a hindrance to deeper relaxation. Given the almost permanent noise level and the overwhelming quantity of the stimuli that characterize our daily lives, silence can be a delight.

If unobtrusive background music seems likely to provide an agreeable opening to treatment and if you use it with the client's agreement, do observe the following:

- The music you choose should not have a melody or rhythm that is too dynamic; it should be restful. After a while, this will assist in slowing the brain frequency and heart rate.
- Instrumental music is more neutral than music with words.
- Music involving too many differences or sudden changes in mood is not so suitable.
- The music should not contain any subliminal messages (the subliminal technique can operate directly on the subconscious via particular frequencies) unless the client has been informed of the fact.

A list of suggested music can be found in the Appendix.

Your inner attitude

Center yourself well before the session begins. Heighten your awareness of your own body, for example, with a few relaxing body exercises, and use gentle energetic breathing exercises to raise your level of awareness and energy. A few craniosacral self-treatment techniques may help in this; for example, you might lie on the treatment table for a few minutes and place your hands on your pelvis (see Self-palpation, p. 58; Self-treatment, pp. 165, 275, and Guided meditation, p. 272, palpate your craniosacral rhythm and its spontaneously generated still point, or invite the still point. Set your own self at rest.

As already stated, it is important for the practitioner to be in a vital state before the treatment begins. This makes it possible to accompany intensive treatments without excessive loss of energy. The basic craniosacral attitude is one in which you do not actively seek to do anything or to produce an effect, but listen to the expression of primary respiration, primarily allowing the fluids and various slow rhythms to operate. These are strengthened by the practitioner's orientation to the slow body rhythms – and so to the expression of health – by means of the practitioner's spacious presence. Instead of adopting a focus that concentrates one-sidedly or solely on the immediate reduction of symptoms and disease, let these remain present in the background – viewing them at the same time in relation to the functional to health and to the expression of primary respiration. This approach supports body, mind, spirit and soul in their natural change to greater balance.

Craniosacral treatment sees itself as supporting the natural rhythms and self-healing forces, as accompanying the universal constant striving of existence to create the greatest possible balance in the microcosmic and macrocosmic realms. I see this approach as important; it differs to some degree from other forms of craniosacral treatment, and fundamentally from other manual therapies. As I understand it, it involves two concerns, to balance the craniosacral system and its rhythm by the use of techniques, and to maintain a safe and protected space for the client so that the 'inner healer' and the body fluids are best able to perform their self-regulatory work. One of the practitioner's tasks is to give the client sufficient space as well as time for relaxation and 'letting go' to take place in the body, for this is how thoughts come to rest and emotions can be perceived more clearly. It is a non-invasive, open attitude that involves allowing yourself to be led by the client's 'inner healing force'. Put your trust in one of the fundamental principles of osteopathy and craniosacral therapy: the body has the ability to regulate itself, to heal itself and to maintain its own health.

So, in craniosacral treatment, the task is to listen to the wisdom of the body, the expression of primary respiration, and how they harmonize our bodies with their own nervous system and relieve the strains on the entire locomotor apparatus. The techniques shown below are performed sensitively and serve as a skilled support to enable the health to develop and establish itself more easily.

You can relax in your role as practitioner. Adopt the most comfortable position at the treatment table, so that your breathing and vital energy can flow freely.

Protecting yourself

There is no doubt that it is helpful to reflect on your own state before, during and after the treatment; however, you should not lay excessive emphasis on the matter of self-protection; otherwise this would reinforce it and cause it to demand too much attention. The best aids to self-protection for practitioners during treatment sessions come with the practical application of the advice given above in this chapter.

You yourself should already be centered, in a state of inner calm, with no pressure to achieve, before you begin to touch. If you feel constantly unwell, disoriented or confused, it is better to remove your hands and distance yourself a little from the client. Experienced practitioners might perhaps examine together with the client whether these feelings are something that currently concern the client and that the practitioner was picking up in this way.

You need to sense and be aware of your own boundaries, especially if the demands of a situation are too great for you, and to insist on them – for your own protection and that of your client.

As a practitioner, I do not start the session until I have connected with my own resources, am in a state of self-perception, and have regulated the distance from the client. My perception is open, wide, and at the same time, I establish the boundaries between myself and the client; I do not identify with the client's process. I exercise empathy, not sympathy – I am an empathetic companion, but not a symbiotic one.

There may be extended periods of silence; by *asking occasional questions*, you can not only perform a 'reality check', a reporting back to assist you as the practitioner in your overall understanding, but also ensure through this interactive support of the client's process that you are carrying out the treatment in the way that is right for the client.

In addition, as well as ensuring that you yourself have an adequate energy level before engaging in touch, it is advisable:

- to establish clear boundaries between yourself as practitioner, and the client, mentally, emotionally and physically, and yet remain present.
- to 'ground' yourself: both feet rest firmly on the floor, if possible with the entire sole. Sense your pelvis, your seat bones, your legs, and your feet on the ground. Distribute your weight downwards.
- to center yourself: once you have established a sure grounding by means of the previous exercise, now at the same time sense your *hara*/ center of power below your navel.
- to energize yourself: Once you are 'grounded' and centered, you should, for example, consciously breathe seven times each into your hara, your pelvis, and your thoracic cage or your heart chakra. Then breathe seven times into all three simultaneously – take time to do this. Then observe your feelings for at least 21 breaths, without changing anything.

Points to note during the treatment

- You can as the person delivering treatment remove your hands from time to time and take a step back from the treatment table.
- You can pause briefly now and then, allowing the client to sense without your touch how things feel at that stage, and whether anything has changed compared with the beginning. During that pause, do nothing, but regulate the distance, remain alert and simply take in your perceptions.
- If you feel irritated or do not know how to proceed next, regulate your inner distance and your physical distance, and allow yourself to pause. Remaining present, you and your client should each individually occupy your own place in the room. Each of you should rest in your center.
- You can apply the points listed above consciously establishing a vertical connection as you do so, e.g., by placing one hand on your hara and the other on the middle of your chest (heart chakra), 'grounding' and centering yourself and making the upward connection with the eternal source of life via your third ventricle and the sagittal suture between your two parietal bones.

Some practitioners use visualization or 'tuning in' to higher energies as their means of self-protection – visualize yourself in a golden cone of light that protects and strengthens you and your aura: allow your heart energies to flow through your arms and hands, vertically upward to the vertex of your head and downward to your feet – take up conscious contact with your power animal, with your angel or with the eternal creator force, to be protected and secure.

At the same time, I think it is important for the craniosacral practitioner not to be in a dissociated (detached) state, at some remove from the world. We should be alert, taking in perceptions, sensitive and present, without 'sending out' anything on our own account, that is, without inspiring or passing anything of ourselves to the client – by visualizing the client or irradiating the client unasked, as it were, with our own energy or love or with prayers, light or chakra colors or in any other way.

Another excellent method of protection for the practitioner (and client) is to approach the 'neutral' state (see p. 244) and to intensify it during the treatment. If both practitioner and client are in the 'neutral' state, which is the ideal, both will have left the personal level behind and body, mind, spirit and soul are experienced as a unity. Give yourself and your client enough time to arrive completely without any expectations in the here and now. Allow thoughts that arise to float by. Client and practitioner approach ever more closely to stillness. It is best to wait until you have taken all the points suggested above into consideration, before beginning treatment.

If at that moment we are present and alert, allowing space as we rest in the stillness, it is easier for us to detect when issues emerge as relevant during treatment: protection, setting limits, or regulating distance, for example. As we gain experience, so we encounter a variety of situations that enables us to learn and grow.

If you find, over an extended period, that 'self-protection' is a difficult issue for you as a practitioner, or if you often feel unwell after treatment sessions, it is wise to look into this. You can explore the underlying reasons together with a professional companion whom you trust, either during your own therapy or in supervision. Although craniosacral treatment is suitable for many people to perform, from many cultures and professions, the simple fact is that it cannot suit every single person or every situation.

The resource-oriented approach

1.11

Establishing a conscious connection with sources of power

The body has the capacity to remember, and non-invasive touch and tension release in a person are precisely the situations that can arouse that person's nervous system and cell memory. The memory (and potential expression) of events, whether amazingly beautiful or traumatic, can happen unexpectedly and suddenly. When practitioners are acting as the companion of another person's process, it is helpful for them to be connected with their own source of power and to sense their own bodies freely, connectedly or fluently.

As a craniosacral therapist, I use the resource-oriented approach for the interactive support of the person's process. If clients have already tangibly and visibly forged the connection with their own sources of power before and during the session, this becomes a supportive element of the treatment, assisting and bearing them up so that they can find confidence, self-empowerment and transformation. It also helps clients in the event of any powerful memories and reactions by the body, so that they can perceive themselves in the here and now re-united with their resources. The ability to draw on this capacity is one of the factors that determine whether the treatment overall is solution-oriented, edifying and strengthening, or whether the old traumas will be repeated and possibly strengthened.

Resources are inner and external sources of power from which we draw strength, trust and self-confidence in unstressed as well as difficult times and situations. Each person's sources of strength are individual, something that they themselves experience and define.

Inner resources in my opinion include:

- a deep-seated trust in life
- a firm faith
- spontaneity; openness to new things
- calmness.

Examples of external resources are:

- nature; pet animals
- fulfilling relationships, with a life partner or with very good friends
- a creative, fulfilling leisure-time activity
- a place where the person feels at ease or safe.

By establishing a link with one's inner and/or external resources, a person can sense *changes in mood and in how the body feels in response* to that mood.

Our resources have an immediate, sometimes involuntary effect on our thoughts and feelings – and ultimately our bodily sensations.
The resource-oriented approach enables us to see the glass as half-full, not half-empty. We have coped before, even in difficult times – things might have been worse, many times. What was it that sustained you then? And what has brought you particular joy and pleasure recently?

A part or region of the body that feels particularly pleasant can also be a resource. Make that conscious connection with your inner sources of strength from time to time, during everyday life as well as before and during treatment sessions. If, for example, you have often had a deep and agreeable sensation of the area of your abdomen around your navel, you can recall this to mind in difficult situations.

- Ideally, craniosacral practitioners should be connected with their own resources before, during and after the treatment and rest in the relaxed experience of the totality of the body.

The client connects with personal resources

At the outset, you should conduct a *resource-oriented dialog*; you can even do this in your initial interview with the client, or in the dialog prior to the session. For example, you could ask about your client's favorite spare time activity. Afterwards, give the client enough time to *perceive clearly the pleasantest changes* in the body, and perhaps also consciously sense the region of the body that feels most comfortable or warm, or senses greatest release and *continue for a while to experience it*.

You can ask about differences from before, to establish a consciousness of these differences. Ask about the region of the body that feels most pleasant, during the treatment (e.g. during the first third of the session, the middle or the last third or at the end), and also in the dialog after the session is over. When you do so, give the client time to experience these feelings more deeply and so establish them neurologically. While all this is going on, you should be connected with your own sources of strength.

If in your role as a craniosacral practitioner you are treating patients with chronic complaints or syndromes, ask which part of the body is least painful, so as not to suggest more than the client can manage at that moment. You could phrase it as a conditional enquiry: 'Which part of the body would be least painful? Where would you be most likely to feel this? How would you know?'

Severely traumatized individuals or clients with an unhappy history should learn to develop resources and to connect with these resources in the here and now. It can sometimes help to treat such individuals seated rather than lying down for the time being, and to give fairly short treatment sessions (around 20–40 min) (see also pp. 217 and 202).

The dialog prior to treatment

1.12

The initial dialog

It is helpful if clients can say as precisely as possible what their expectations are and have a clear treatment task in mind that they want to have addressed. This dialog can be a verbal one and will usually take place at the first session, and afresh at the beginning of each session.

This is also the time to explain again the form of treatment, the cost and the likely duration, if you have not already done so in sufficient detail at the time of making the appointment.

Explain to the client that the effects of craniosacral treatment can be different each time. Symptoms can sometimes be experienced more strongly, stabilizing after a while and then disappearing completely. The practitioner is responsible for providing the safe therapeutic context, for treatment itself, plus a concluding phase for integration, and for the brief closing dialog. Clients have a responsibility to themselves for their own integration and healing process, which is usually harmonious and apt, though not always or exclusively pleasant. The issues that may arise in the initial dialog do not need to be given too much weight and take up too much valuable time; however, it does help to run briefly through these and establish clarity for all concerned.

Bear in mind, it is also helpful and important to enquire about the resources that clients have (areas of life from which they derive strength, or hobbies that they enjoy), and to sense these resources. Give your clients enough time to *realize consciously the changes in the body that they can experience* by calling on resources.

It is helpful for practitioner and client to agree together on certain minimum expectations, for example before the start of a session or before a treatment series. These agreements, along with other matters (such as treatment time, or where the client does not wish to be touched) form the external framework of a treatment session or series. They are essential for any professional work with people and provide the security of a set framework for both practitioner and client.

The initial interview

I recommend carrying out a detailed initial interview with each new client.

- Personal details, date of birth, address, telephone number.
- Present and previous professions.

- Reason for visit, specific treatment task, expectations, aims and partial aims of treatment: What do you want from this treatment/therapy?
- Present complaints/illnesses; recent operations, accidents.
- Notable events in the last 3 months.
- Known complaints/illnesses, past operations, accidents since childhood/since birth.
- Is there any current medical or psychological treatment? If yes: the relevant treating institution should be informed about the treatment; you can then indicate your readiness for professional cooperation.
- Is the client taking any medicines? If yes, which, how often and at what dose?
- Is there anything that might be important in terms of the treatment or for the practitioner that the client wishes to mention?
- What does the client know of craniosacral or other kinds of therapy? Is the client receiving parallel treatment?
- How does the client feel at the moment?
- What sources of strength/what resources does the client have? Hobbies? Encourage your clients' awareness of what they are feeling as they describe their sources of strength, e.g., 'What do you sense in your body now, as you talk about this?' (The same question could be asked about their last good holiday.)

Next, you should carefully examine the contraindications (see p. 64). Your duty of care will require you, if in any doubt, to request further exploration of the matter by a conventional medical expert or to consult with the treating physician or psychologist who referred the case to you for treatment.

Enter all the data on a client record card, which must be stored away securely after the session, in a place to which others do not have access (together with the treatment record as necessary).

For the well-being of the client, you should:

- decide whether you can treat the client in a safe context
- form a clear idea of the approximate length of treatment.

This depends on:

- the client's state of health
- the client's individual history and means of dealing with it
- how soundly connected the client is with sources of strength
- your own experience in acting as a companion of the process of severely traumatized people.

The treatment task

It can happen that the specific treatment task is changed during the course of the treatment. This change may either be requested by the client or come about as a result of the process. The practitioner should recognize and address this. Experience gained from the dialog with the client is important in this respect.

Encourage the client to give you feedback from time to time during the treatment. This is important for you as the practitioner if changes occur on the physical or emotional level. It is also helpful to agree with the client on some particular word – maybe simply 'stop' – that can be used if the client feels any discomfort or unease during treatment, or wishes you to pause.

1.13 The treatment record

Experience has shown that it is helpful to make a record of each craniosacral session, summarizing the treatment given. These patient notes will record information on matters such as the free flow of the craniosacral rhythm or any restrictions of the craniosacral system and of the body, about the course of the session as a whole and how the client felt at the end of the treatment. Practitioners usually keep a record of each session. This documents the individual treatment session, and once several sessions have been completed, the records provide an overview of the course of treatment as a whole. Practitioners can use these records for their own quality control, to reflect on their own performance, and for supervision purposes.

You can use your treatment records to discuss the treatments in greater detail together with the client if wished and as necessary. The dialog should emphasize the positive and take the resource-oriented approach rather than picking out aspects that are not ideal; e.g., 'The right side seems to be allowing free flow; the craniosacral rhythm there is strong and can be detected across a wide area', is much better than 'the left side is very restricted and no craniosacral rhythm can be detected there'. In other words, we direct attention to what is free and healthy; to use the same comparison as before, we see the glass as half full, not half empty, and express ourselves accordingly.

If you are working professionally in the field of craniosacral therapy, you can use your treatment records to produce a summary report on the course of treatment at any time, if this is required by the prescribing physician or service provider such as a healthcare scheme or insurer. The act of maintaining these records is also helpful to the practitioner after the treatment has been given, as it can be used for a careful review of the session and so is an aid to deeper learning and understanding.

The results of whole-body assessment (see p. 106) at the beginning of a treatment session and in the first quarter of the session can be noted down on the record sheet in one color. At the end of the session, listen to the tissues and the slow motions/rhythms. It is then a good idea to enter this assessment in another color so that you can instantly see the difference between 'before' and 'after' from the differently colored entries.

Another helpful approach to client records is to make a brief note of the most significant events and results, in writing, after the session. You can also note down which parts of the body you might need to include in a subsequent session or some other information that might be important for the next session.

If record-keeping is new or fairly new to you, do not be afraid to pause briefly for up to a minute after palpating the 'listening stations' or after 'tuning in' to the tissues and rhythms, and also before and after giving treatment to the head. Clients then have time to sense their bodies again while you record the main points in the suggested shorthand form on the front page of the record sheet and in brief outline on the back (see p. 334). With a little practice, you will find that your attention and awareness during the session are so great that you do not need to take notes until after the client has left the room. Do not let this stress you: this record-keeping is intended as a stimulus and an aid to learning. As you gain your own experience, attend courses, and give and receive treatment, you will sense more as a practitioner, and maintaining the records will become easier.

Another helpful use of this method is whole-body assessment of one person by several practitioners (*multiple hands-on*), as part of *instruction and training*. This can be followed by team comparison of the results you have each recorded, and then by comparing notes with the person being assessed.

It is not always easy to describe what you sense or to capture it in words – but it is enormously useful and important for reflecting on the sessions. Recording your notes and describing perceptions also helps you as a therapist to reflect and learn from each session. This will help you to develop the ability to discuss matters competently with other students and practitioners of craniosacral therapy, and other experts.

Important points

Your task when making these notes is not to evaluate the client, but rather to describe the *state of the client's body at that moment and the body's capacity for change* toward greater self-regulation.

What the client feels is valuable both to the client and to you. Ask from time to time during the treatment session how the client feels (see Therapeutic dialog I, p. 90). This will provide you with feedback about the treatment, and you can note down the most important points on the back of your treatment record.

You will find a copyable *craniosacral treatment record* sheet at the end of the book in the Appendix.

1.14 Position

Observe the body posture of the person seeking treatment, even while conducting the initial dialog and while the person is lying on the treatment table. Note any unusual features, but avoid overestimating their importance. If the client is supine, make sure that this position does not impose any pressure or strain. Enquire whether this position feels comfortable.

If necessary, you should *support the client's head and cervical spine region* and relieve the pressure in this area, using a slightly raised support. A towel folded to the right thickness or a small cushion would be suitable: when the person is supine, the head should not tip forward so that the chin is angled toward the breastbone, nor should it be overextended backward, but reasonably straight with the neck in an easy, relaxing position.

When palpating and treating the occipital bone, this head support can get in the way; in that case, you should remove it while attending to the occiput and replace it afterwards.

The cushion can be essential, particularly when your client is in the side-lying position.

If necessary, you can relax the abdominal region and also the *lumbar and sacral regions* by placing *a support under the hollow of the client's knees*. Use fairly large towels or blankets that you can roll to the required dimensions and place under both knees. Various kinds of knee roll bolsters are also available to buy. For individuals with a tendency to sciatica, lumbago or herniated disk, use of a knee roll or blanket is essential (Fig. 1.14.1A, B).

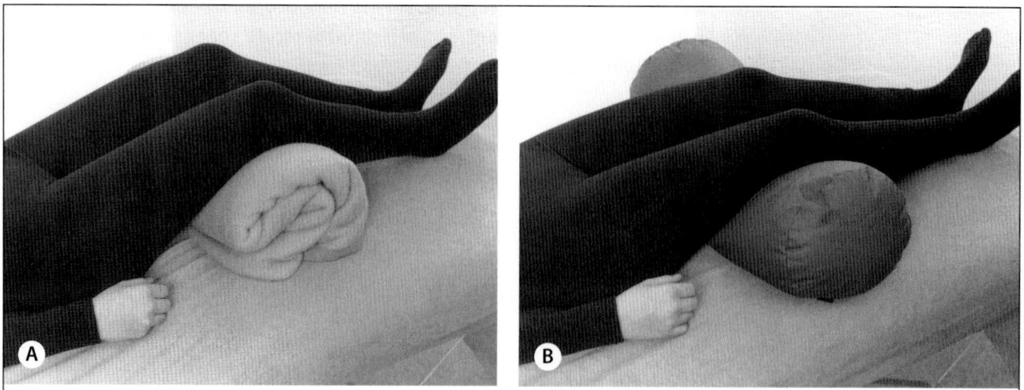

Figure 1.14.1
Relieve the pressure on legs and torso with (**A**) a blanket or (**B**) a knee roll bolster.

Always ensure that your own position is relaxed and does not place stress on your back.

As the practitioner giving treatment, you should be able to adjust your sitting position at the table *at any moment* (by height adjustment or by moving closer to or farther away from the treatment table) to ensure you are comfortable and relaxed and able to palpate without strain.

The following method will enable the client to lie down and sit up without putting strain on the back:

- As a first stage in lying down, the client should sit on the treatment table, then roll *sideways* onto the padded surface, first putting down one side of the body, and then turning to lie in the required position, e.g. supine.
- When sitting up from a supine position, the client should first turn over into the *side-lying position* and then get up *sideways*.

1.15 Therapeutic dialog I

Why dialog in craniosacral treatment?

One of the basic differences between craniosacral therapy and osteopathy is, as stated previously, the use of therapeutic dialog.

Resource-oriented communication and questions from the craniosacral therapist enable clients to gain an experience of the self in a protected place in the here and now. The act of reporting back verbally benefits the client because the new, more relaxed sense of the body becomes 'anchored' neurologically as experience.

Craniosacral therapy begins by applying touch mainly at the physical level of the client's body. Body, mind, and spirit are a unity, which cannot be divided into separate levels. This means that physical touch is also capable of touching the client's mental and spiritual level, in other words, render it more conscious.

The mental–spiritual level is addressed through the body – and this happens precisely because the body level does not need to put up a defense against the gentle, careful touch. The limbic system is then activated; one of the effects of this is to link the sensory impressions of the moment with memory and recognition. If awareness through touch occurs during the craniosacral treatment, and if the treatment is for the most part supported in a resource-oriented way, an inwardly-directed deepening of the perceptions can take place. This reduces, perhaps even removes, the need for activity in the external sphere. The body or the person as a whole is given the opportunity to relax more deeply, to regenerate and heal itself and maintain its state of health. This relaxation can promote intensified self-perception and enhance well-being.

It may happen that, during the self-regulation and regeneration or through the touch of the therapist, parts of the body are addressed which have stored up some unpleasant experience or traumatic memory. If so, these locations and/or the memories associated with them may re-enter the consciousness (see p. 249). Even if the memory does not become conscious, apt and 'harmonious' touch can activate the connective tissue, various fluids, and so the cell memory, with the consequence that deep healing processes are set in motion. For the practitioner to accompany these in a resource-oriented way, it helps to be skilled in the use of dialog and working as a companion in the process and able to apply these approaches reliably at any moment.

One of the integral aspects of the holistic application of craniosacral therapy is a touching of the whole with all its various levels (physical, emotional, mental and spiritual, the soul, and the transpersonal level). In the protected space, all that stands in the way of lightness, balance and improved self-regulation can be changed into something positive. Many corrections come about of their own accord and in a way that does not necessarily require the associated story, such as breaking a leg 25 years ago, to be remembered. If the client does become conscious of some ancient trauma, perhaps an accident that caused significant damage, this can now – with the aid of this resource-oriented dialog – be released from the 'cell memory' without re-traumatizing the client.

The therapeutic rapport and appropriate support by the practitioner as companion of the client's process, by means of dialog and by the practitioner's presence, are of fundamental assistance to the client; the person may perhaps experience powerful processes, but this time experiences them in a different way: not overwhelmingly but more mildly. This happens at a manageable tempo in a safe here and now.

The emphasis of the treatment you give as a practitioner is a matter of your own personal style and professional knowledge; consequently, you may work in a mainly body-oriented, psychotherapeutic, systemic, spiritual way, or a synthesis of all of these. Appropriate questions and your therapeutic dialog assist the client in the attainment of consciousness and integration of the session. It is the task of the practitioner to support the client in a respectful way. The way this is done will suit the particular situation, depending on whether the person lying on the treatment table is in a state of pleasant, deep relaxation or engaged in resolving a memory of trauma.

Proven methods of therapeutic dialog include neurolinguistic programming (NLP), voice dialog, focusing and transaction analysis. Dialog with the 'inner child' and elements of Gestalt therapy can also be used supportively.

Self-reflection on the part of the practitioner is important to the therapeutic dialog. Ask yourself the following questions from time to time before committing yourself to words:

- Why do I want to say or ask this?
- To what extent does what I want to say or ask have to do with me?
- Does this question really help the client; does it weaken or strengthen the client?

The dialog must never be used in a manipulative way. The rule is the same as elsewhere: it is primarily your clients who set the pace, decide which themes they wish to address and which they still want to exclude. They for the most part decide for themselves what is good for them. Practitioners should be essentially restrained, with a fundamental trust in the process – even when, as sometimes happens, they believe that they know what might help the client (see also Chapter 1.12).

The practitioner should be able to use the dialog for therapeutic intervention at any moment (see p. 96)

Some tips on dialoging

- Intonation, volume and speed are all very important. You should adjust them to suit the particular situation.
- In your role as therapist, you should ask 'open' questions – questions that cannot be answered with a simple 'yes' or 'no,' but call for the client to *describe the state* they are experiencing; open questions help develop an awareness of the body and an understanding for inner processes.
- Open questions are important as a way of enabling you to check such things as the intensity of touch or determining how the course of treatment is to proceed. They enable you as the therapist to assess the physical, emotional, mental or spiritual state of the client, addressing whichever level is concerned.

The following are 'open' questions:

- **What?**
  — 'What is happening at this moment?'
  — 'What do you feel at the place where my hands are resting?'
  — 'What do you feel here, and what do you feel in your body overall?'
- **How?**
  — 'How would you describe the impressions you are receiving now?'
  — 'How do you feel at the moment?'
  — 'How does that feel?'
  — 'How does this touch feel?'
  — 'How does it feel at the place where my hands are resting?'
- **Whereabouts?**
  — 'Whereabouts do you wish to be touched next?'
  — 'Whereabouts in your body feels especially pleasant?'
  — 'Whereabouts in your body do you feel …?'
  — 'Whereabouts is this evident?'
- **Where to?**
  — 'Where is your attention being directed now?'
- **In what way?**
  — 'In what way could you … (e.g., create more space for yourself)?'
- **Explain; how do you know?**
  — 'Explain how you know that it feels good.'

If the client cannot cope with open questions, but you still want feedback to help fine-tune the therapy, e.g., to know about the intensity of touch, you can use a straightforward enquiry. Asking the client to express a judgment, e.g., about your touch, helps create a better rapport between you and the client (you can respond to the answers by varying the quality of touch):

- more or less?
- better or not as good?
- pleasant or not so pleasant?
- pleasanter than before?

If a client's state has clearly persisted for some time (whether in professional or private life, or before, during or after the treatment) it can help to ask *'if' and 'would be' questions*. It is a way of re-engaging with the solution-oriented approach, it restores flow to what had become static and so enables development to occur once more.

Examples of 'if' and 'would be' questions:

How *would it be if* ...? What *could* ...? What/where *might* ...?

'If this part of the body could speak, what would it tell us?'

'If you could choose the best solution in this situation, what would it be?'

'What might help this to develop naturally in a way that would improve it?'

'If you could make things easier for yourself, how would that be? What would it be like? How would it feel?'

'How would you know that things are becoming easier?'

As you hear what the client says, let that tell you which level of the senses the client is presently at:

- visual/seeing
- auditory/hearing
- kinesthetic/touching, feeling or moving
- olfactory/smelling
- gustatory/tasting.

Ask further questions on that same level.

During the craniosacral treatment, you are a kind of *companion on the journey* for the client who is lying on the treatment table, sensing and perceiving. It is a basic principle for us as practitioners that we go with *what in fact is*, rather than what we think we see or what seems to us to be important. Never forget transference and countertransference; if these occur, the fact that the practitioner is aware of it makes a significant difference. You can be confident that the *client's system* already carries within it the answers that are the key to resolving symptoms or problems, and knows them. These answers can become conscious, given the assistance of dialog conducted with empathy and clarity. When, for example, physical symptoms, situations, conflicts, health, the inner child, and the like are given the opportunity to communicate, this aids the process of arriving at consciousness.

The aim of craniosacral therapy is not in my view psychotherapy, regression, or even a symbiotic blending of therapist and client. It is more a matter of physically re-experiencing something of that issue from the past, in a secure context; at the same time experiencing it in a state in which the individual is connected with personal resources in the here and now, so that the perception of it is anxiety-free.

Perhaps the inner healing force, the client's inner healer, wishes to express itself and suggest solutions. If means to resolve the problem do emerge, it is important to *sense how the body feels*. Invite the client to seek out practical opportunities to apply them in everyday life, so as to convert the insights into action. It is not you who find the solution for the client.

Your role is not to bombard the client with interfering questions, but to be a constant and adequate companion through the course of the session, accompanying it with dialog suited to the situation.

When you ask 'open' questions, this assists and deepens clients' self-awareness, so that they can make contact with their fundamental needs. They become able to set new priorities, leading to greater self-reliance, self-empowerment, and self-determination. The resource-oriented seeking out of the new sense of the body by means of feeling, combined with the process of formulating and expressing it, especially at the end of the session, 'anchors' the new more successfully both mentally and neurologically: old sensations or traumas can seldom be completely extinguished, but they can be overwritten by pleasant, new experiences.

There are specialized courses available to provide training in the art of dialog in craniosacral sessions. It helps to attend at least one such course. It is after all not only the hands that 'speak' in craniosacral treatment; words too have their effect.

Interactive work as the companion in the process

1.16

Basic principles

We are linked with our unity of mind, body, and spirit through the medium of our bodies. Attuned, apt and 'harmonious' touch touches us. Through gentle craniosacral treatment, it is possible to perceive physical levels and levels beyond them; we can accompany sensations and processes of development in a more conscious way. This carries within it an enormous potential of healing power.

The experienced practitioner is present in a spacious manner, allowing space to the client and guiding the person through the treatment as a companion in the process. The practitioner accompanies the course of the treatment session at each moment in a direct and immediate way suited to the situation and the needs of the client. If the intensity that develops during the session becomes too great, perhaps through a high level of trauma activation, the practitioner knows ways of intervening therapeutically (slowing down, for example, or sensing resources) that can be used to protect the client from re-traumatization, and uses them. Experience gained in the art of dialoging is very important here.

Clients have a need of some change or improvement; otherwise, there would be no sense in coming for treatment. There is often a subconscious agreement between client and practitioner to be careful in dealing with processes and to allow only so much to become an issue; no more than the individual can bear or integrate at the time. The first task is usually to find out the client's present state. Next, you can look together for constructive, positive elements that can be reinforced and 'anchored.'

The integrating and concluding phase, approximately the last third of the session, is always important. Questions to ask then are, e.g., 'What impression do you have now?'; 'What has changed?'; 'What are you experiencing?' or 'The session will be over in about ten minutes; what do you need to round off the treatment in a pleasant way for you?'

A particular feature of the treatment lies in accompanying tension release and the integration of these releases. Do not provoke anything. In your role as therapist, you should monitor and regulate the distance throughout the session, be present and aware of your own boundaries – and also of the degree of intensity you yourself can bear and are able to accompany. Be conscientiously aware whether transference and countertransference are occurring. You should not identify with the client's issues. If you are greatly touched by these issues, it is often very revealing to look back and reflect after the session or at the end of the treatment day. You should process your own issues in your own sessions or supervision.

Being a companion in a process is a path of learning and experience, just like the conduct of dialog and other elements of comprehensive craniosacral treatment. You can acquire knowledge for the purpose, but it is only any use if appropriately applied. Knowledge can lead to 'thinking instead of feeling' and get in the way of spontaneity (which would be a hindrance). Therefore, in order to accompany a process in a fitting way, a great deal of individual experience and clarification of your own history are important, as well as practical application of these things in the secure context of a training course.

Being an interactive companion in a process also involves intuition, presence and the kind of understanding that comes from the heart – and, as the idea of something 'interactive' implies – an immediacy as you travel the road with the client and a co-operative structuring of the session or of the way it develops.

Therapeutic intervention

The practitioner places a fundamental trust in the way the session evolves and the degree of intensity that develops. However, there are situations and moments in which the practitioner has to assume active leadership. For example, if clients begin to lose themselves in lengthy, prolonged processes, clear therapeutic intervention is advisable. The practitioner would use dialog to recall the person from that dissociation and reside more in the sphere of *sensing and perception in the here and now*. It might be possible to identify some basic topic area, and sense, look at and accept it. Then you may be able to find new, positive, solution-oriented pathways (see also Therapeutic dialog I, p. 90 and Therapeutic dialog II, p. 267).

If the client is involved in processes that place excessive demands on you as practitioner, you should respond by realizing this and setting clear boundaries. Ask the client to proceed more slowly and above all more carefully. Regulate the distance again, and the level on which transference is happening. Remain on the conscious level and in contact with your own sources of strength.

If the treatment develops in such a way that the demands placed on clients' own strength are too extreme (or if they find themselves in the midst of such overwhelming physical or emotional sensations that they risk re-traumatizing themselves), it can be helpful to ask them:

- to slow down or speed up
- to be/remain in the here and now
- attentively and consciously to sense the moment and the touch applied to their bodies
- to sense their entire body, its weight, and the padded surface on which they are lying

- to open their eyes and:
  - consciously take in the room around them, and orient themselves afresh
  - consciously make eye contact, so as to re-establish (social) contact with the external world.

If, as the practitioner, you feel that the pace and intensity of a process continues to overwhelm you, you can tell the client so.

Tips

It can sometimes be more helpful if clients sit for a while, rather than remain lying down, on the treatment table. As they sit there, ask whether it would be welcome for you to touch them, and if so where (e.g. you might give support on their sacrum, back or occiput).

If they are breathing rapidly, they should breathe more slowly: breathing is often very rapid during powerful processes. If their breathing is slight, allow your own breath to flow and ask them to concentrate awareness on their own breath, and, if necessary, to breathe more deeply. Suggest that they should observe what they sense as they do this.

Another aid to integration is for clients to adopt a side-lying position and sense their bodies again after powerful processes, and to relax in a kind of fetal position (see p. 202).

Divide the treatment period into sections: when giving treatment, be sure to allow the last third of the session – the final 10–15 min at least – for you to round off the treatment and enable integration.

You might 'listen' at the client's occiput and sacrum, to discover whether the client's craniosacral system and craniosacral rhythm overall is more balanced, and what has changed as compared to the start of the treatment. You can end the session by 'listening' (e.g. on the feet) and with a still point – if the client does not give an answer to your open question as to where touch would be welcome at the close.

Section 2

Treatment and balancing of the craniosacral system

2.1 The art of gentle touch

You will find it easier to sense the expression of primary respiration after you have experienced the quality of touch and its effects yourself in several craniosacral sessions. Self-palpation of the various body rhythms and performing some craniosacral treatments on yourself will extend your capacities of perception.

Before you begin to apply touch, regulate the distance and remain for a few moments in stillness.

Whenever you place your hands onto the body of the person lying on the treatment table, remember: your touch must be light and soft. You should already be attentive and centered before you apply touch and you trust your perceptions.

Ensure before you begin to touch that your hands, your forearms and your shoulders are utterly relaxed; now begin the gentle touch; it must be very light. Exert no pressure as you place your hands on.

Once you have placed your hands onto the client's body, reduce the weight in such a way that you retain clarity of contact. Allow your hands to follow the line of the part of the body you are touching, adopting the same shape as the body – not the other way round!

'Listen' with your hands to what the client's body is telling you. The wisdom of the body can reveal a great deal to you as you gain in experience, telling you for example about the permeability of the connective tissue and thus its conductivity, and about the quality of motion of the various body rhythms.

Your hands should 'tune in' to the various kinds of motion happening in the body, as in the self palpation (see p. 58): the subtle motions that you can sense over the entire body, mainly through the connective tissue, motion caused by the respiratory rhythm, the pulse generated by the heart, and the craniosacral rhythm. Attentively palpate and observe the different slow kinds of motion, perhaps beginning with the respiratory rhythm and following this for a few cycles, then moving on to the slow-motion, subtle craniosacral rhythm.

While you are administering treatment, lay aside the intention that says you have to bring about some effect. The easiest way to palpate the craniosacral rhythm is for you to be as grounded, centered and relaxed as you can.

Practice the skill of giving treatment using your hands' *sense of touch* rather than using pressure. You can listen deep down using your numerous different receptors, without increasing the pressure.

Do not become too technical. There is nothing for you to achieve or force to come about. You support the client in the releases of tension. Your receptive passivity, your attentiveness and respectful presence during the treatment are the best fundamental attitude to enable you to sense the craniosacral rhythm and assist its harmonization.

2.2 Golden rules before you begin

'Tuning in' before commencing treatment

Being relaxed yourself

As the practitioner, you (too) should allow yourself to relax, before, during and after the session. Your state of tension or relaxation during the treatment affects your perception and the success of treatment.

Grounding and centering; self-awareness

Sense your feet on the floor and perceive your body as a unity.

Then, sense your pelvic region as a whole, together with your seat bones and sacrum.

- Perceive your sacrum, vertebral column and head.
- Take several deep breaths, right down into your chest, and breathe out through your slightly open mouth. Observe your breath, with no compulsion to do or change anything.
- As you do so, consciously ground and center yourself.

Regulate the distance – establish your own presence

Before you apply touch and also during the session, the matter of *regulating the distance* is a fundamental one. It concerns all levels. Appropriate distance ensures that we are not too close to our clients, but allow them space; otherwise, it could be a reason for them to feel unease or an inability to relax. In that case, the practitioner is neither 'neutral' nor permitting enough space. Clients may feel uncomfortable or under pressure if the practitioner has paid too little attention to ensuring the right physical, emotional, or mental distance.

Do not begin to apply touch until you have determined for yourself that you have regulated the degree of distance and your own presence. This gives clients *sufficient room for their individual process*. Another benefit of right distance is that it enables the practitioner to perceive more as a whole.

Neutral

Before starting the treatment, give yourself enough time to apply the above advice. Free yourself of all expectations. Set yourself inwardly at rest, more and more, and make contact with the *stillness*. Remain in this stillness for at least 1 minute before beginning to apply touch. This precious time gives the client too a chance to arrive consciously on the treatment table and become attuned to the treatment that is to follow (see also Neutral and Stillness, p. 244).

Note concerning the treatment sequence

- The structural sequence in this book should be regarded as a guide and does not need to be followed absolutely or observed every time. If in your practice you have used this basic treatment dozens of times, as routinely as you use the alphabet or a musical scale, you should not just continue out of habit. Your fund of experience, your trust in your palpation skills and perceptions, your intuition and instinct, will all help you to support the craniosacral system and its rhythm during the treatment sessions at the right time and in the right place. Advanced craniosacral courses and craniosacral supervision are enormously helpful here.

Arranging your position at the treatment table

Check that you have made all the necessary preparations before each treatment session to ensure the best possible conditions. Arrange the room and equipment as well as you can (see p. 74). Your ability to sit comfortably, in a relaxed position at the treatment table, has a significant effect on your ability to listen to the craniosacral rhythm and body tissues. You should therefore make sure that you are sitting at the right *height* and at the right *distance* from (or nearness to) the *treatment table*. If your position at the table is too cramped, you will find it difficult to palpate the subtle motions of the craniosacral rhythm. Nor is it right if a craniosacral session, whose purpose is to help the client to release tensions, has the effect of exhausting your energies, maybe causing you to sit awkwardly and finish in need of treatment yourself.

Any excessive tension on the part of the practitioner can affect the well-being of the person receiving treatment. Do therefore ensure that you sit at the right height in relation to the table (Figs 2.2.1, 2.2.2). You can use cushions or blankets to adjust the height.

You yourself act as a pivot point or fulcrum, and so does the position in which you rest your arms and hands. It is important for you to be able to avoid putting stress on yourself as you arrange your position to provide these pivot points, and this requires skill. The pivot points need to be free and flexible, not inert, rigid or slightly unsteady.

It is entirely permissible for the practitioner to relax as well; in fact, it is essential. It is important not to have to impose any strain on your pelvic region, back, shoulder, neck or arm regions; instead your position should be easy and relaxed.

- If you do feel any tensions in your own body during the treatment and if these are hindering you, it helps to remove your hands, move away from the table, and relax. You can then re-establish the optimum position at the treatment table.

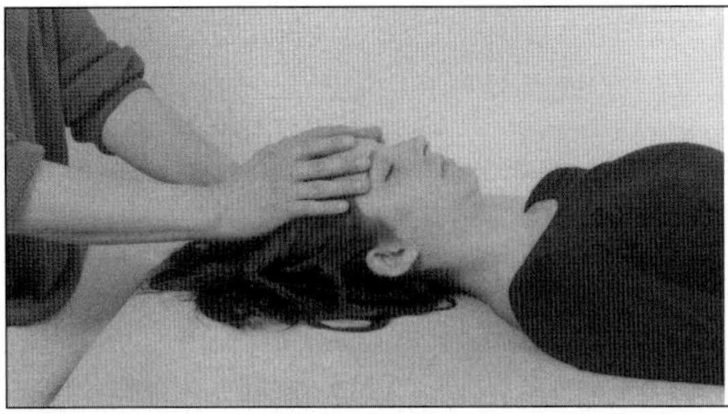

Figure 2.2.1
Too high in relation to the table.

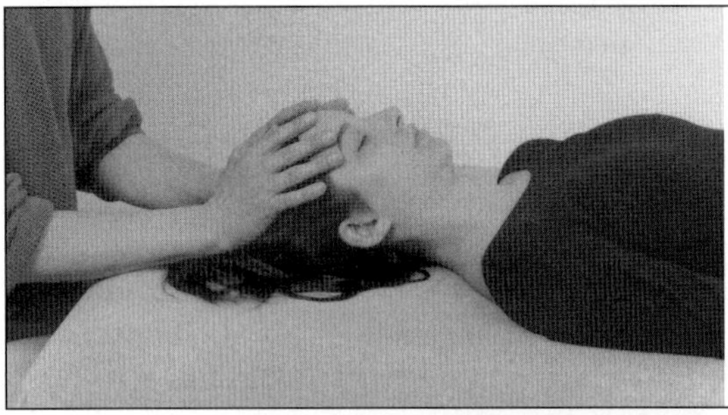

Figure 2.2.2
Correct position in relation to the table.

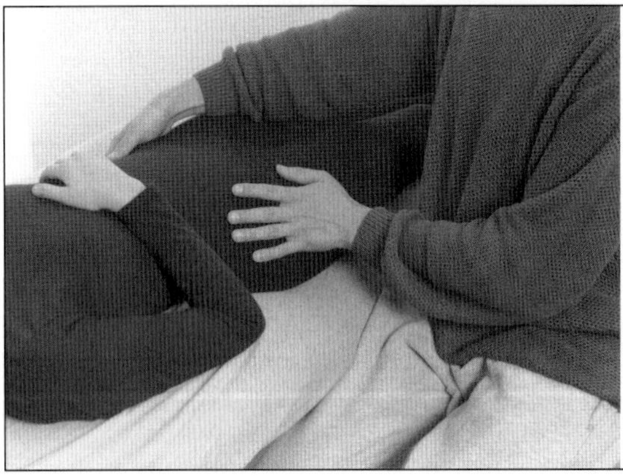

Figure 2.2.3
Seated by the table.

Correct position when working beside the treatment table

Seated by the table: You may need to ask the person lying on the table to move towards you slightly so that you can be near enough to your client's body (Fig. 2.2.3). If the distance between you and the client is too great, that can sooner or later lead to strain. Sit at the correct height in relation to the table, ground and center yourself. Your pelvis, legs, and feet in particular should be in conscious contact with the ground. *This is recommended as the preferred position.*

Standing by the table: Again in this case, you should ask the person lying on the table to find a position close to you, so that the separation distance is not too great (Fig. 2.2.4). Ground yourself by consciously

Figure 2.2.4
Standing by the table.

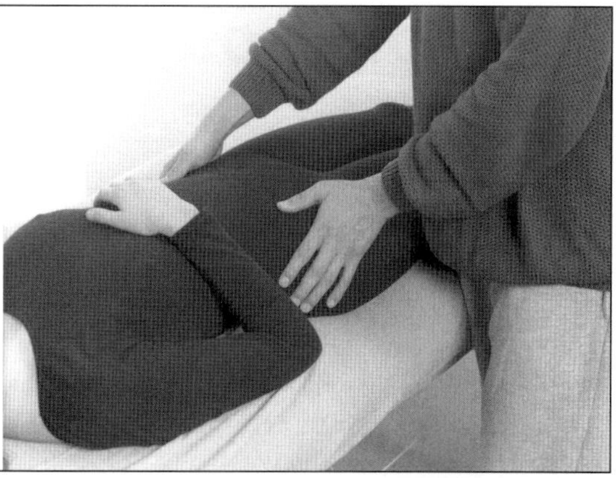

Figure 2.2.5
Seated on the table.

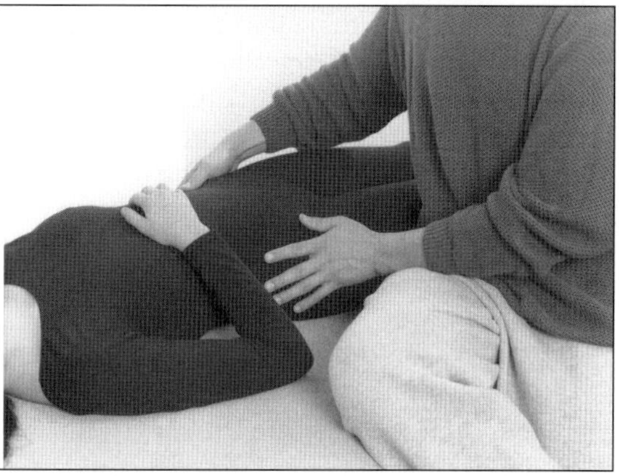

establishing the contact of your feet on the floor. Remain supple and flexible in your ankle joints, knees and hips, and centered in your abdominal/pelvic region. It will take the weight off the lower part of your body if you place one leg to the side, supported on a chair.

Seated on the table (if the treatment table is a wide one, measuring more than about 80 cm [approx. 30 inches]): Ask the person to move across as far as possible to the other side of the treatment table (Fig. 2.2.5). This will create room on your side of the table for you to sit or rest one leg at an angle on the table.

Tips

Make sure that your client's head is always in view while you are applying touch from your position at the side of the table. If your positioning means that you are facing the client's feet, simply change over the position of your left and right hands. That will rotate your body so that you turn more to face the person on the treatment table. You then have a direct view and can see such things as the respiratory rhythm in the region of the rib cage, and other body signals, especially the person's facial expression and non-verbal signs such as tears or joy.

2.3 Whole-body assessment

Once the initial dialog is over and the client is established in the best position on the treatment table, we begin with whole-body assessment. In craniosacral treatment, we do not determine a diagnosis, as this could narrow the focus of our treatment. Diagnosis is the province of allopathic medicine, and something that craniosacral practitioners need to take into account with respect to the contraindications.

For the craniosacral practitioner it is *whole-body assessment*, also called whole-body evaluation, which provides the first contact with the body of the person receiving treatment. One welcome side-effect is that it assists the development of our capacities of perception.

A short visual assessment (what is immediately noticeable; what differences are there?) is followed by an examination in which the practitioner senses, through the client's clothing, the texture and elasticity of the skin, connective tissue, muscles, and joints. This provides the first important impressions, e.g., concerning the basic muscle tonus and conductivity of the connective tissue. These impressions, and in particular evaluation of the motions of the craniosacral rhythm, give indications as to where any body structures are free or to any degree restricted, and which structures are involved. We should take a mental note of these, or write them down in brief. We may encounter patterns and interrelationships that operate across the entire body and show how and where the body has compensated, and gain an impression as to which locations may need to be included in the treatment.

During the course of the session, we sense changes in the body, the slow rhythms, and the overall atmosphere in the room. I advise approaching the listening stations and techniques listed below by first listening for the slow rhythms working in the functional manner, as in the Three-step healing process (see p. 246). If, when you do so, you find a reduction in self-regulation or that a structure appears particularly restricted in its function, there are many options available to provide gentle release.

In the closing stage of a treatment session, you can listen again briefly at individual sites, palpating and recording in your notes the changes between 'before' and 'after' (see pp. 86, 199, and 334, The treatment record).

- With increasing experience, palpation/evaluation and treatment will no longer be separate procedures, but will merge fluidly into one another.

Palpation of the craniosacral rhythm

The craniosacral rhythm can be palpated over the entire body, through the medium of the connective tissue as well as other means. By tuning in to the slow motions of this rhythm, we can listen to its strength, amplitude, symmetry, and the number of cycles/min (see p. 51).

The craniosacral rhythm can be detected particularly clearly when the craniosacral system and its associated structures, such as the many layers of the connective tissue, are free of any kind of restrictions. Although the rhythm can be felt all over the body, there are certain locations where this is easier, and where its motion enables us to conclude which areas of the body are free, inhibited or restricted. These places are called listening stations (or palpation sites).

Tips

1. At the beginning, it can be easier to palpate the slow body rhythms if you occasionally close your eyes. Trust in the fact that thousands of receptors of various kinds in your hands are becoming activated and that you will develop deeper and more subtle sensitivity every time you palpate.
2. With your eyes open, you can watch the motion of the client's breathing at any time and check whether you are listening to the motions of respiration or of the craniosacral rhythm. This 'reality check' will train and extend your palpation skills.
3. Once you have more experience of palpation and you have developed a clearer and more differentiated ability to feel, it is advisable to palpate mainly with your eyes open and your gaze focused into the distance. Some practitioners find that what they sense when their eyes are closed is too much 'of themselves'; they may lose themselves in this, dissociate (i.e. separate themselves from reality), or find that they are neither 'neutral' nor present. The visual level too can inform you of many physical changes that you can take into consideration in shaping the further treatment.

The following are the most important listening stations, working upward from the feet:

- feet
- knees or thighs
- pelvis/sides of the iliac crests
- costal arch/inferior thoracic aperture
- shoulders/superior thoracic aperture
- head (various positions).

It is helpful for beginners to work in this order. The sequence can be varied, shortened, or extended with the use of advanced techniques as your experience grows through courses and actual practice.

Palpation of the craniosacral rhythm on the feet

Begin with the palpation of the craniosacral rhythm at the feet. There are two hand positions that can be used; of these, the one in the seated position is recommended as the preferred option:

Position seated at the lower end of the treatment table: Starting from a point on your client's legs, slide your hands laterally under her heels, so that the client's heels rest in the palms of your hands. Your fingers should rest gently on the heels/posterior part of the feet (Fig. 2.3.1).

Position standing at the lower end of the treatment table: Place both hands from above onto the anterior part of your client's left and right foot or ankle, approximately level with the instep. Ensure, by asking the client, that your touch is clear but gentle, and not felt as being firm or restricting. If you are standing, your hips, knees and ankles should constantly remain supple; your pelvic region and your shoulder and neck region should remain flexible (Fig. 2.3.2).

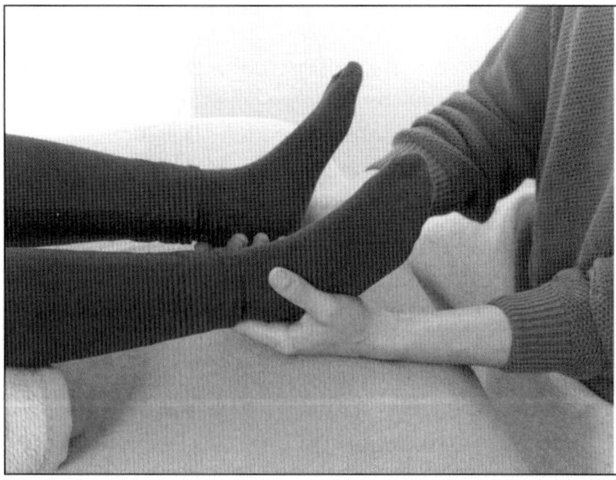

Figure 2.3.1
Hand position when seated at the client's feet.

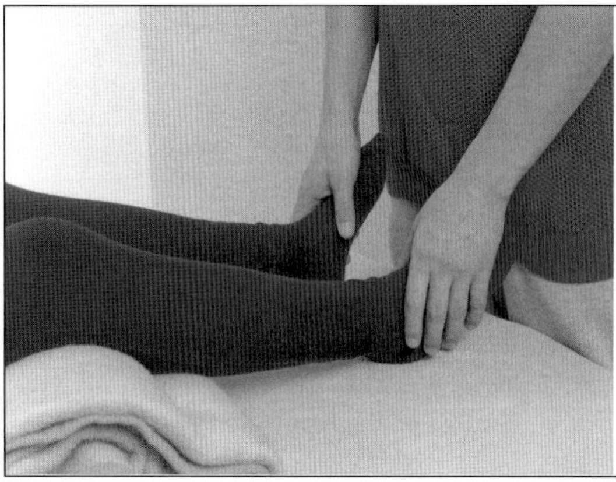

Figure 2.3.2
Hand position when standing at the client's feet.

Palpation of the craniosacral rhythm on the knees

This is the first listening station for which you take up a position at the side of the treatment table. Place your hands, exerting no pressure, on your client's knees at a point where you can feel the kneecap and the entire knee beneath your hands.

When working from the side, make sure that you *keep your client's face in view*, once your hands are in place. If you are facing your client's feet, simply change over the position of your hands. That will have the effect of turning you to face the person (Fig. 2.3.3).

Palpation of the craniosacral rhythm on the thighs

Take up a position at the side of the treatment table. Rest your hands gently on each of your client's thighs. 'Tune in' to the motions of the tissue.

Palpation of the craniosacral rhythm on the pelvis

Take up a position at the side of the treatment table. It is a good idea to begin by palpating your own iliac crest, sensing its shape and upper border. After a little practice, you will know how different the height of the iliac crest can be in different individuals. Place your hands gently on the side of your client's pelvis, on the iliac crest. You are not touching just the level of her clothing and skin; rather, through them you are slowly blending with deeper levels of the tissue, so that here – depending on the qualities – you can also palpate the *bony structure* of the iliac crest (Fig. 2.3.4).

Figure 2.3.3
Hand position when palpating on the client's knees.

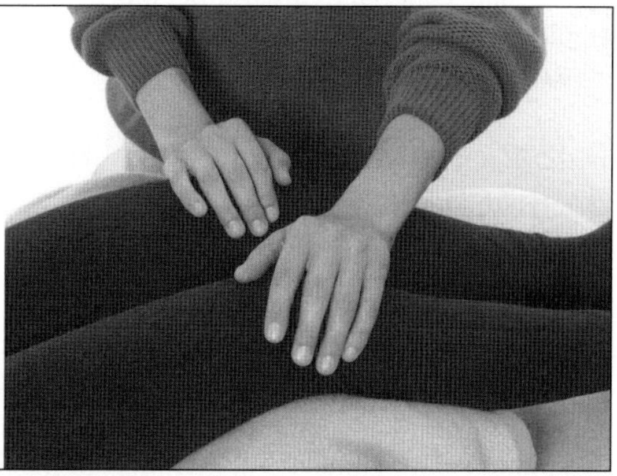

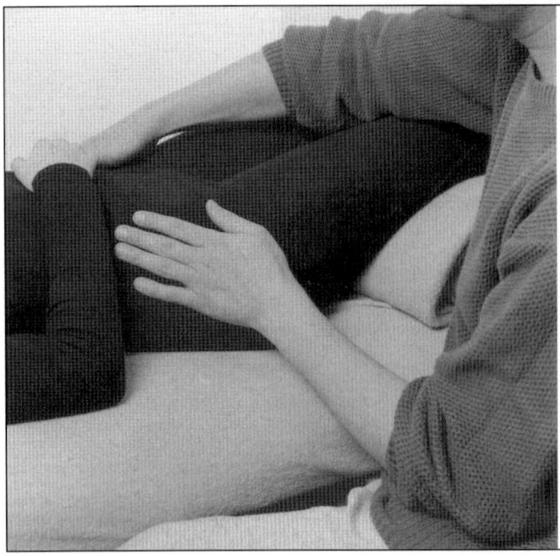

Figure 2.3.4
Hand position when palpating on the client's pelvis.

Palpation of the craniosacral rhythm on the costal arch

Take up a position at the side of the treatment table. Place both hands gently on the costal arch/inferior thoracic aperture. The motion of the respiratory rhythm is very dominant here because the diaphragm, the main respiratory muscle, is located beneath the costal arch. The respiratory motion makes it more difficult to palpate the craniosacral rhythm, so you should not despair of your palpation skills if you cannot sense any craniosacral rhythm in the costal arch area. Listening with your hands to the respiratory motion for a few minutes is a useful palpation exercise, however, especially for beginners. It helps to do this with your eyes open and also with eyes closed. Is there more abdominal breathing or more thoracic breathing? Does the breathing change? If so, how?

Your gentle touch supports the respiratory flow of the person receiving treatment and so perhaps draw the person's attention to the place where your hands are resting; this in itself can assist relaxation. The craniosacral rhythm can be palpated in parallel to the respiratory rhythm, at about half the rate (Fig. 2.3.5).

Palpation of the craniosacral rhythm on the shoulders

Take up a position at the top end of the treatment table (near your client's head). Place a hand on each shoulder of the person lying on the table. Palpate the motions you can feel: at the shoulders, you can clearly feel the motion of the respiratory rhythm, which tends to move your client's shoulders toward you on inhaling and toward the torso on exhaling. The motion of the craniosacral rhythm is different in that it tends to be a subtle, slow external and internal rotation (ER/IR) (Fig. 2.3.6).

Figure 2.3.5
Hand position when palpating on the client's costal arch.

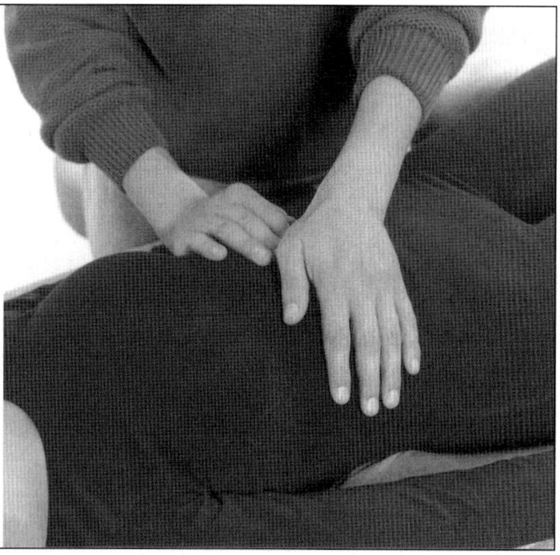

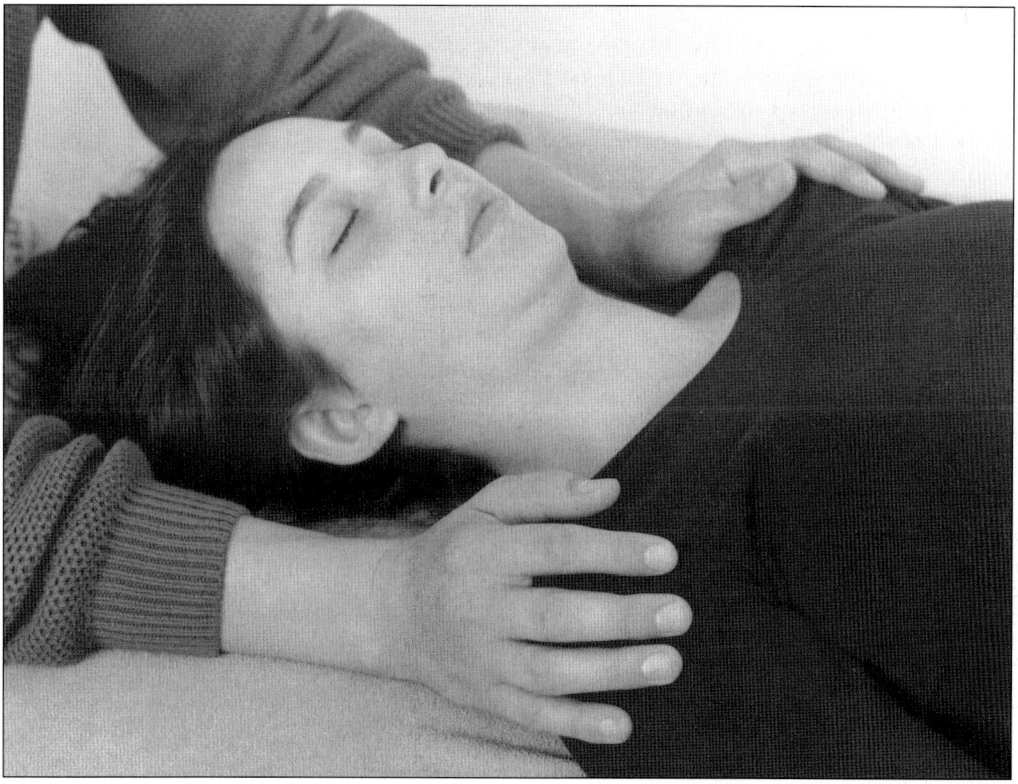

Figure 2.3.6
Hand position when palpating on the client's shoulders.

Palpation of the craniosacral rhythm on the head

When working at your client's head, you need enough room to rest your forearms, so that you can palpate in a relaxed way, with no trembling. It is advisable to be able to place around half the length of your forearm on the treatment table, so that it is stable and supported. This creates a pivot point (fulcrum).

You might need to ask the person to move down a little further toward the lower end of the table, keeping her heels on the table. Alternatively, an extension can be used to lengthen the table, or you could place a blanket on your lap in such a way that it provides an extra area of support for your forearms.

In principle, assuming that the craniosacral system is free, the craniosacral rhythm can be palpated more or less clearly on all the cranial bones. Two requirements are necessary here: anatomical knowledge of the individual bones of the cranium, and precise positioning and touch. Recall this consciously to mind from time to time and put it into practice: keep your palpating hands and fingers supple, and set aside the sense that you have to 'do' something. Make contact with the stillness and let the motions of the craniosacral rhythm come to you.

Take up a position at the top end of the treatment table (near your client's head) – with both hands on the frontal bone. Place the entire surface of the fingers of both hands on the frontal bone, without exerting any pressure. Your palms should not unintentionally touch the cranium. You should not restrict your client's head or compress the coronal suture (Fig. 2.3.7).

Take up a position at the top end of the treatment table (near your client's head; if necessary slightly to one side – one hand on the frontal bone and one on the occipital bone, in combination). Move a little to the left or right of your client's head to enable you to place one hand under her occiput, lengthwise or crosswise. Once this hand is in position in the right place and without restricting the head, place your second hand gently down from above onto the client's frontal bone. You can place this hand lengthwise or crosswise, whichever is most comfortable for you and the person receiving treatment (Fig. 2.3.8A, B).

Cradle hold

Take up a position at the top end of the treatment table (near your client's head) – both hands under the occipital bone. This listening station on the occiput owes its name to the fact that you 'cradle' the client's head in your hands.

Place your slightly cupped hands together side by side with your little fingers almost touching. A helpful way to find the correct position for your hands on the occipital bone is to bring the hold upward underneath the occiput with both hands, working sideways up the neck from the direction of the client's shoulders, with your open palms facing upwards. The tips of your fingers should rest gently in the region of the occipital ridge and the muscles in the upper neck region.

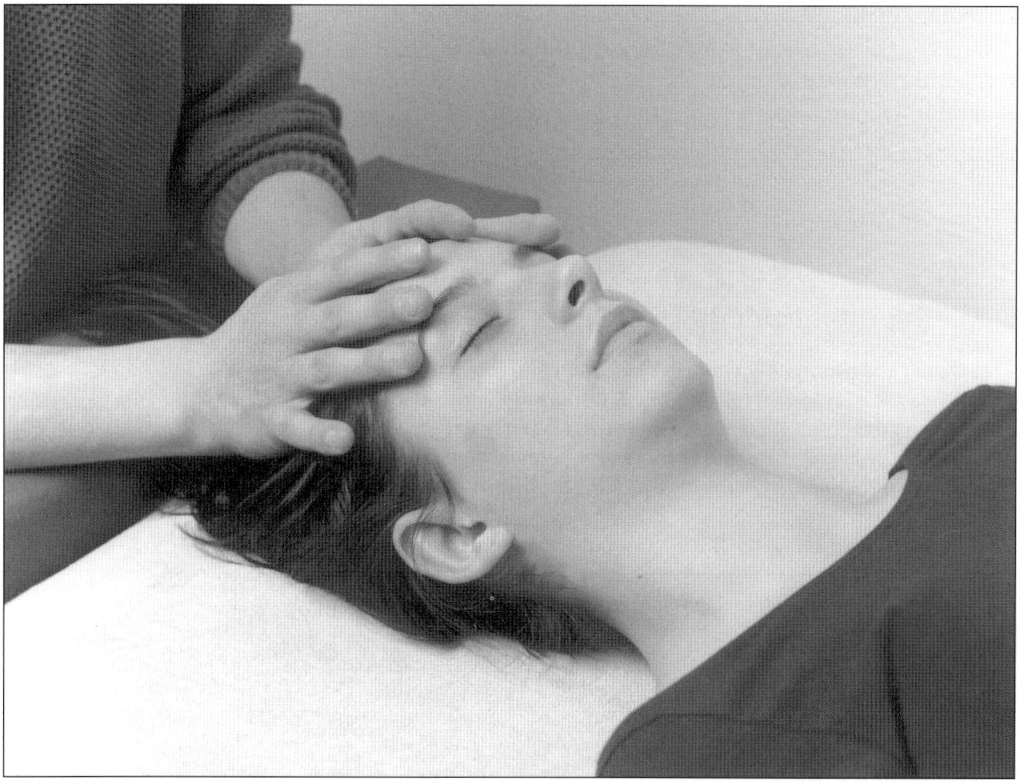

Figure 2.3.7
Listening station on the frontal bone.

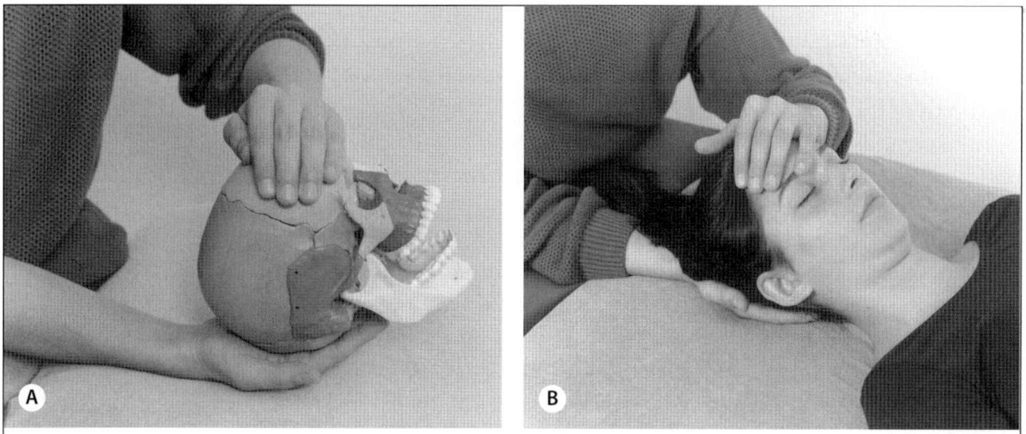

Figure 2.3.8
Listening station on the frontal and occipital bones combined: shown on (**A**) model, (**B**) client.

Another method is to draw both hands, open and facing upwards, toward your client's head from each side and then use sight movements to left and right to bring them slowly into the middle and position them under the occiput.

Important points

The thenar and hypothenar eminences of your hand should not be restricting to the head; it is important to allow enough space. Beginners should check and adjust this from time to time, based on their own judgment and also by asking their clients. Nothing – listening or treatment – should be done in a forceful or restricting way; it is not in the nature of the treatment approach presented here.

The cradle hold allows the person lying on the treatment table to rest the whole weight of her head in your hands, in an act of handing over. This also gradually releases tension in the region of the shoulders, neck and cranial base.

Take care that you do not push your hands down towards the body of the person lying on the treatment table; this would restrict or compress the cervical spine and neck area. Distribute your weight perhaps just slightly backward; do not exert any traction that can be felt as such; just a subtle hint – the aim is to take the weight off the whole region and give it more room. Then sit upright again, check the amount of distance in front of you, between you and your client, and by doing so, in a relaxed manner, create a free fulcrum.

In the cradle hold (Fig. 2.3.9A, B), which is pleasant to both client and practitioner, use the soft contact of your supple hands and fingers to sense the hair and scalp of your client's head, exploring its firmness or mobility. Next, sense the bony occiput. If you are fully relaxed and passive, you might sense the craniosacral rhythm with your hands on the occipital bone. In flexion, this moves the occipital bone toward your hands (Fig. 2.3.10), that is, toward the table and also slightly caudad (toward the client's feet). In flexion, you feel the occipital bone becoming fuller; it also becomes broader laterally. What are the qualities of the craniosacral rhythm like at this moment? Do you sense it more distinctly when you widen your perception to the level of the meninges and cerebrospinal fluid?

- The other listening stations on the head are described in 'Treating the head/ releasing the cranial bones' (see p. 170).

Figure 2.3.9
Listening station on the occipital bone:
(A) Frontal view using model. **(B)** Lateral view shown on the client.

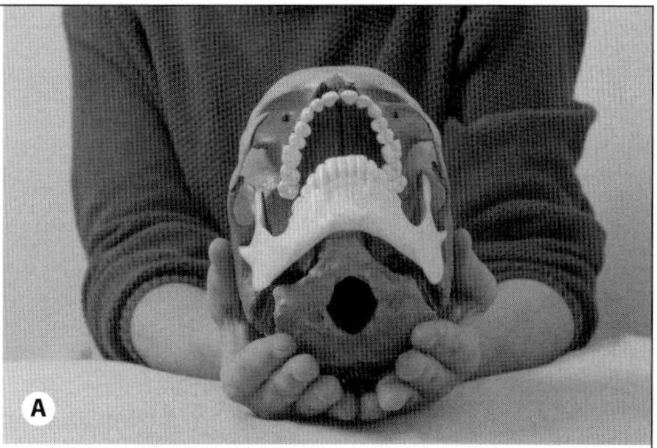

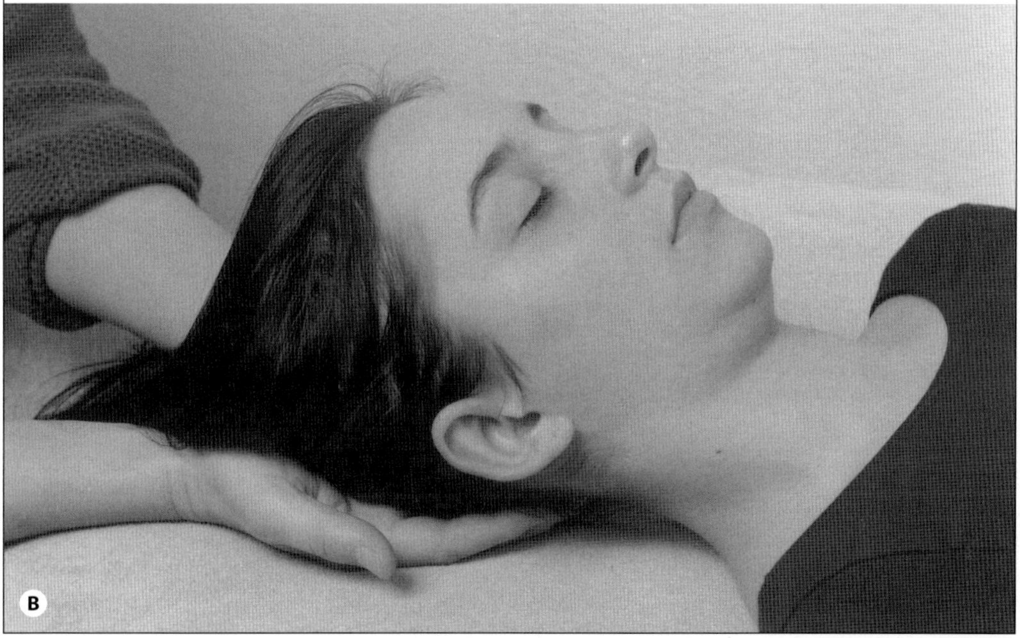

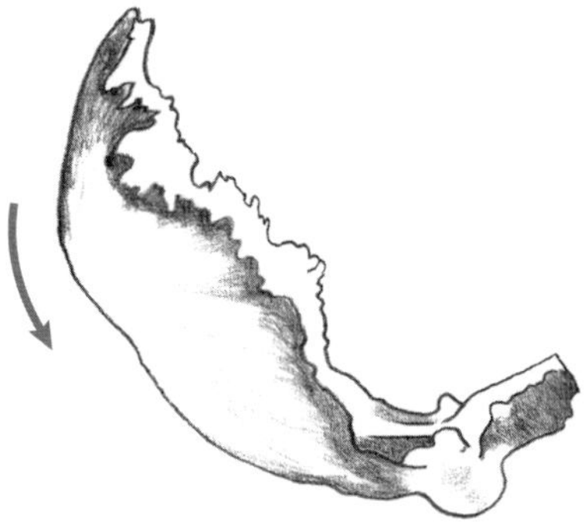

Figure 2.3.10
Direction of motion of the occipital bone in flexion (simplified).

Testing the fasciae by fascial glide

The fascial glide method of testing the fasciae provides another technique for whole-body assessment and release of the connective tissue.

Fasciae are made up of collagen fibers and nets of elastic tissue forming an envelope around individual organs, muscles or muscle groups. Body fasciae surround the musculature as a whole everywhere in the regions of the face, neck, torso and limbs, making them a kind of 'enveloping organ beneath the skin'.

Fascial glide on the torso or limbs enables the practitioner to tune in, first of all to the level of the skin, and then the layers of connective tissue beneath it, working by means of touch applied to the client's clothing. The next step is to apply constant, gentle traction, *without sliding over the surface*; this might for example be done in the longitudinal direction first of all, working upward, then later downward, and to right and left. During this gentle gliding and moving of the uppermost layer of connective tissue, your attention should focus entirely on detecting the free tissue or the skin resistance in these different directions. Your intention, as you slowly move the skin and the layers of connective tissue and fasciae lying beneath it, is devoted to finding free (or inhibited or restricted) tissue. You must be ready to follow the direction of ease (greatest possible mobility), both longitudinally (toward the head and toward the feet) and transversely (across, laterally; to left and right). Fascial glide gives you a sense of the places where the connective tissue is freely mobile and where there is lack of movement.

Tips

If the resistance of the tissue increases or the fascial glide stops completely because of tissue resistance, wait there. The tonus of the tissue will probably change of itself after a while. If that does not happen, glide with the fasciae in another direction that is free.

After some practice, when craniosacral treatment has trained your sensitivity for subtle changes in the body and in specific tissue layers, you will be able to distinguish free and inhibited or restricted areas of the body in a matter of seconds, using this fascial test. Fascial glide can be used both as a method of evaluation and as a treatment technique used to make various tissues more supple, and more flexibly interconnected.

Fascial glide is often combined with the release of the transverse connective tissue layers (see p. 119).

Functional version: Remain in the area that is free, without confronting the tissue with the barrier. As you do so, tune in to the tissue tension and leave the release to the motions of breathing and craniosacral rhythm. The Living Matrix (the connective tissue) then seeks and finds a new balance.

Self-treatment: You can also try performing the fascial glide technique on yourself. This is best done lying down. You can also use it regularly as a self-treatment method.

Free/reduced craniosacral rhythm and whole-body interrelationships

This calls for a spirit of enquiry on the part of the practitioner. The expression of primary respiration is unique to each individual and the state that it reveals is that of the moment. The results obtained from palpating the motions of the craniosacral rhythm and from the fascial tests provide valuable information about free and inhibited or restricted structures. You can then evaluate using your whole-body assessment to find out about compensatory interrelationships or patterns of any restriction across the whole body.

Explore the locations and regions in the body that are free and also those where there is any resistance – also take an overall view and include the results of the whole-body assessment that you have just carried out. Reduced motion of the craniosacral rhythm reveals impairment to the structure, perhaps caused by trauma, a fall, shock, accident, operation, stress or faulty posture. You might carry out a release of the connective tissue at that point and then listen to the craniosacral rhythm again. As we know, structure and function influence each other.

Figure 2.3.11 shows how this can appear in practice. The left leg followed the motions of external and internal rotation according to the craniosacral rhythm, which was detectable to a slightly reduced degree higher up on the left iliac crest. On the right foot, knee and thigh, the craniosacral rhythm could be palpated as inhibited in strength and in ER/IR. At the other listening stations higher up, the craniosacral rhythm was well detected and balanced, except at the right shoulder. Another noticeable feature was the tendency of the person's head to turn to the right in the cradle hold.

The fascial glide test showed the left leg to be free and revealed some restriction running from the right knee to the pelvis on the left-hand side of the body, slightly above the left iliac crest; from there the tissue was free apart from some restriction exerting a pull running to the right shoulder.

Overall, such results enable us to draw conclusions about patterns of connection and interrelationship affecting the whole of the body. In this case a line of slight restriction could be traced diagonally across from the right shoulder to the upper part of the iliac crest and down from there to the right thigh. The next question might be which of these areas of restriction is the oldest, the strongest or the most important, and which others are compensatory, having come about as a result.

When you are performing the release of tension in the transverse connective tissues described below, it is important in every case to include both the areas detected as being free and those identified as at all restricted. If you treat a main point of such restriction (a primary inertial fulcrum), i.e., a location that is related to a number of other areas where there is also any restriction, then other interrelated or linked areas of restriction begin to be resolved. If treatment of the main restriction is

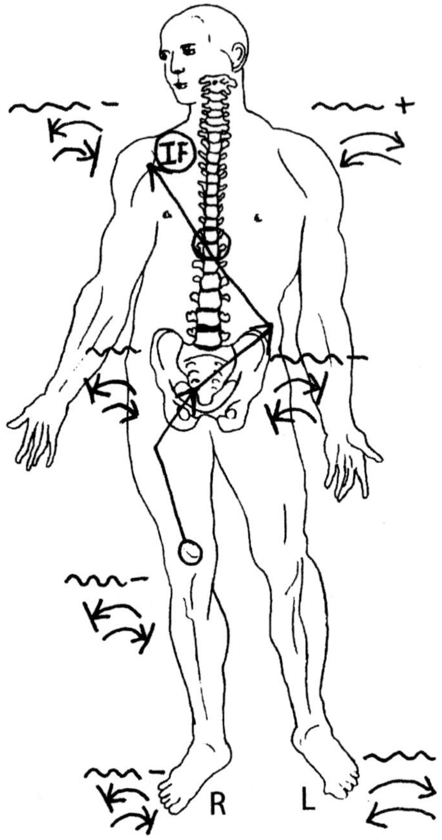

Figure 2.3.11
How structure and function influence each other. (Sample of treatment record; original on page 334)

unpleasant or painful for the person receiving treatment, even though you are placing minimal weight on the tissue and are regulating the distance, you can in that case treat indirectly, in other words you can treat via other, more distant points in this whole-body pattern.

Working by the functional method, there is greater emphasis on promoting what is healthy: instead of releasing restrictions, you listen and draw into the process the motions of respiratory rhythm and craniosacral rhythm. Your main task is to support the areas of the body that are already free.

2.4 Release of the transverse layers of connective tissue

The connective tissue speaks

The first description of the connective tissue in the west was given by Theophile de Bordeu in 1767. Today, we know it to be an active physiological system – an interactive organ, in its own right. The connective tissue is a whole-body matrix endowed with a high degree of intelligence. Its capacity for conducting energy and transmitting information is more rapid than that of the nervous system, as has been described at length by authors such as James Oschman in his books and lectures (see Further Reading). This 'Living Matrix' is an energetic communication system that integrates, organizes and energizes the body as a whole, in such a way that every tiny part is able to communicate with every other. It includes all the fibrous systems in the body. Structures belonging to the skeleton of the cell operate through the membranes of the cell and the nucleus, forming a link between these and the extracellular matrix, the connective tissue. These connections enable mechanical and bio-electromagnetic forces to be transmitted through the body as a whole.

The human body, with a water content of around 70%, can be sensed via the medium of its connective tissue as a living being that is capable of conduction. The aspect of fluids in the connective tissue should not be underestimated. Humoral physiology is important in ancient Hippocratic medicine as well as in traditional Indian and Chinese medicine. The human body is to an extent a cosmic 'resonance body', because the body fluids within it are also affected by macrocosmic influences such as temperature, the weather and seasons. Electromagnetic fields in and around the body, the earth and the cosmos, which today we are able to detect, influence human health. Our bodies even radiate a small amount of light, by means of biophotons. The connective tissue and its fluids are important transmitters of processes; they can also store and recall events.

The functions of the connective tissue are to provide support, conduct, separate, and bind together. At the same time, local connective tissue provides a link for us with our bodies as a whole. Even a slight injury can affect other parts of the body via the medium of our connecting tissue. Free and inertial fulcrums in the body, affecting for example the locomotor apparatus, can be sensed through the connective tissue.

Once you have carried out the whole-body assessment, you have an initial impression of various parts of the body that are free and others where there are restrictions of the craniosacral rhythm, the connective tissue, and the muscles, ligaments, and fasciae.

The next step is the release of connective tissue layers. This is mainly done in areas of the body that have *transverse* layers of connective tissue and muscle, which provide especially good support and stability. These are mainly responsible for our posture as a whole and have to *compensate* in their own way for any *imbalance*.

Transverse connective tissue is found at every location in the body where there is a *transition* (from wide to narrow or narrow to wide) and where there is a particular need for a great deal of support and freedom of motion, for example the pelvic floor and the shoulder and neck region. These areas of the body, where there is a large amount of transverse connective tissue, are often particularly tense or felt to be constricted. If the connective tissue layers experience release locally, this can have a relaxing effect on the whole body segment, on neighboring segments and also on the entire body.

It is the connective tissue that provides the link with the depths of the body and allows us to sense it, when we take up contact with our sensitive hands and slight contact weight: with sufficient practice you can sense and *differentiate* the layers, through the clothing to the skin, from there via the conductive connections of the connective tissue to the fasciae that surround and protect the muscles and organs, on through the muscle to the bones. As you do this, you are able to detect and distinguish free or inhibited tissue structures.

When we release tension in *transverse connective tissue*, this has a considerable effect on the *longitudinal connective tissue* and *body posture*. Our organs are also given more room when the surrounding connective tissue relaxes.

We also place hands on the natural *transition zones* such as the pelvic/abdominal region or the superior thoracic aperture/neck region; this means that by this simple technique we also support the balancing and integration of this part of the body with neighboring regions, since areas that had been isolated from each other because of excessive tension, connect better with each other once more. The person is enabled to experience the body more as a whole entity.

When transverse connective tissue relaxes, this usually increases the ER/IR or the quality of the craniosacral rhythm. When longitudinal connective tissue relaxes, this improves the flexion and extension motion or the longitudinal fluctuation. This explanation assists our functional understanding; in actual practice, each release of one structure automatically also helps bring about a change in all the structures that are linked to it: the whole-body matrix will then balance itself anew, of itself.

Methods and sequence of treatment

Procedures and intention in treatment to release the transverse connective tissue of the torso: There is a simple way to help tensions and restrictions in your client's body to 'melt' and resolve. Instead of provoking tissue resistance by applying a forceful manipulative technique, slowly and consciously take up the contact with the tissue tension that reveals itself.

'Harmonious' touch

Once you have placed your hands in position, check that the touch you are applying with your upper hand is experienced by the client as soft and light. Use your own capacities of perception to examine your quality of touch and correct as necessary; then, if you wish, ask your client how the touch feels, and adjust it according to what the client tells you. Your lower hand should be soft and supple, and should also listen to the tonus of the connective tissue and muscles. Your touch should be gentle, with enough clarity so that the structure you are touching, along with the tension in it, can sense itself and then – brought about by the warmth and spaciousness of your hands, the fascial glide and the slower body rhythms – release happens.

Version 1

Apply gentle, yet distinct touch and remain listening at the surface until the tissue expands of its own accord to meet your hands and fingers, and relaxes. Some of the signs that this is happening are that it becomes softer, warmer and more relaxed. Continue to listen as, after a while, the tissue spontaneously relaxes, through your respectful, harmonious touch. The better you regulate the distance and the more you are present, allow space, and at the same time, remain in clear contact to enable perception, the better the client's body as a whole is able to regulate itself. The warmth of your hands and the permission to 'let go' in the protected space of the treatment room, and not be obliged to do anything during the treatment, begin the first stirrings of the release.

Version 2

With your hands, slowly take up contact with the deeper levels: through the client's clothing to the level of the skin, and below that to the connective tissue and the muscles. Focus your attention to sense deep down, without significantly increasing the pressure. Take up contact with the first level of the tissue that feels firm or where you detect any resistance. This is where we encounter tissue tension, and we accept it as a natural barrier, a place where we have to stop. Pause there, listen, and be open for all body signals. Is there any change?

After a while, you also begin to sense deep down with your other hand. There, you slowly take up contact again with the 'stop' point and slowly adopt the same tonus, as if you are 'docking' at this level of tension. Try to sense the nature or quality of this resistance.

This happens without applying any firm pressure and without provoking reaction in the tissue. Simply use your attention and a 'three-dimensional sense of touch' *to slowly take on the same intensity of tension as the tissue*. Maintain this contact and wait. Is there any change?

- What do you perceive with one hand, and what do you perceive with the other?
- How do you perceive *the space* between your hands?
- What is your client's breathing like, overall; is it detectable locally, in the place where your hands are listening?

It often happens that after a while, the tissue releases its tension. The tissue perceives that the intensity supplied by your hand from outside – slowly and supportively instead of quickly and in an interventionist way – is almost the same as its own. The tissue no longer has to put up a protective defense and can release tension: a release takes place. If the practitioner then listens, attentively and quietly, without actively doing anything, the connective tissue then seeks and finds a new 'state of balance'. As a result, the craniosacral rhythm also becomes more balanced.

Once the uppermost inhibited layer has been released, keep the contact there with your hands on this location and sense what is happening beneath your hand. Try to sense the quality of this resistance and what is happening beneath your hand.

Do you perhaps want to seek out the next layer of tissue tension below that, and support and release it? If so, take up contact again in the depths of the tissue with your palpatory awareness, until you stop just before the next level of resistance. You follow the same process of distinct 'docking' again, and the clear contact with this stopping point. Sense and reflect the same degree of tension as the tissue and continue as described above.

As you do so, note what your other hand detects, what changes it perceives when an area of resistance is released, or once it has experienced release.

When this release of transverse connective tissue layers occurs, you could also simultaneously administer gentle fascial glide with one hand. However, this should be done very carefully, step by step. You should not slip into a mode of constant activity. Give the tissue time for self-regulation. Do not disturb it with numerous or forceful impulses from you, but trust and listen.

Version 3

Place one hand on the front and one on the back of the client's body (or on the two sides of her body) and *sense the space between your hands*. Now, apply clear and spacious contact to invite all the layers between your hands increasingly to relax.

Apply your touch with the intention that the various body segments should relax more and more and spontaneously connect with each other, through the agency of your gentle touch and spacious presence and the non-invasive way in which you listen to the tissue.

Before you start

The following techniques are intended for gentle tissue release, so supporting the body's own process of self-regulation. They are *all* carried out within the comfort zone, *well below the 'activation zone'* at which the intensity of touch or pressure prompts the body to protect itself by a natural and instinctive reaction of tensing involuntarily. Once the tissue has relaxed and established a new balance, you can move up to the next position.

You can combine release and fascial glide over the whole of the torso, especially those places where there is a great deal of transverse connective tissue.

Transverse connective tissue of the torso

The following regions of the body are important sites of transverse connective tissue:

- The pelvis (pelvic floor; transition between the pelvic and abdominal regions).
- The costal arch/inferior thoracic aperture (diaphragm region; transition between abdominal and thoracic regions).
- The superior thoracic aperture (shoulder/neck region, transition between thoracic and neck regions).

In the structural basic treatment described here, the release of connective tissue layers is explained working from the pelvis toward the head, so supporting the freeing of the craniosacral system working upward from below. In actual practice, this happens in any order.

The release of the connective tissue of the torso is extremely important for the craniosacral system, because important muscles and ligaments pass upward from the torso through the neck to the head, with attachments to the cranial base. If there is too much resistance in these muscles, the tensions in them affect not only the locomotor apparatus but also the craniosacral system and its rhythm. An excessive or one-sided 'pull' originating from the torso can have a considerable effect of restricting the craniosacral motion of the cranial bones, leading to compensatory dysfunctions of the cranial bones and meninges. This can be expressed in a number of possible problems.

It is therefore sensible to begin the release at the torso, using the following sequence and allowing yourself enough time for this before you begin to release the cranium and its membrane system.

Take up a position at the side for this treatment. The time needed to perform a release at these locations on your client's body is often more than you would need for palpation of the craniosacral rhythm alone, so it is important to be comfortable. Ideally, you should be seated, and position yourself as comfortably as possible at the table. The person receiving treatment should normally lie supine.

The treatment sequence

When a change or process of release begins at any particular place on the body, you might ask your client to describe the feeling at that location and whether you may continue giving treatment there. If the (release) process is fairly complete, you can continue to the next position or you might involve your client and ask where she would like you to apply touch and treatment next.

Release at the pelvis

The entire pelvic region benefits from the release described below. The change in the pattern of forces relieves strain from the spinal column and the whole locomotor apparatus. This supports organs and their functions.

An impairment or dysfunction in the pelvic region is usually transmitted upward to affect other body segments and their fulcrums.

The pelvic region is important for a number of reasons, including the legs, excretion, experiencing fulfilled sexuality, and reproduction. Pelvic flexibility is important in pregnancy and especially in childbirth, to both mother and baby.

Take up a position at the side of the treatment table

Positioned at the side of the treatment table, place one hand under your client's sacrum. With your cranial hand (the hand nearer your client's head), lift up the knee on the side away from you. Pass your other hand under your client's knee, with your forearm angled upward at 90° so that it lies parallel to the torso, next to the client's pelvis (see Fig. 2.4.1).

With your cranial hand, raise your client's pelvis on the side away from you. Place the other hand – the one that is already alongside your client's pelvis – *under the sacrum*. Then carefully set the client's pelvis back on the treatment table. With your free hand, carefully put the knee you raised at the beginning back down onto the table.

Watch for non-verbal indications as to whether the position of your hand on the client's sacrum feels agreeable, or ask how it is. You should be able to feel the full extent of the sacrum in your hand: the lower end against your thenar eminence (at the ball of your hand) and the upper end of the sacrum against your fingers. Do not hesitate to adjust the position as necessary, e.g., to shift it more deeply so that there is no pressure from the ball of your hand.

Sit close to the table in a relaxed posture and relax the hand under the client's sacrum. *Place your other hand* gently from above onto the pelvic/abdominal region, *above the pubic bone*. If this is difficult to find, ask the client to feel for her pubic bone and show you where it is. Then place your hand in a position above this bone. As you do so, keep both hands, arms and shoulders and your torso including your pelvis relaxed, and consciously ground yourself. You may wish to raise the thumb of your upper hand slightly, to make sure that you are not touching the genital

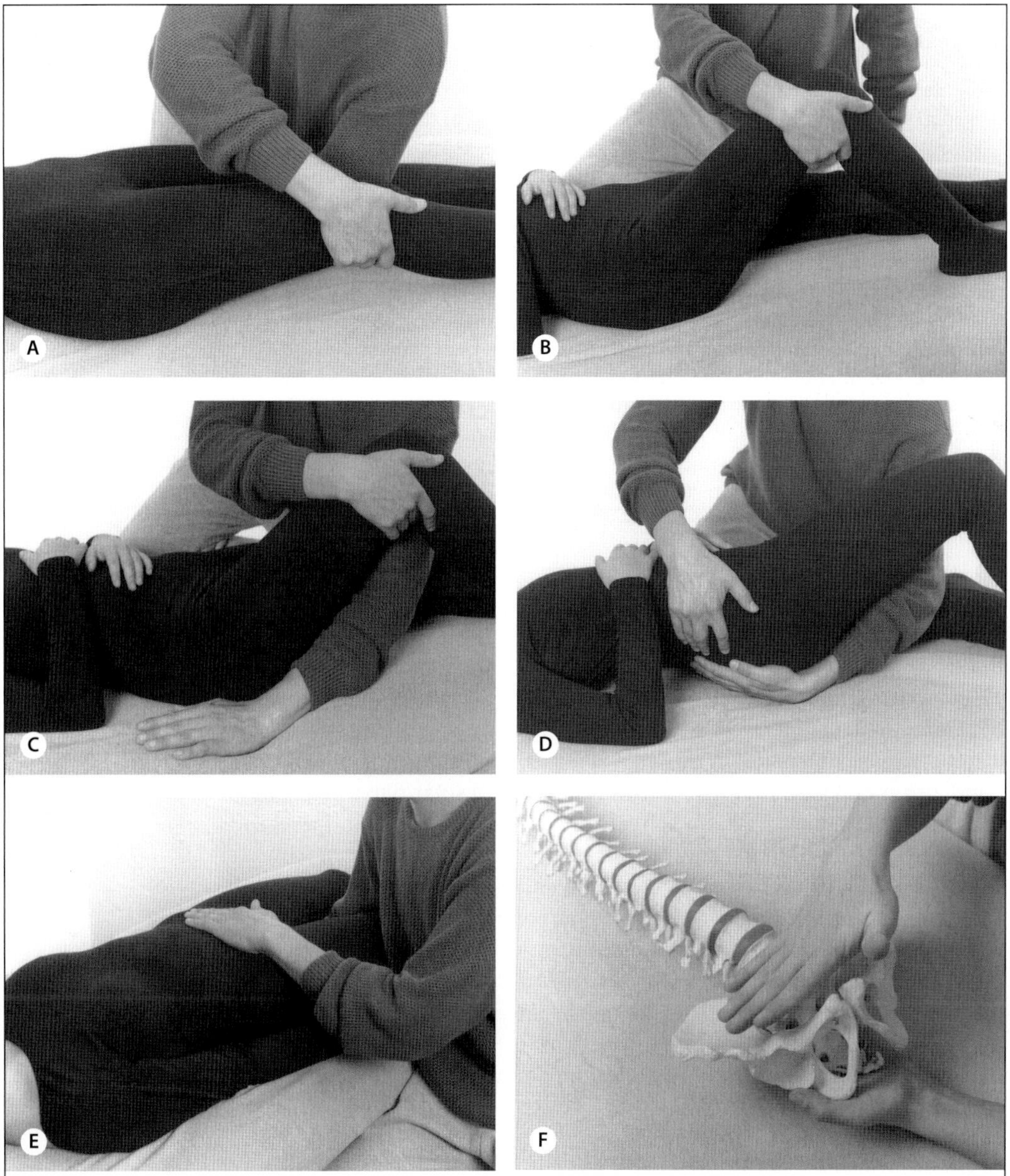

Figure 2.4.1
(**A–F**) Approach to the hand position for treating the pelvis.

area; alternatively, you can simply shift the position of this hand a little higher.

If you are relaxed and have taken up a position that is agreeable for both you and your client, begin the release of this region as described above in Version 1, 2, or 3 (Figs 2.4.1A–F).

Tips

Before you use this hand position on the pelvis (and the positions described below) you need to tell your client what you are going to do. The client then knows where you are going to touch, and this creates trust.

In the first session, you might begin with the release of the transverse connective tissue in a more neutral area such as the costal arch and inferior thoracic aperture in the diaphragm region, and only then proceed to treat the more intimate region of the pelvis.

If your client has previously suffered unpleasant sexual experiences such as sexual violence, it is wise to postpone this position. One possible way of preserving confidence is for the client to place her own hand above the pubic bone; you put your hand on top of that. Then you ask your client if it is acceptable for you to place both your hands on the pelvic region in the way described above. Following this release, you listen from one position higher, at the costal arch, to detect changes, and then move on to the next position, at the superior thoracic aperture.

Release at the costal arch

The main respiratory muscle, the diaphragm, is located in the region of the costal arch. It separates and links the thoracic and abdominal regions. Careful release of tension in this area is extremely important. Your upper hand also maintains contact with the stomach and solar plexus. Tension release at the diaphragm allows breathing to become more fluid, and this has a positive effect on the energy in the body and on the metabolism. The release of tension in the diaphragm means free respiratory motion, which also 'massages' our organs in the abdominal and chest regions.

The diaphragm retains at the autonomic level the imprint of shocks received in childhood, as does the solar plexus; the latter also reacts directly to nervousness and to sensations such as joy, anxiety, pleasure, and pain.

This release connects and integrates 'heart and stomach', feelings and spontaneous impulses.

Take up a position sitting at the side of the treatment table

Seated at the side of the treatment table, place the hand that is nearer your client's head, palm uppermost, under her body; it should be approximately beneath the lowest thoracic vertebra and the top two lumbar vertebrae. If you position the 'wrong' hand here, this will tend to turn your body to face your client's feet and make it less easy for you to keep her face in view.

It may help locate your hand in the right position along the person's back if you simultaneously lift this slightly with your other hand, roughly at the bottom of the rib cage. Position the middle of your hand approximately in the middle of the spinal column.

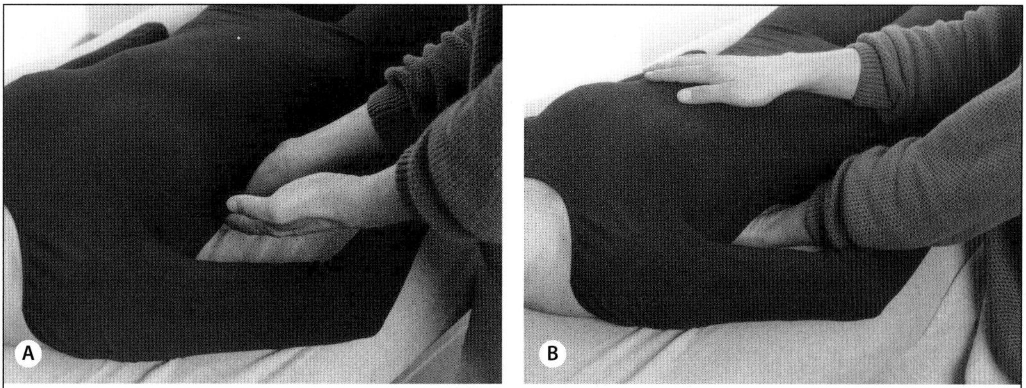

Figure 2.4.2
(**A**, **B**) Approach to the hand position, and hand position on the costal arch.

Place your second hand gently down from above, in the middle of the body, in the region of the costal arch, so that the upper part of your hand touches the lower end of the rib cage and the lower part of your hand the superior border of the abdomen (Figs 2.4.2A, B).

Have you checked for yourself the quality of touch of both your hands? Ask your client if this touch feels agreeable, and begin the release of this region as described above under Version 1, 2, or 3.

Release at the superior thoracic aperture

Most people today suffer from tension in the shoulder and neck area. As you tune in to the tonus present in the upper chest region, you often palpate slight resistance and tension. However, gentle touch can release connective tissue layers and the affected muscles. A large number of ascending muscles link the thorax, sternum and clavicles anteriorly with the cranium, and posteriorly many muscles pass over the shoulder blades and through the shoulder and posterior neck region, again to link with the cranium. In the region of the superior thoracic aperture, for example, the two sternocleidomastoid muscles link the clavicles and sternum with the mastoid processes of the temporal bones. Some muscles and ligaments run upward from the superior thoracic aperture at the neck to the hyoid.

The release of the peripheral muscles also has the effect of reducing the tonus in the deeper-lying muscles, tendons and ligaments, which in turn attach to deeper-lying bones and joints such as the clavicle, sternum, shoulder blades and spinal column.

One of the effects of the layer-by-layer release of the region of the thoracic aperture is to assist the upright posture of the body and freedom of breathing. Seen from the bioenergetic point of view, the vital energy rises from the pelvis, to be expressed higher up via the arms, hands and voice, for example.

Emotions and feelings are perceived in the region of the lungs (exchange/connection between interior and exterior) and heart. In this region, which is also called the heart chakra, emotional pressure can become conscious and can be transformed into the healing power of the heart.

Lymphatic drainage is assisted particularly by the release of the tissue in the region of the clavicle; the transition of the lymphatic system into the blood circulation occurs beneath the left clavicle.

You can combine palpation at this location with fascial glide. Apply your touch slowly and carefully and ask about the quality of touch.

Take up a position sitting at the side of the treatment table

Seated at the side of the treatment table, as before, extend and relax the hand that is nearer your client's head, placing it under the body of the person on the treatment table. Position this hand, palm uppermost, in the region of the top thoracic vertebra and the seventh cervical vertebra. In order to position your lower hand, push this hand under the person's body between the neck and shoulder, *at an angle of about 45°*. Press your hand down into the padded surface of the treatment table until the middle of your hand is at the person's spinal column, approximately between the superior borders of the shoulder blades. By doing this you will also contact the region of C7/T1.

Now spread the thumb and index finger of your other hand as far apart as you can without strain, and with them explore your client's clavicles. Place your outspread thumb and finger on the two clavicles. Then lay your hand flat on the client's rib cage *with as broad an area of contact as possible*. If your client is female, take care not to touch her breasts; if necessary, you can slightly raise your little finger and the lower part of your hand (Figs 2.4.3A, B).

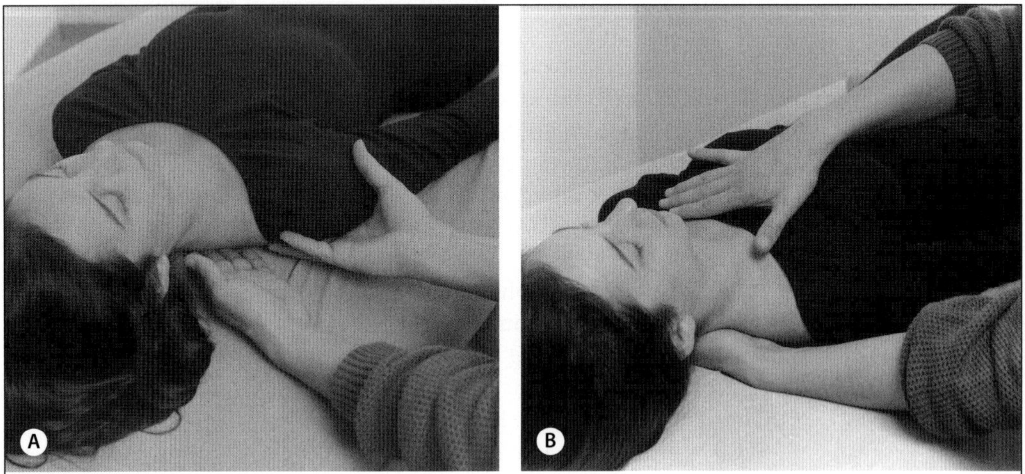

Figure 2.4.3
(**A**, **B**) Approach to the hand position, and hand position on the superior thoracic aperture.

Ask your client how your touch feels. Begin the release of this region in the same way as described above under Version 1, 2, or 3.

Tips

Make sure that the thumb and index finger of your upper hand rest either precisely on or immediately below the clavicles, and that they do not touch or restrict the neck area.

Your lower hand must not put any pressure on the spinal column or shoulder blades. There is an easy way to ensure this: the key is to adopt the right position relative to the treatment table (height and distance) and also to use a soft padded surface on the table.

Release of the neck by means of the hyoid

The neck is a narrow region of the body. A great number of muscles, ligaments, tendons, and fasciae are involved in controlling the posture and movement of the head and neck. Touch applied to the hyoid, and especially subtly lifting this bone, addresses the tonus of the whole musculature of the neck and connective tissue and invites it to release. This particularly benefits the flow of lymph, since there are around 170 lymph nodes in the neck region, and, as mentioned above in connection with the superior thoracic aperture, it benefits the transition from the lymphatic system to the circulation of the blood behind the left clavicle.

The gentle touch of your lower hand, applied without pressure in the neck area and around to the nape, automatically encourages the flow of energy in the spine. This relaxed touch molds itself to match the curve of the posterior neck region; it supports trust and 'letting go' and the linking of 'head and heart' as well as physiologically supporting the transition from the shoulder and neck region to the head.

One effect of the release of the muscles of the neck is development of the voice and of free, spontaneous expression overall. This treatment also helps the client with the swallowing reflex, any sense of narrowing in the throat and any associated emotional issue, and things that are unspoken or psychologically 'undigested', as she is enabled to perceive and transform them.

Take up a position at the side of the treatment table

The hyoid (*os hyoideum*) is a horseshoe-shaped bone, lying freely in the upper part of the neck (superior to the larynx and inferior to the mandible) and surrounded by the musculature. The muscles and ligaments that have their points of attachment on the hyoid run upward to the floor of the mouth, laterally to the base of the skull and downward (to the shoulder and neck region), where they are linked with the larynx, breastbone (*sternum*) and shoulder blades (*scapulae*) (Fig. 2.4.4).

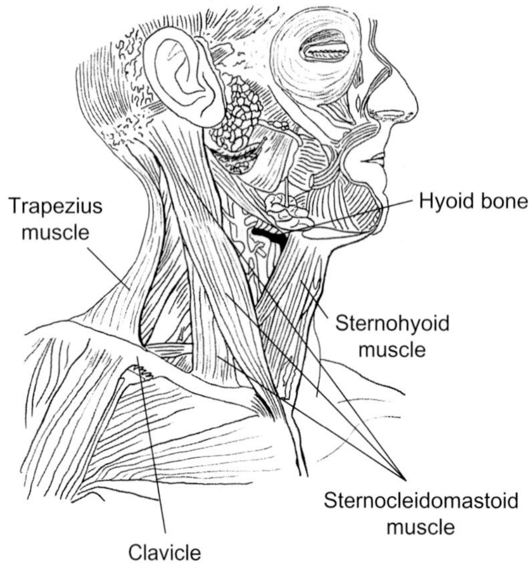

Figure 2.4.4
Muscles in the neck region.

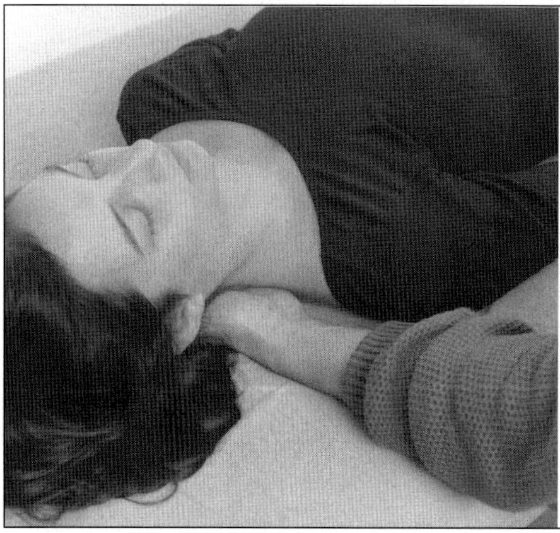

Figure 2.4.5
One hand loosely under the cervical spine.

Before beginning to touch, *check that your sitting position is high enough;* this takes the strain from your shoulder region and makes treatment easier.

Slowly slide your cranial hand (the hand nearer to your client's head) under the client's head, using either the flat of your whole hand or just that of the fingers. This provides support from below to the muscles of the neck, but without exerting any pressure (Fig. 2.4.5).

Tell the person that you are now going to palpate the hyoid bone in the area of the neck. To do this you should place the thumb and index finger of your other, free hand gently on the left and right side of the client's neck, in the upper part of the neck between the mandible and the larynx (Fig. 2.4.6). You will find it easier to locate the hyoid accurately if you ask

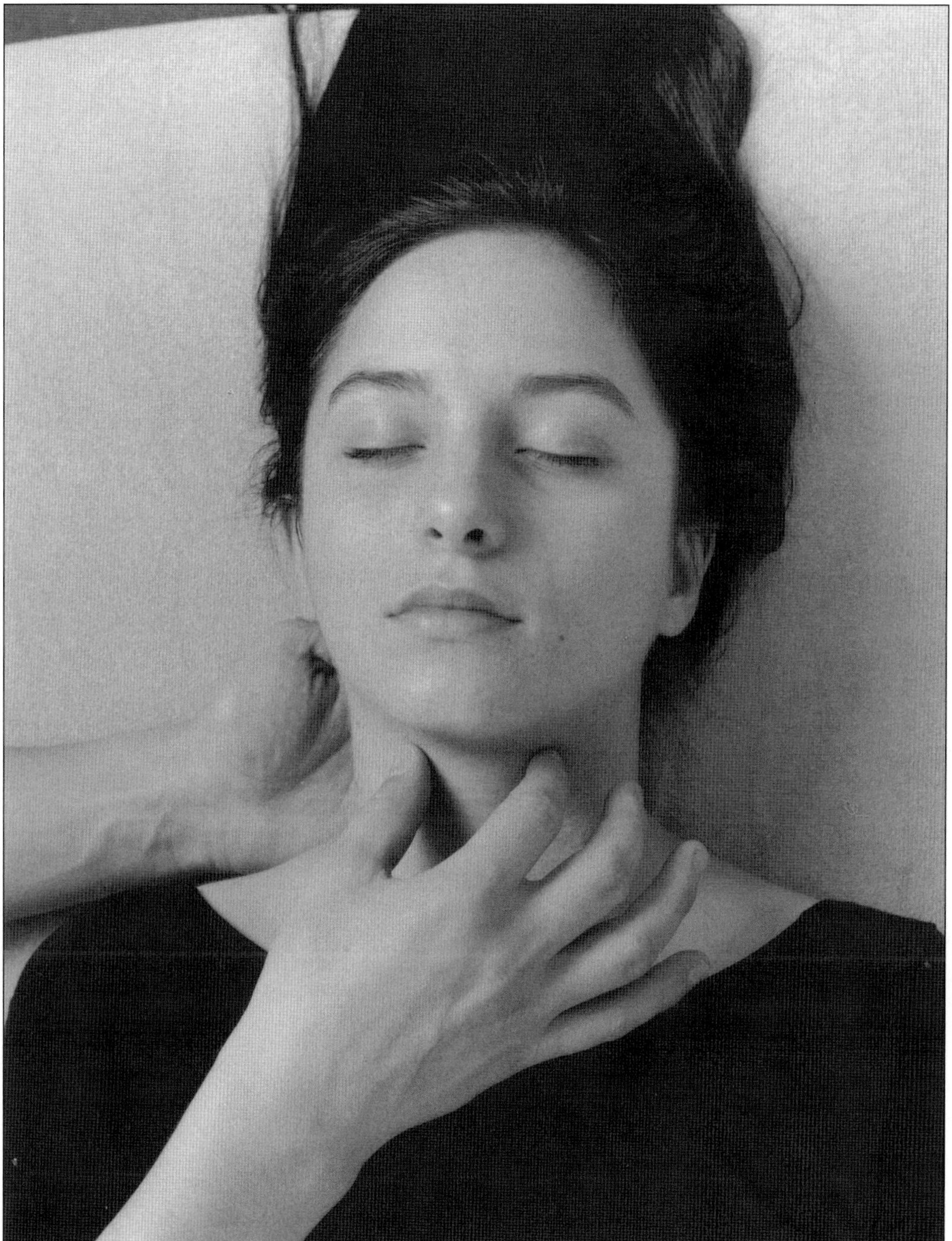

Figure 2.4.6
Position at the hyoid.

your client to swallow briefly just after you touch the person's neck. This causes the hyoid to rise and fall.

As you maintain this contact, your fingers should remain relaxed. Make sure that you are not applying any pressure to the hyoid and that your arms, shoulders and pelvis all remain relaxed. Ask your client how the touch contact feels, and reduce the intensity if necessary, still maintaining the clarity of contact with the tissue. Check that your height and distance from the table are correct, and that you continue to regulate the distance between you and your client.

Now begin to slowly explore the mobility of the hyoid. Remaining centered and relaxed, you should prepare to carry out a very subtle test in which the minutest sensations (of the free flow or slight resistance of the tissue) are extremely important for successful evaluation and treatment.

1. Slowly move your thumb and index finger to the minutest degree in one direction and then back to the center; then similarly in the opposite direction and back to the center again. Note which direction allows greater motion and, which is more inhibited or offers more resistance.

   One possibility at this stage is to invite the tissue to release by using a combined indirect and direct technique. *The movements should be merely hinted at*, rather than performed in any manipulative way:

   First, move the hyoid gently and bit by bit *in the direction of ease*, and pause briefly when you reach the limit of the tissue resistance, the 'stop' point, to show the tissue around the hyoid how much movement is possible here. Then glide slowly back with the hyoid as it returns to the central position, and immediately move on in the opposite direction until you reach the limit, where you pause. Wait there and invite the tissue again to release its tension.

   Every time, you must accept the tissue's indication to 'stop' when you reach the limit. Pause and wait there. The resistance may resolve, so that you can then slowly continue the lateral movement until you reach the next resistance. Then, follow the hyoid gently back to its central position, which will very probably be different and feel generally freer than before.

2. The next step, following this combined indirect and direct technique, is a straightforward, *gentle raising of the hyoid in the ventral direction* (if the person is supine, that would be in the direction of the ceiling). Allow yourself sufficient time. As you carry out this slow, continuous, merest hint of movement, listen attentively for the tissue's message to 'stop' and pause there, yet allow an infinitesimal suggestion of continuous, subtle upward traction toward the ceiling to remain. This continuous raising of the hyoid should last around one minute. Then release your contact on the hyoid, lift away the contact of this hand and remove the contact of the hand at the nape of your client's neck by sliding your hand out to the side. Allow the client to sense her body.

Tips

The treatment you apply on the hyoid should be very gentle. If your thumb and index finger slip off while you are lifting the hyoid toward the ceiling, simply replace them on the hyoid and re-establish the connection between *the receptors* in your thumb and index finger and the horseshoe-shaped hyoid, through the skin and connective tissue. Even if the touch you apply to the hyoid is incomplete, the muscles concerned will sense the subtle invitation to widening and release of the tissue will take place.

If you are unable to keep your hand steady for the few minutes it takes for you to explore the hyoid with the fingers of that hand, ask if your client would mind you resting the outer edge of your hand gently on her sternum. Another approach would be for you to use a blanket or cushion between you and the client to create a stable support high enough to rest this arm on. That will provide you with a fulcrum which will not only be more comfortable for you while you administer the treatment, but will also prevent you from transmitting the minute motions – however subtle – of your own arm and torso to the client.

Pause

The time has now come to take your hands away from the body of the person lying on the treatment couch, if you have not already done so. Observe a few minutes' pause, distance yourself consciously from the treatment table and take a quick look back over the course of the session so far. What is your impression now? How does your client feel now? How has the session been so far for the client?

You might wish to take a drink of water and stretch yourself, maybe to move or loosen up your body a little. For you as the practitioner it can help to loosen your hands, arms and shoulders, and also your breathing, but do not stand close to the table as you do so; you do not want to disturb the client lying there. You can stand aside from the table in stillness for a while, sensing your own body and once more regulating the distance.

Your client too can continue to relax and sense her body, and the treatment taking effect – even in the absence of your touch – now that no hands are resting on the body. If you can talk to your client (if the client is not in a deep trance), ask how she feels and what changes have taken place since the session began. You can also make good use of short pauses for noting down information for your written records.

The sensations that occur during and after whole-body assessment and the release of transverse connective tissue layers can be very different and varied. They can be expressed on the physical, emotional, mental or spiritual level, and the client can tell you about them at any time according to individual needs. Open questions from you from time to time help develop the client's consciousness.

Release for the upper end of the spinal column

The atlanto-occipital joint

Previously, you released the entire region of the torso, working upward from below. As stated already, hypertonus of the muscles, connective tissue, tendons, ligaments and fasciae in the cranial base region can have a considerable effect of restricting the craniosacral system and craniosacral rhythm, as many of these structures run upward from below to the cranial base and have attachments here. Many people experience tensions in the neck area, and these can be resolved using the treatment explained above, and using the following method (Fig. 2.4.7).

Release in this region is particularly important. Here, at the upper end of the spinal column, the spinal meninges (the dural tube) pass over into the cranial meninges. The dural tube is attached at the foramen magnum of the occipital bone, again in the region of cervical vertebrae C2/C3, and then not again until the attachment at the sacrum.

Each stage of treatment described here for the atlanto-occipital joint (also called the A/O joint) frees the transitional region between the cranial and spinal meninges a little more, and this gives greater flexibility overall to the sheaths covering the nervous system. It improves the communication running each way between the brain and the body. Once this area is free the cerebrospinal fluid can flow down better along the spinal cord, benefiting the torso and the organs there; as a result, the craniosacral rhythm can be sensed better everywhere. There is more

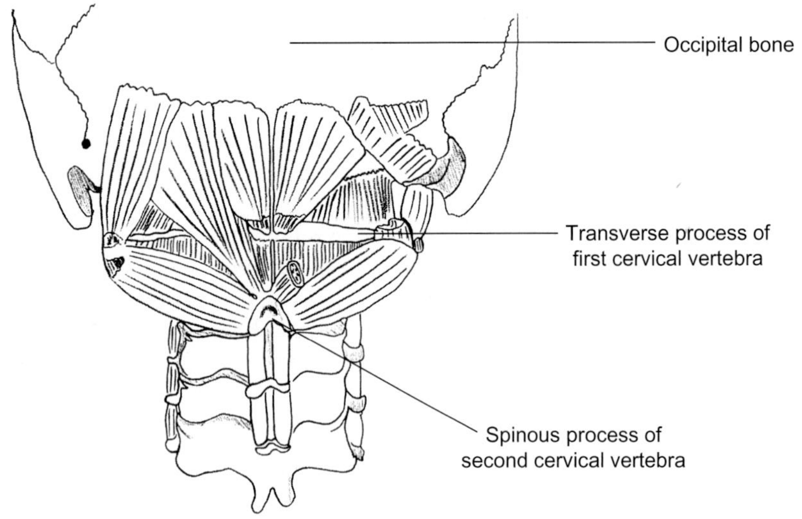

Figure 2.4.7
Muscles of the atlanto-occipital joint.

room for the cranial veins and arteries and so for the blood to circulate, and more room in particular for the cranial nerves that have their exit points at the cranial base.

This joint is the place where the occipital condyles, the ends of the occipital bone, meet the articular surfaces of the first cervical vertebra, the atlas, and enables the nodding movement of the head. The interaction of the first and second cervical vertebrae enables turning of the head.

When using these hand positions at your client's head, you will need sufficient room to rest your forearms; you also need to be at a sufficient distance from the table, so that you can treat in a relaxed way and without trembling (as advised previously for the palpation of the craniosacral rhythm on the head). It helps when working at the head to be able to rest approximately half the length of your forearm on the treatment table. It can be helpful if the person lying there moves up or down towards the foot of the table, as long as the person's heels stay on the table. Another method is to use a table extension or to place a blanket on your lap to rest your arms on.

The forms of treatment shown here for the release of the A/O joint and cranial base are extremely gentle.

Although gentle, these release methods are not indicated within a period of around 6 months of a whiplash injury or fall; sometimes people who have suffered this kind of injury may continue to find the treatment unpleasant for some years afterwards, so that it should still be avoided. Even beyond that time, treatment of health problems by release of this area should only be carried out after thorough examination and clearance by allopathic medical means.

Touch in this region is in general very slow and gentle. Never exert pressure on cervical vertebrae and never manipulate them. Readers with a great interest in the technical-structural aspect will find further techniques for atlanto-occipital release (also called A/O release or release of the cranial base) in the advanced specialist literature.

Tips

As you will mainly be using your fingers to achieve the release of the muscles at the occipital ridge, it helps if you shake to loosen them before you begin. Remember that your own fundamentally relaxed, open attitude helps determine the success of the treatment. Give your client enough time and space, both during the various stages of treatment and in short pauses in between, which you can both use to silently sense how the body feels through the treatment so far.

Begin and end the following hand positions and actions slowly and carefully. If there is a support under the head of the person lying on the treatment table, carefully raise her head and remove the head support; you can replace it once the treatment is finished.

The release is introduced and accompanied in several phases

- preparation phase
- release phase
- minimal traction/decompression
- assistance by the client
- 'rounding-off' with before-and-after comparison of the craniosacral rhythm.

For all the techniques described below you should take up a position sitting at the top end of the treatment table, near your client's head.

One aim of this treatment is to enable relaxation, easy space and room to be created between the occipital bone and the top cervical vertebra and all the neighboring structures.

Preparation phase

Before beginning the actual release phase and the minimal traction/decompression it is important to prepare the entire affected region at the occipital ridge.

The preparation phase includes

- cradle hold
- motion testing of the nape of the neck and the head
- palpation of the craniosacral rhythm on the shoulders and head
- exploring and gently massaging the scalp on the occiput
- exploring and gently massaging the muscle attachments on the occipital ridge
- effleurage of the muscles on the occipital ridge (a gliding massage stroke applied to the muscles).

This order can be varied.

Cradle hold

Relax both hands and place them underneath the occiput. Do not let the ball of your thumb and hand restrict the head at all, but allow plenty of room. Regulate the distance and check your own posture (see Listening stations, p. 107).

Palpate the individual shape of the occipital ridge with the pads of your fingers, without applying any pressure. This will give you a clear idea of the anatomical details so that you can work accurately and carefully as you proceed. Can you sense the craniosacral rhythm at the occiput in the cradle hold? If so, how does it feel?

Motion testing of the nape of the neck and the head

Place both hands under the occiput. Sensing in a relaxed, present manner, let your hands follow every motion *that arises spontaneously*. If, as may happen, your client's head shows that it is relaxing by moving slightly in a particular direction, follow every slow movement and gently support it, listening. If the motion stops, you too should immediately pause and wait, listening.

You might tune in to the next free level you can detect, or to the next level where you find any resistance in the layer of connective tissue and muscle. Sense this level where the tension is, wait attentively, remaining relaxed and in close contact with this level. You will possibly be able to sense which direction of motion of the head experiences less resistance. Which side is freer – the left or the right? Or does your client's head tend to be drawn to the opposite side by some strain?

Support every spontaneous motion impulse of the head, attentively follow every movement and pause every time the tissue tells you that you have reached a 'stop' point. Optionally, you may invite the slow movement to left and right by giving a brief, slight impulse to motion with one hand and then with the other.

It can be helpful to take note of your client's respiratory rhythm from time to time, e.g., each time you reach a limit to motion, and periodically ask the client to take a few deep breaths, breathing out through a slightly open mouth. Yawning or uttering a sound can also indirectly help relaxation.

If you have followed the client's head to one side and then the other, you can seek out the mobility in the middle region. Pause there so that your client can sense her body.

Then deliver a slight motion impulse for your client's head to move slowly to the other side – only ever as far as is possible gently and without resistance. In this turning motion of the head you should again sense the quality of the motion (or of the slight resistance) and follow the motion that voluntarily occurs. Once you have the impression that the client's head has reached the farthest point of rotation, pause for a few moments, and carefully deliver a slight motion impulse to invite it to return to the middle.

This slow left-right motion will probably have shown you which side is freer or more restricted, and given you an overall impression of the tensions in the neck and cranial base region (Fig. 2.4.8A–C).

Palpation of the craniosacral rhythm on the shoulders and head

Take up a position at the top of the treatment table (near your client's head), and proceed as described above for palpation of the craniosacral rhythm (p. 110).

Exploring and gently massaging the scalp on the occiput

Place all your fingers underneath the occiput. You can explore the scalp at the occiput, displace the skin slightly, and massage it with circling motions.

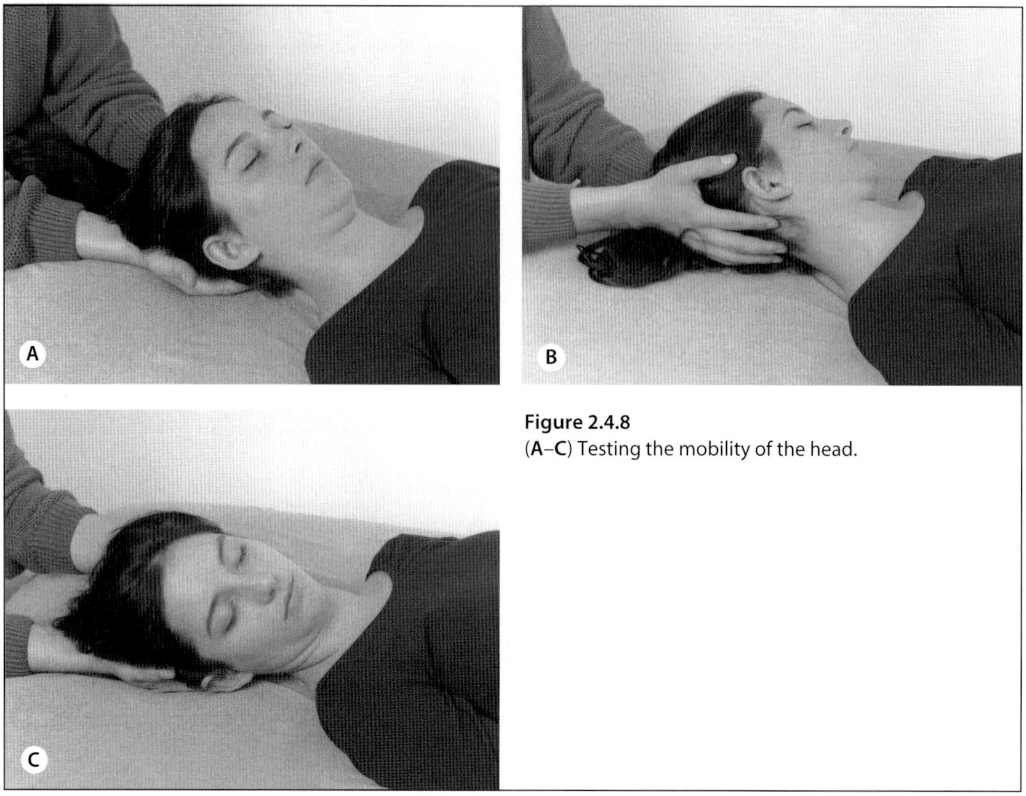

Figure 2.4.8
(**A–C**) Testing the mobility of the head.

Exploring and gently massaging the muscle attachments on the occipital ridge

Place the palms of your hands under your client's head, with all the pads of your fingertips on the occipital ridge. Starting from the cradle hold on the head, position your hands so that the *pads* of your fingertips on the occipital ridge are touching the *attachments of the neck muscles to the occipital bone*. Then explore and massage the muscle origins with slow circling motions. Vary the speed and intensity to suit the client's wishes.

Effleurage of the muscles on the occipital ridge

From time to time, you can apply *a gentle, lateral* (sideways) *gliding massage stroke* to the muscles along the occipital ridge between all the phases of the release.

To do this, place your hands under the client's occiput in the cradle hold. Position your fingertips toward the middle of the occipital ridge, with your ring fingers and middle fingers both slightly touching each other. Take care to start from the middle, so that you relieve the strain indirectly on the foramen magnum and the more deeply-lying fibrous ring of dura mater: begin by moving the fingers of both your hands slowly away from each other in a lateral direction. As you do this, explore the muscles on the occipital ridge with the pads of your fingertips and apply a gentle gliding massage stroke toward the side. Then once more reposition your fingers in the middle and repeat the massage stroke.

Important points

Ask your client how the touch and the gentle massage feels. The sensations experienced by the client are the important deciding factor here. Take care that your hands and fingers *remain relaxed and exert no pressure* as you loosen and release the muscle attachments on the occipital ridge. Your fingertips should remain in constant contact with the occipital ridge – you must on no account let your fingers shift to a position lower down, in the delicate region of the cervical vertebrae.

Release phase

Your fingernails need to be as short as possible for this procedure. Loosen your hands, fingers and wrists. Position both hands on the client's occipital bone so that the pads of your fingertips explore along the occipital ridge. Check to make quite sure that you do not touch the cervical spine at all during this release phase, and do not put any pressure on it or manipulate it in any way at any stage. Position both your hands as for the cradle hold. The sides of your hands and little fingers should touch in the middle but otherwise play no part. Using the index, middle, and ring fingers of both hands, explore the occipital bone exactly along the occipital ridge. Now bend the joints of your fingers so that the phalanges point upward toward the ceiling and toward the cranial base of your client at an angle of 90°, and let the very tips of your fingers sink into the structure of muscles, connective tissue and ligaments close up against the occipital ridge (Fig. 2.4.9A–C).

Important points

It is very important to observe the *correct degree of intensity of touch* as your fingers sink in along the occipital ridge. The client should experience this as pleasant, neither too weak nor too strong, so it is best to ask an open question, e.g. 'How does this touch feel?' Alternatively, you could slowly increase the intensity a little and then ask whether this feels more agreeable.

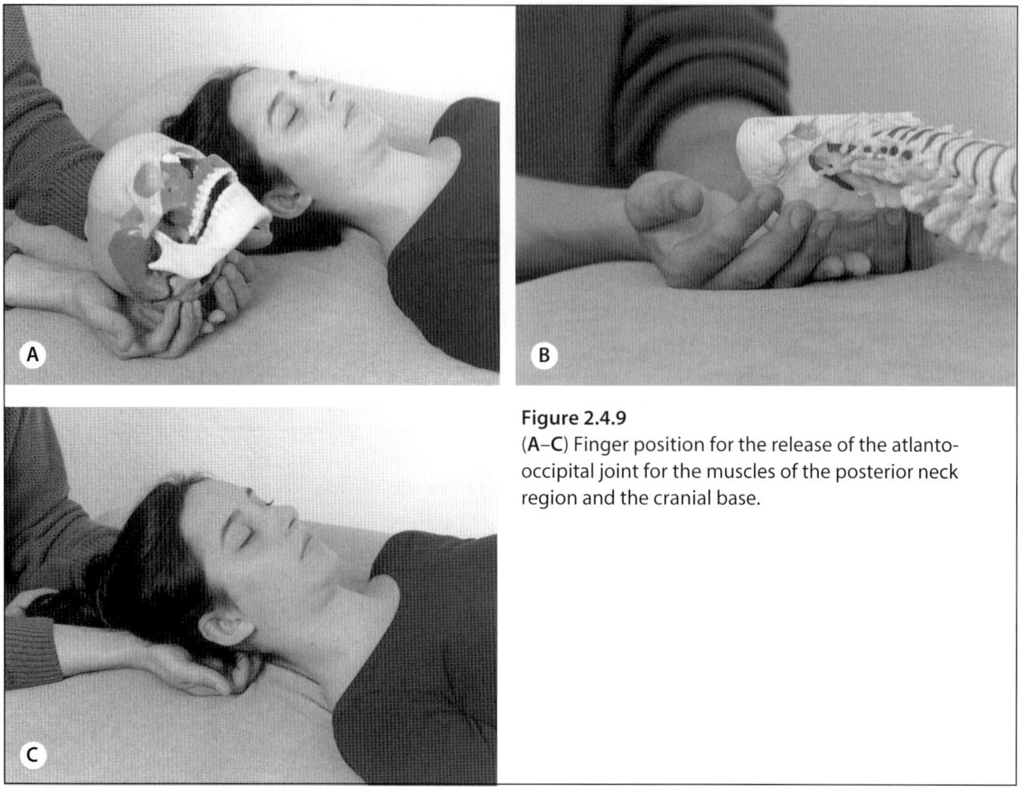

Figure 2.4.9
(**A–C**) Finger position for the release of the atlanto-occipital joint for the muscles of the posterior neck region and the cranial base.

Tips

You can bring about a very subtle change in the resting pressure of your client's head (caused by its own weight and the release that is occurring): as the ends of your fingers slowly implant themselves along the occipital ridge, you can raise the client's head slightly on the ball of your two hands. This reduces the pressure of your client's head on your fingertips and so also reduces the pressure on the client's occipital ridge. Ask how this touch feels and what the intensity of it is like, and either reduce or increase the intensity in response to the answer.

It is important for you as the practitioner to keep your forearms, hands, fingers and the various joints you are using relaxed. *Let the pads of your fingers become meltingly soft so that the way they sink in along the occipital ridge is as relaxed as can be.*

If you find your fingers sinking in by some distance as the release at the occipital ridge occurs, your fingertips must follow the bony outline of the occipital bone; this is important. You must *not* let your fingers slip down toward the client's neck. *Maintain the clear contact between your fingertips and the occipital bone* at all times so that when your fingertips have finished sinking into the muscles along the occipital ridge, they still point upward in the direction of the ceiling.

Minimal traction/decompression

This widening or decompression phase does not begin until you have given enough time to the preparation and release phases and your fingertips have sunk into the muscles along the occipital ridge. Here as before, there must be no pressure or manipulation to the bodies of any vertebrae. Not only is this forbidden; the pressure and manipulation are not necessary in craniosacral treatment, which operates on a quite different basic principle. The form of treatment given here delivers valuable impulses to release. This release works inward from the periphery of the body to bring about a profound 'letting go' – even releasing quite considerable restrictions – at the same time exerting a positive effect on the individual affected parts.

This gentle widening assists the affected muscles, the tendons and ligaments and the upper end of the spinal column by creating more room, especially in the area between the upper vertebrae and the occipital bone.

Following the release phase, maintain the position of your hands, especially that of your fingers, which will have sunk inward as a result of the release at the occipital ridge, *and continue straight away with the minimal traction/decompression*:

Keep the finger position produced in the release phase on the occipital ridge. Continue to support your client's head in the cradle hold, and to make sure that the ball of your thumbs and hands do not restrict the client's head. Now slowly begin to apply a hint of gentle traction (minimal traction of around 1 g) in the cranial direction (toward your client's head) *with the part of your fingers along the occipital ridge, gliding slightly toward you*. Listen to the structure as you do so, to detect when and by how much it can let go and disengage *of itself*. Take time when doing this; sufficient time is needed both for you and especially for this sensitive part of your client's body.

The very slight, constant, subtle traction should be almost imperceptible to your client, and should not produce any defensive counter-reaction by the tissue involved. Once more the rule is that 'less is more': although almost imperceptible, this very gentle traction is continuous over an extended period, to communicate a sense of more room, more space, release and 'letting go' to the affected parts.

If, following the preparation and release phases, the region involved in the release of the atlanto-occipital joint is already very relaxed, an invitation to disengagement exercised in the cranial direction with all your upward-angled fingers is sufficient.

Differentiated listening during minimal traction/decompression

As you deliver this gentle suggestion of cephalad traction, listen for any *differences in release and resistance on the left and right sides*. For example, it may feel at first as if release is happening on both sides in the affected region at the same time, but then there is slight resistance on one side (simply perceive this; on no account should you increase the minute hint of traction) while the other side continues the release and stops at a certain point – and later on, further release occurs on both sides. Possibly the release in the tissue might occur precisely because of further relaxation by the practitioner, and also breathing assistance by the person receiving treatment, who is asked to breathe more consciously in the thoracic region.

Assistance by the client

The client can provide assistance during each phase in the atlanto-occipital release by supporting the release from inside.

Eye movements

The client should perform slow eye movements from time to time, with eyes closed. Ideally this should be done spontaneously rather than mechanically and involve a wide range of motion for both eyes; for example your client could trace out a continuous figure-of-8 with eyes closed. The practitioner can usually sense these eye movements very slightly in the muscles on the occipital ridge; they have the effect of 'massaging' these muscles from inside. You should then ask your client to relax both eyes completely, letting them settle down in their sockets to rest like a pair of dormice slowly curling up to sleep in a cozy nest.

Deeper breathing, with the emphasis on thoracic breathing

Many muscles with attachments at the superior thoracic aperture and cranium pass through the region of the occipital ridge. Muscles also run from the shoulder blades to the occiput. The free, linked breathing in the thoracic region moves and gently massages the affected neck area and its muscles, tendons and ligaments. Clients can further assist the release by relaxing the lower jaw and breathing out any tensions they are aware of, through a slightly open mouth.

Before-and-after comparison of the craniosacral rhythm; overall evaluation

The preparation and release phases and the minimal traction/ decompression often bring about a state of deep relaxation in the person lying on the treatment table, as well as a heightened sensitivity. As a result the client may well experience a deep level of 'letting go' during or following the release phase and minimal traction/decompression and feel subtle body sensations such as warmth, the flow of energy in the body, or a pleasant lightness or heaviness. Give your client time to sense her body. Ask about the client's feelings during the session so far.

Differentiated listening following atlanto-occipital release

Continue to support the client's head in the cradle hold. Now compare what you find with the situation before the atlanto-occipital release: what are the changes? Can you perhaps sense the craniosacral rhythm at the occiput better now? Listen to the motions for several cycles: are they clearer, stronger and more even than they were at the beginning? Does the craniosacral rhythm here at the occiput seem inconstant, or can you palpate its slow motions evenly over several cycles?

You could slowly perform a suggestion of gentle traction toward you by slightly transferring your own body weight backward. Do you sense a difference in the elasticity and suppleness in the neck region and dural tube, compared with previously?

Finally, remove your hands by lifting them carefully away. Loosen your fingers, hands, arms and shoulders and allow yourself and your client to take a short pause to check and sense the effects on her body.

You might listen again to the craniosacral rhythm on the client's shoulders and head, for example using the cranial vault hold (p. 196). Do you sense any difference in the qualities of the craniosacral rhythm as compared with before?

Now step back from the table enough to distance yourself and think

- What overall impression do I have, compared with the beginning of the treatment?
- Do I see any changes in the client on brief visual assessment?
- What is the atmosphere in the room now?
- How does the client feel?
- Which parts of the client's body feel good?
- Where in the client's body has there been a change?

Release for the lower end of the spinal column

The lumbosacral joint (L5/S1)

Once you have established release of the cranial base at the upper end of the spinal column, it is advisable to assist the release of the lower end of the lumbar vertebrae (at the transition to the sacrum). This transition zone is called the lumbosacral joint or L5/S1 region. Considerable strains and compression are often found here.

The following release methods reduce this compression and slight resistance at the lower end of the spinal column. They relieve not only the body of the vertebra but also the intervertebral disks, muscles and ligaments in the lumbar and pelvic region, with a beneficial effect on the upper end of the spine, the forces acting on it and its flexibility overall. The dural tube becomes freer in the entire region, also relieving tension in terms of the forces acting on the meninges, especially on the falx cerebri and falx cerebelli and the tentorium cerebelli. The release enables

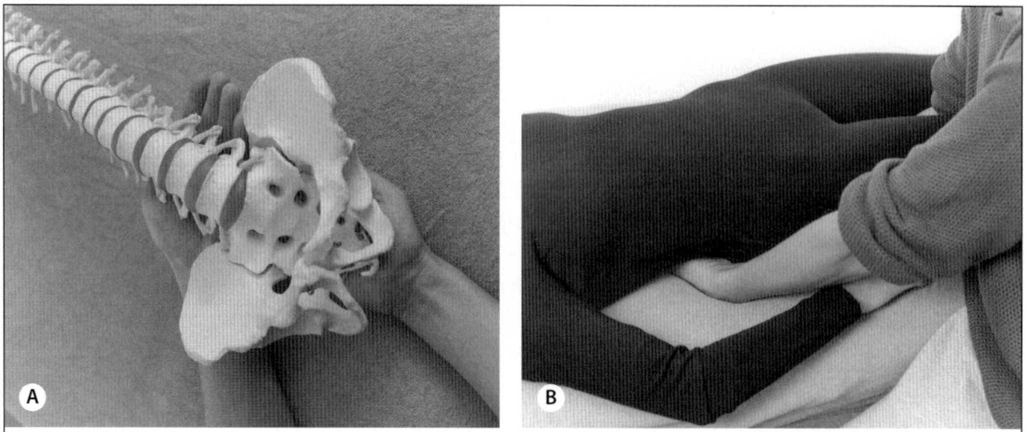

Figure 2.4.10
(**A**, **B**) Release in the lumbosacral region.

the sacrum to oscillate more successfully in the craniosacral rhythm, which then develops more freely in the lumbar and pelvic regions. In craniosacral practice, compensatory patterns of resistance are mainly encountered not only in the lumbosacral region, but also at the atlanto-occipital joint and sphenobasilar synchondrosis. Comprehensive basic treatment will therefore release all three regions.

The body of the vertebrae and the intervertebral disks in the lumbar region are very large, but they have to take up and compensate for strains coming both from above and from below. Tensions in the lumbosacral region restrict the mobility and in time lead to sciatica, lumbago, slipped disk and other painful conditions.

People whose work involves sitting for long periods, for example in the office or while traveling by car, train or plane, are especially likely to be familiar with the unpleasant effects such as a sense of too much resistance, tension, pressure or a slight, dull pain in the lumbosacral region, sometimes radiating out to neighboring parts of the body.

Release of the L5/S1 region also improves the mobility of the pelvis and legs. It helps the whole locomotor apparatus (Figs 2.4.10A, B).

Take up a position sitting at the side of the treatment table

1. Place the hand that is nearer to your client's feet (when sitting at the side of the table, facing the client) *under your client's sacrum* (as in Release at the pelvis, p. 124). Ensure – also by asking the client – that this hand position on the sacrum is comfortable for both you and the client. As the practitioner, you should feel the entire expanse of the sacrum in your hand, with the lower part, the apex of the sacrum, in the relaxed ball of your hand (thenar eminence) and the upper part resting on your fingers. Check your position at the table so that you are sitting at ease, and relax the hand under your patient's sacrum.
2. Now stretch out your other hand, the one nearer the client's head, and place it *sideways* under the person's body just above the pelvic

region. You can press your hand down into the padded surface of the treatment table to help you position your hand more easily. Bring this hand under the lowest lumbar vertebra in the middle of the person's body, so that you can palpate *the muscles of the back* either side of the lumbar spine *with the ball of your hand and your fingers*. Leave this hand too in position and relaxed, regulate the distance and check your own posture.

3. Direct your attention alternately to what you sense with the hand under your client's sacrum and to your other hand in the region of the lumbar spine, without changing anything. Palpate both places attentively:
   - Can you feel the sacrum moving in harmony with the craniosacral rhythm?
   - Can you sense the different contact points synchronously, in both hands at the same time?
   - How does the lower part of the lumbar region feel through that hand?
   - What is the muscle tonus like?

   With the hand that is positioned across the client's lumbar region, sense attentively deep down into the tissues, without applying any firm pressure. Take up contact with the first level where you can sense any resistance and then relax your hand again, without losing the contact with this level. You might think of your intention as being to sense the tension present in the tissue and to invite it to release. This clear intention alone, along with the warmth of your hands and your own fundamentally relaxed attitude invite the tissue mentally, physically, and energetically to release.
4. While the tense musculature of the inferior lumbar spine region slowly relaxes (the options here are the same as for the release of the connective tissue, p. 119), you can slowly shift the position of your own body by moving down toward your client's feet. This has the effect of automatically delivering the very slightest degree of caudad traction (i.e. towards the feet) to the sacrum. This slight, gentle hint of stretching is delivered to the sacrum, gradually increasing in strength, while your other hand, the one positioned higher up and crosswise under the client's body, stabilizes the area. This subtle stretching therefore operates mainly on the transition from the fifth lumbar vertebra to the sacrum (L5/S1), also extending more widely in the inferior lumbar region and pelvic transition area. Release this caudad traction to the sacrum after about 1 min.
5. Having released the wider lumbosacral region using the position described above under points 3 and 4, you next proceed to *a more precisely targeted release* of the lumbosacral joint, the L5/S1 transition.

   Your caudad hand should remain under your client's sacrum. Place your other hand flat underneath the client's body, superior to the pelvic region (as described above under point 2). Again you can press your hand down into the padded surface of the table to help you position it easily. Keeping the first hand under the person's sacrum, move the hand in the lumbar region into the middle, carefully feeling for the *spinous processes* of the three inferior lumbar vertebrae with your index, middle and ring fingers. Having done this, place the tips of your fingers on the spinous processes, without exerting any pressure, and stabilize them. This hand too should remain relaxed.

Now shift your body position again so that you move nearer to the person's feet, automatically applying *caudad traction to the sacrum*. This slight, gentle stretching applied to the sacrum at the same time as you stabilize the third, fourth and fifth lumbar vertebrae, de-stresses the lumbosacral joint in a very precise, targeted way. This form of decompression happens slowly, constantly and subtly. Apply this slight caudad traction on the sacrum for about 1–2 min, after which you should slowly decrease and finally cease the traction. Listen: what do the sacrum and lumbar region feel like now? Can you sense slow motions at the sacrum? What does the craniosacral rhythm feel like? Are the motions of this rhythm continuous and stable or very irregular?

Once you have palpated the qualities of the craniosacral rhythm on the sacrum, slowly remove your hands.

6. Alternative versions are to remove the hand under the lumbar region once you have performed stages 2 and 3 and to place it *on top of* the person's body in the pelvic, abdominal or thoracic region, as for the treatment of the transverse connective tissue; or to lay this hand flat *underneath* any part of the torso or spine.

   Then deliver the merest hint of gentle caudad traction to the sacrum, at the same time sensing upward along the dural tube. As you gain in experience you will be able to sense those places where the dural tube, and with it the spinal column, is experiencing release from below and becoming freed of adhesions (see Releasing the dural tube, p. 204).

   Listen: can you sense the craniosacral rhythm at the sacrum now? If so, how does it feel?
7. To end this element of the treatment, go to the lower end of the treatment table. Tell your client what you intend to do; then take hold of her feet and lift her *legs* with the intention of also providing more room *inferiorly* for the expansion created in the lumbar and pelvic region (Fig. 2.4.11). Then place the client's legs and feet back down on the treatment table.

Release of the sacrum

After you have completed the release of L5/S1 (or independently of it), you can carry out the following: leave your hand under the client's sacrum and tune in to its motion in the craniosacral rhythm – Can you sense the motion of the sacrum? If so, what does it feel like? Can you feel the flexion or the extension motion more?

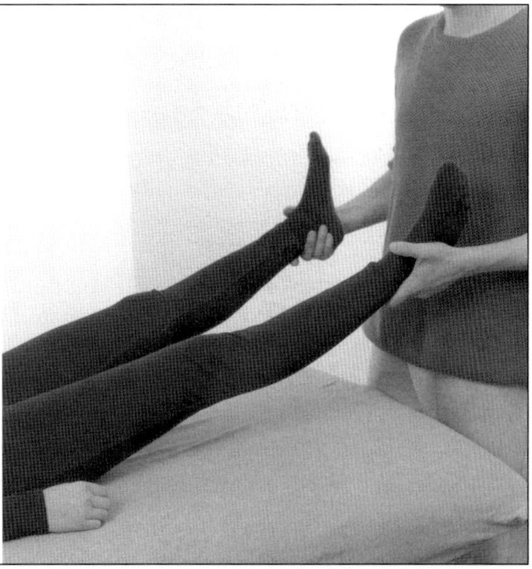

Figure 2.4.11
Widening of the lumbar and pelvic region.

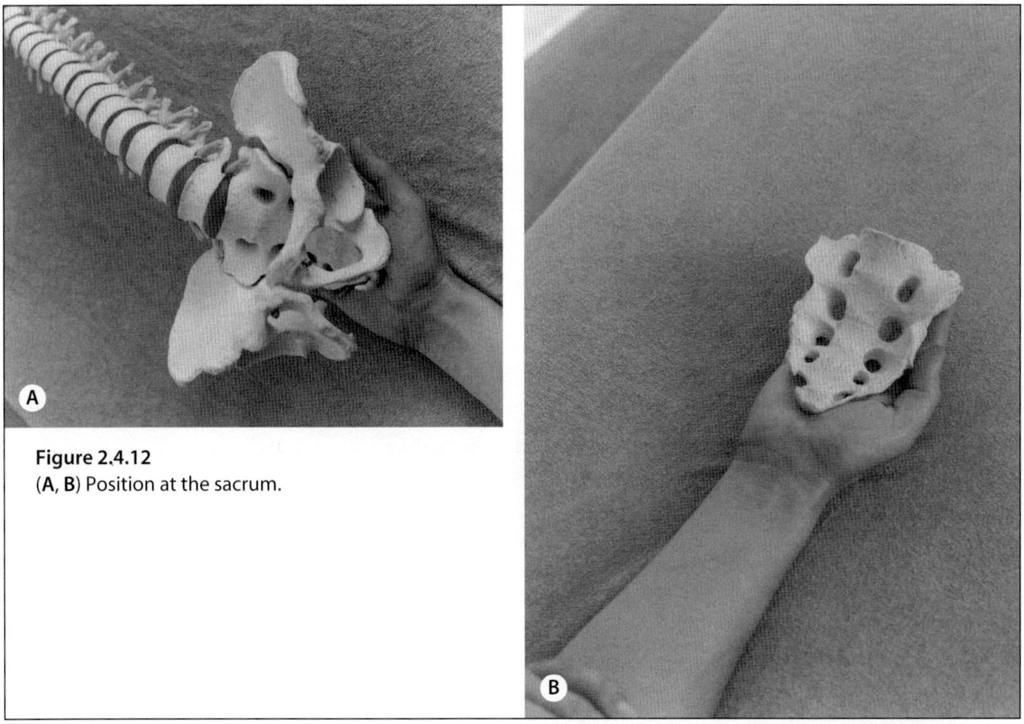

Figure 2.4.12
(**A**, **B**) Position at the sacrum.

The sacrum may possibly want to move more freely as a result of the previous release you have induced, or because of the softness and warmth of your hand, and may begin unwinding motions. Support this by attentively following these slow motions of the sacrum. After a while, you can invite these motions to become wider and stronger and more balanced, but you must do so *with your intention and not by applying any pressure* (Fig. 2.4.12A, B).

Palpatory exploration and gentle massage of the lateral border of the sacrum

Take up a position at the side of the treatment table

This can be used as a pleasant preparation to precede treatment or before specific release techniques, especially before the release of the sacroiliac joints. Place the pads of your fingertips on the lateral border of the sacrum as shown (your thumbs are not involved here). It may help you find the lateral border of the sacrum if you think of the sacrum as shaped like a triangle with its broad base at the top and then tapering down towards its apex, where it joins the coccyx. The client should lie supine (she is shown in the side-lying position in Figure 2.4.13 simply in order to demonstrate the hand position).

Explore the sacrum from the side, using the four fingers of both hands. The sacroiliac joints are located in the superior third of this border, *at the side of the sacrum*. Avoid letting your touch extend too far down the side of the sacrum, so that you do not encroach on the region of the coccyx. When you have finished massaging the border of the sacrum on one side, do the same on the other side.

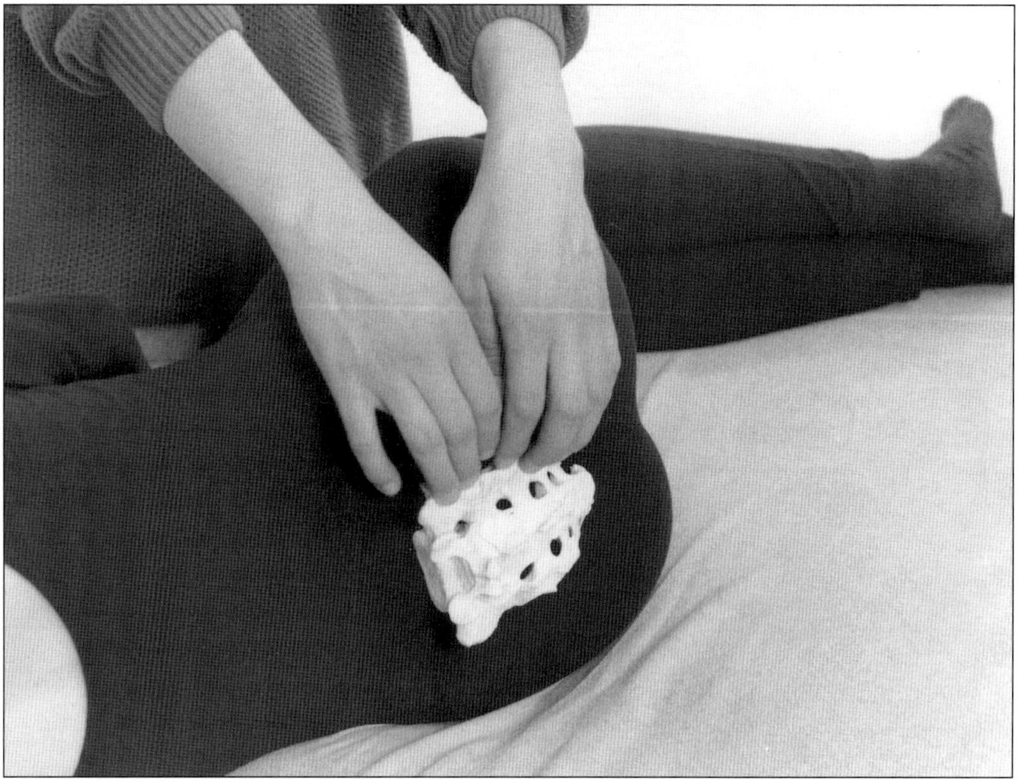

Figure 2.4.13
Use 3–4 fingers of each hand at the border of the sacrum.

Method

When you have found a satisfactory position on the border of the sacrum for the ends of your fingers, slowly turn your fingertips to point upward toward the ceiling. Make sure that it is the soft, fleshy part of the end of your fingers that sinks into the tissue, and not your fingernails.

Your own fingers, hands, wrists, arms, shoulders, spine, and pelvis (including your own sacroiliac joints) should remain relaxed. If you sense any strain, you can dissipate it down through your hips, legs and feet, away to the floor.

Your fingertips should be meltingly soft; allow them to sink into the tissue of the client's body at this point of touch and invite this region to release. The weight of the pelvis is quite sufficient; you can vary the intensity of touch *by varying the height of your upturned fingertips*. Ask your client to tell you how it feels, and adapt your touch to comply with the client's wishes.

After a few moments, you can also begin to move the tips of your fingers in slight circling motions, but without slipping out of position.

After this gentle massage of the sacroiliac transition, stretch out your fingertips again so that your hands – especially your fingers – touch the place you have just massaged and can sense the quality of the tissue. Keep your fingers, hands and arms relaxed and in position.

Release the contact after a while and slowly lift your hands away to the side. Loosen your arms, wrists and fingers. Then take up a position on the other side of the treatment table and perform the release again.

Release of the sacroiliac joints

The ilium and sacrum meet in the pelvic region, forming the sacroiliac joint on the left and right lateral borders of the sacrum. These are very important for the elasticity of the entire pelvic girdle. The firm ligaments enable the sacroiliac joints to play a stabilizing role; these joints are at the same time relatively mobile, although there may be some degree of restriction or even inflammation on one or both sides. Free, flexible sacroiliac joints are important to provide resilient support to the spine and so indirectly also to the head. They play a role in creating an efficient, pleasant gait.

The mobility of these two joints is extremely important in cranial osteopathy and the craniosacral concept, because the craniosacral rhythm must be able to express itself freely from the cranium to the sacrum, and also in the reverse direction. Otherwise, if there are restrictions of any kind, these often produce a compensatory effect on the cranial base and the meninges, and especially on the horizontal and vertical membranes.

The *3-dimensional awareness phase* in the pelvic region, as its name suggests, assists palpatory awareness of the entire pelvic region, enabling better perception of muscles, ligaments, tendons, connective tissue layers and the fasciae that envelop the organs, and enabling their better release. It particularly helps the sacroiliac joint achieve greater flexibility, and especially helps in the case of problems with bones, joints and organs in the pelvic region or spine, assisting the removal of stress affecting them.

The next stage, *sacroiliac widening by minimal traction/decompression*, delivers an impulse to gentle stretching and expansion specifically to this area, the transition and articulation of the sacrum and pelvis. This is often experienced as very soothing by the person receiving treatment. This sacroiliac widening phase (the arm bridge with traction) significantly increases flexibility in the pelvic region, and this is particularly stress-relieving for the locomotor apparatus (Fig. 2.4.14A–C).

These two techniques can also be combined with the release of the transverse connective tissue in the pelvic region and lumbosacral joint. These techniques are typically used to ease problems of painful menstruation, chronic inflammation (e.g., cystitis) or before and after operations in this region.

If there is considerable lack of movement in the pelvis in general, the sacroiliac joints are also to varying degrees inhibited or restricted. In this state, the sacrum is inhibited by the sacroiliac joints, hindering its natural motion in the craniosacral rhythm. This significantly affects palpation of

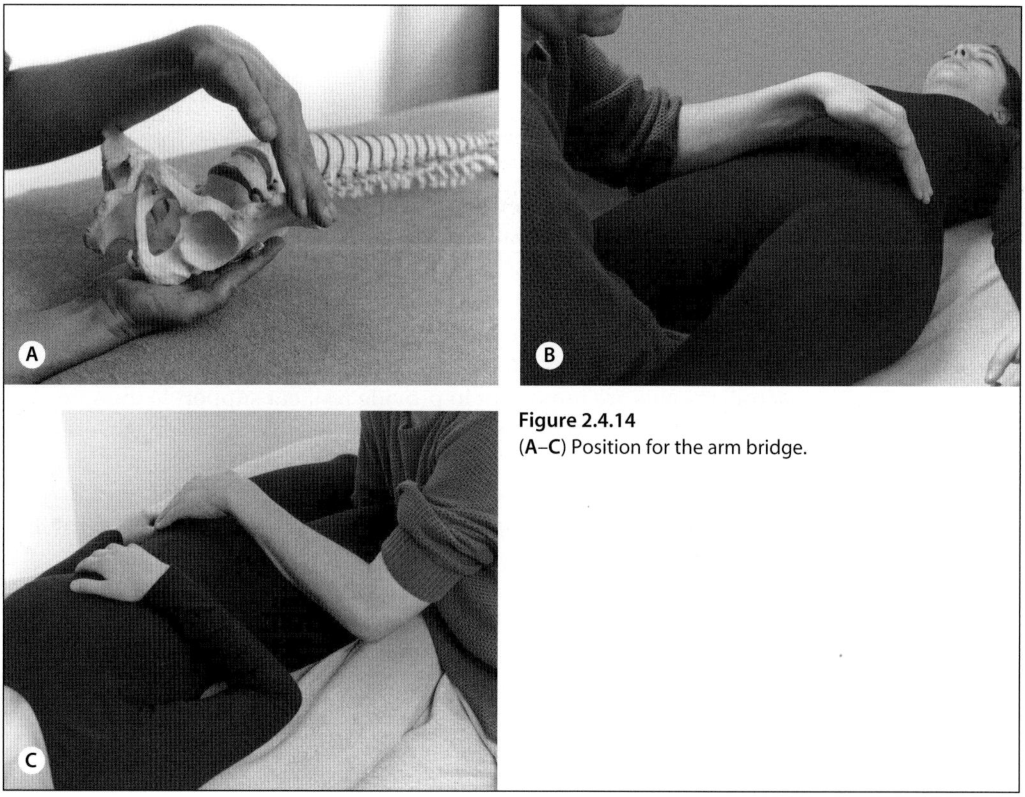

Figure 2.4.14
(**A–C**) Position for the arm bridge.

the craniosacral rhythm at both sides of the pelvis, at the sacrum, feet, and legs, and even at the occiput.

3-dimensional awareness in the pelvic region (arm bridge without traction)

Begin by exploring the superior border of your client's pelvis, especially the two sides of the pelvis, the left and right anterior superior iliac spine.

Sitting beside the table, place the hand that is nearer your client's feet under the client's sacrum. Place the end part of your fingers (the distal phalanges) of the hand nearer your client's head gently on the iliac spine on the other side of your client's body, and hook the fingertips in place around the side. Then rest part of your forearm on the iliac crest on the nearer side. Your wrist should be slightly bent, with the outer angle of the wrist joint uppermost, but without imposing any strain on your shoulder. Ensure that the intensity of touch is equal on both sides; there should be clarity of touch, but no downward pressure (i.e. in the direction of the table).

The forearm and fingers of the same arm are now simultaneously in contact with the left and right iliac crest. Your other hand should meanwhile lie beneath the client's sacrum, relaxed and ready to support any release or the motion of the craniosacral rhythm.

As the practitioner you should relax, adopting the most comfortable position you can at the table, in particular relaxing your hands, arms and shoulders. Now sense deep down *in the spatial sense* into the pelvis through your three points of contact (on both sides of the pelvis and on the sacrum), without changing anything: you can train your capacities of '3-dimensional sensing' of the body and so perceive more *overall*. Invite spatial release in the pelvic region and apply your touch with the intention of permitting the tight ligaments and muscles, and all the joints and organs, increasingly to release.

If you did not tell your client about the form of contact you intended to use, the contact of hand and forearm on the iliac crests together with that of the hand on the sacrum can feel like the contact of three hands. Do not be surprised if the client looks up to see where this third hand has come from. It helps if you inform the client in advance about where you intend to take up the contact.

Tips

If your forearms are not long enough or if the particular client has a particularly broad pelvic region, so that you cannot reach both iliac crests with your forearm and fingers, remove the hand from underneath the client's sacrum and lay the palms of both hands on the iliac spine/superior border of the pelvis, hands parallel. (This position is the same as that for the palpation of the craniosacral rhythm at the pelvis, p. 109.)

Sense and analyze:

- What do you sense with the hand under the client's sacrum?
- What do you sense with the forearm and fingers on the sides of the pelvis? Can you sense the ER/IR of the craniosacral rhythm here?
- Does this change after you have listened for one or two minutes? If so, how?
- Is more room established in general in this region?

You can now perform the arm bridge with traction, described below, or you can conclude the contact with the sides of the pelvis and use your free hand to carry out a release of transverse connective tissue.

Sacroiliac widening by minimal traction/ decompression (arm bridge with traction)

This is performed immediately after the 3-dimensional awareness in the pelvic region. Your hand position is the same as described above. Now, with the fingertips hooked around the opposite iliac spine and the forearm on the iliac crests, deliver *slow, gentle traction to both sides simultaneously in an inward and upward direction* ('upward' being toward the ceiling).

As you do this, you will find that you angle your wrist more acutely upward. Make sure that this subtle inward, upward traction to the iliac crests is *equal on both sides*; in particular be sure to maintain it continuously, for about 1–2 min as necessary.

Your intention as you apply this constant, slight inward and upward lifting is for this traction to extend on through the two iliac crests and the muscles and deep ligaments attached to them, arriving as a subtle stretching in the region of the sacroiliac joints. If you deliver the widening impulse for too short a time, or if you use no more than a hint of traction, you will achieve no more than a suggestion of an effect – it would not produce a comprehensive release of the sacroiliac joints. The continuous, even intensity and direction of traction sends an ever-clearer message to the region to widen and release. This widening by minimal traction/decompression is not done in cases where the sacroiliac joint is hypermobile.

You may find that after performing this traction for a while, your fingers and forearm slip off; if so, replace your fingers and forearm on both sides of the client's iliac crest and continue to lift as before.

Sense and analyze: look at the qualities you studied after the 3-dimensional awareness in the pelvic region (see p. 151), just as you did then, comparing the qualities before and after.

When you have completed the widening by minimal traction/ decompression you have two options: one is gradually to reduce the inward and upward traction and follow on with touch (=3-dimensional awareness in the pelvic region), during which you allow the person to sense her body. After a few moments, remove your superior hand, and then the hand under the sacrum.

Or: you can continue the gentle inward and upward traction until a point where you intentionally let your hand and forearm slip off, up toward the ceiling, so concluding the sacroiliac widening phase. Then slowly remove the hand under the sacrum.

Integration of the release in the torso region

Craniosacral therapy, as I understand it, is not only concerned with the local release of individual structures belonging to the body segments or cranial bones, to give them a greater capacity for motion in their own right (motility), but at the same time with their capacity for motion in general (mobility), in other words to ensure their optimum integration with neighboring structures and with the body as a whole.

The integration of the release in the torso region, for example, is aided by touch and listening in the following locations:

- Middle of the torso: costal arch/diaphragm/solar plexus (p. 126).
- Simultaneously in the superior and inferior parts of the torso: double arm bridge (p. 209).
- Pelvis: 3-dimensional awareness in the pelvic region (p. 151), sacrum (p. 146) or both sides of the pelvis (p. 109).
- Thighs, knees or feet: palpation of the craniosacral rhythm; before-and-after comparison (p. 107).
- Invite a still point (p. 155).

What is your overall assessment now? What is the craniosacral rhythm like now, compared with before? Has there been any change in your client that can not only be felt but also seen, compared with the beginning?

Ask how your client is now, how her body feels and whether anything has changed as compared with the beginning of the treatment; if so, what, where and how? Which locations feel most comfortable now?

Why release these regions before treating the head?

It is advisable to observe the order of release given so far as closely as possible, before carrying out craniosacral treatment of the head. The reasons for giving treatment in this order are first, that it increases the overall well-being of the client, especially in the region of the torso – and it is very important for the complete release of the craniosacral system, which of course runs from head to sacrum and can also be restricted in many places in the periphery, apart from the head. If we bear in mind the fact that our connective tissue 'speaks' and that tensions and restrictions in the body can be reduced or resolved by treating it, we can clearly see that structural treatment of the head cannot be as comprehensive, and is often not as effective, if it is not preceded by treatment of the torso. We should also bear in mind that areas of muscle, connective tissue, ligaments and fasciae that are tight or tense can extend their effect upward to include the head and act as a restriction of the craniosacral system; therefore release in the region of the torso is crucial. These structures also have their attachments from below at the occipital ridge and cranial base, where they can lead to compensatory patterns of motion and dysfunctions.

Release and general balancing of *transverse* connective tissue layers automatically has a positive effect on the *longitudinal* layers of connective tissue and on all the physical forces acting on the body. The sacrum, the dural tube and the fibrous ring of dura mater surrounding the foramen magnum all relax. There is better exchange of information between brain and body, harmonizing all body functions. Release of the adhesions, torsions and intense strains of the spinal meninges has a simultaneous effect on the forces acting on the cranial meninges and intracranial membranes, as these together form a single unit.

2.5 Inviting and inducing still points

Basic principles of the still point

On the basis of my many years of experience, I can say that there are many, very different, still points – on a whole range of levels. A great deal more detail could be given on the fascinating subject of the still point, but this would exceed the scope of the present book, which is intended to be introductory. The following is therefore a summary of the most important information for the beginner.

Every still point occurs in a direct, spontaneous way and is unique. It must be the sheer variety of still points and their origins and effects that has led to differences in emphasis and application in the teaching of still point techniques over recent decades. The skills required to bring about a direct, invasive stopping of the craniosacral rhythm at the level of the bones are different from those required, for example, to invite the still point on the fluid level. Craniosacral practitioners use a still point at an appropriate moment to support their treatment in various ways according to their treatment approach, character and experience.

The craniosacral rhythm and the still point are highly central, powerful elements in the body's intrinsic self-regulation. I therefore recommend all readers with little or no training or practical experience in craniosacral work not to induce still points actively at first, but to invite them. You need to respect the inner healer and should not disturb the craniosacral rhythm, as the expression of the Breath of Life, by incautious, manipulative intervention. First, you should train your palpation skills by differentiated listening to the craniosacral rhythm and the body's spontaneous still points.

What happens during a still point?

As explained previously in the chapter 'The craniosacral rhythm' (p. 46), the craniosacral rhythm can suddenly stop during its ebb-and-flow motions in external and internal rotation (ER/IR), or flexion and extension. This is called a still point (or 'stillpoint').

A still point can last 20 seconds or even 3–4 min. It should not be confused with the short pause that is a preliminary to moving on, or the brief halt at the changeover from flexion to extension motion or ER/IR.

Still points occur of themselves, spontaneously generated by the body. They can also be induced by external means. The wisdom of the body decides whether and when our invitation to a still point will be accepted and made a reality, and how long it will last.

During a still point the entire craniosacral system, and with it the entire body, has a chance to reset the balance and organize itself, subtly and outward from within, for example orienting itself on the body's midline. Homeostasis is improved.

A spontaneous still point is an important indication of changes occurring in the body and in the consciousness of the client at that moment. A still point can also spontaneously occur in the release phase following natural unwinding motions (p. 255), for example as the body seeks or establishes a new inner point or state of balance.

If a still point occurs, a change can often be observed in the person concerned, e.g., in the person's breathing or tissue or the atmosphere in the room, and the person usually also slips into a state of agreeable, deeper relaxation. Still points can be described as a great 'stillness in the deepest ocean of the body' and allow the person as a whole to plunge into great relaxation on the level of body, mind and spirit.

When the craniosacral rhythm re-emerges after the still point, usually more strongly than before, the central nervous system is once more bathed in fresh, vitalized cerebrospinal fluid. The increased exchange of fluids cleanses the brain and spinal cord better of impurities, at the same time bringing fresh nourishment. One role of the still point is therefore to act as a kind of fluid drainage for the brain.

Externally induced still points have a positive effect on:

- the qualities of the craniosacral rhythm – strength, amplitude, symmetry, frequency (cycles) – which often become more clearly detectable and more even
- the longitudinal fluctuation of the CSF and craniosacral rhythm
- the improved exchange of all body fluids
- greater emphasis on the parasympathetic part of the autonomic nervous system, and so a greater degree of ease in the autonomic sphere
- the tonus of the connective tissue, which is reduced
- the balancing of the whole-body matrix and its natural and compensatory fulcrums
- most involuntary processes of the body, especially the endocrine system
- the integration of the release during the craniosacral session
- integration after powerful physical, emotional or psychological processes
- the best possible integration of the session as a whole in the period following the treatment
- uterine contractions and the process of childbirth.

No list of specific indications is given here because the effect is highly individual. The effect in principle is to encourage greater balance.

Contraindications for still points are:

- serious injuries to the body and to the head
- serious injuries in the head region; skull fractures
- the risk of cerebral hemorrhage; immediately following cerebral hemorrhage; cerebral aneurysms
- in the first and final trimesters of pregnancy, as a precaution (see Indications and contraindications, p. 63).

Listening to the craniosacral rhythm and spontaneous still points

As stated above, at the beginning of this chapter, the first requirement is to develop palpatory skills and assurance as regards the craniosacral rhythm and spontaneous still points, so that these skills can then be used to invite still points for the client's benefit, or – more actively – to be able to induce them.

You should therefore take the time you need, listening to the craniosacral rhythm and the qualities of the rhythm (p. 51). If you palpate in a relaxed way for about 15–30 min, you will automatically come to recognize the shorter pauses in the craniosacral rhythm (approx. 1–10 seconds) and be able to distinguish them from the longer, spontaneous still points (from 20 seconds to several minutes) generated by the body. This practice in palpation alone, if done regularly, can teach you a vast amount about the craniosacral rhythm, spontaneous still points and self-regulation.

Inviting or inducing the still point at the sides of the body

The places on the body where still points can best be externally induced are those where the craniosacral rhythm can be palpated clearly as external and internal rotation (ER/IR)

- The feet
- The thighs
- The iliac crests/sides of the pelvis
- The shoulders.

The following ER/IR technique can be used on the sides of the body wherever it is possible to sense the craniosacral rhythm as a motion of external and internal rotation (ER/IR).

Version 1: Inviting a still point by slowing the craniosacral rhythm

If you can detect the craniosacral rhythm for several cycles at the sides of the person's body, you can also invite the still point by *slowing and shortening ER*: follow the whole of IR for about 15 cycles, but as soon as

ER begins, reduce its *rate and amplitude* a little more with each cycle. If the craniosacral system is willing, a still point will occur after about 15 cycles. Listen for another 2–3 min after the still point to sense whether the craniosacral rhythm now feels more even, or whether still slower rhythms can now be detected. This version is recommended as the preferred method of the three described here.

Version 2: Following IR; then inducing the still point

1. Place your hands gently on the left and right side of the part of the body you have selected, and palpate the craniosacral rhythm. Follow the craniosacral rhythm in external and internal rotation and note its qualities.
2. After a few cycles, make the decision to follow the *internal rotation phase* attentively, support it evenly with both hands, and *hold it at its innermost point*.
3. By *continuously holding* these paired parts of the body at their innermost point of internal rotation (IR), you prevent the motion of *external rotation* (ER). This holding back initiated by you is transmitted on through the connective tissue, muscles and joints to the craniosacral system, temporarily restricting the system in its ER. The consequence is often that the *still point* occurs, after *5–15 cycles*. You will possibly sense a subtle resetting of the balance by the body, but no more ER/IR motions. As the still point begins, your hands will sense a reduction in the tendency to lateral motion into ER until this finally stops altogether and the rhythm becomes still.
4. As soon as you detect the stillness that indicates the still point, your hands should soften and *stop holding the sides of the person's body in the medial position of IR*. You now listen and do not need to do anything more.
5. *Wait, listening in a spacious manner; until the craniosacral rhythm resumes,* between about 20 seconds and 3 or 4 min later. This can usually be felt as a lateral ER motion. *Palpate the qualities* of the rhythm for a few cycles – strength, amplitude, symmetry, frequency (cycles). Are there any *differences* as compared with before the still point? Is the rhythm more even? How have the qualities of the craniosacral rhythm changed since the still point?

These two versions assume that you can sense the craniosacral rhythm.

Version 3: Bring into IR; induce the still point by stopping the motion

If you cannot yet sense the craniosacral rhythm, guide the paired parts of the body slightly farther inward (into IR), stop and pause there for about 3–4 min. If the craniosacral system is willing, a still point will be induced. After about 3–4 min, you should stop holding the system back but maintain the contact of your touch. Listen for another 3 min to sense whether you can now sense the ER/IR motions of the craniosacral rhythm, and the qualities of these motions.

Inviting or inducing the still point at the occipital bone

Begin by listening to the craniosacral rhythm in the cradle hold (p. 112). Finish the following technique by listening again to the craniosacral rhythm in the cradle hold and make a before-and-after comparison.

Take up a position at the top end of the treatment table (near the person's head)

The best place to induce a still point on the head is at the occiput. After a while, the pressure produced by the positioning of the practitioner's thenar eminences and the *weight of the head itself* gradually reaches the fourth ventricle of the brain, via the occipital bone. The continual gentle compression so caused to the fourth ventricle at its apertures brings about a still point.

You should practice the following hand position (1–3) on your own to begin with, before applying it under the occiput of the person on the treatment table. At the end of this section, you will find two alternative versions to point 6.

1. Open both hands, palms uppermost, and place your fingers across each other.
2. Draw the *inner surfaces of your two thumbs* together until they touch each other. This will also bring the thenar eminences closer to the middle, so that they almost touch (the distance between your thenar eminences should be from one to three centimeters (half an inch to just over an inch), depending on the size of head the person has).
3. Check that *the soft part of your thenar eminences is uppermost and presents the largest possible surface for the person's occiput*. Make sure that you do not have the bones or joints of your fingers uppermost, because this would create a bone-on-bone contact, which would be uncomfortable for the person receiving the treatment (Fig. 2.5.1A–D).
4. Now put your hands, in this position, underneath the occiput of the person on the treatment table. One way to do this is to put your hands, palms uppermost, on the treatment table and draw them up to their position under the occipital bone from the direction of the neck and shoulder region. A slight shifting of your thenar eminences to left and right at the ball of your hands will enable you to draw your fingers across each other, and then to bring the thenar eminences closer into the middle at the ball of your thumbs. This is easier if there is a soft padded surface on the treatment table, as you can press your hands down into it, and do not need to lift the client's head too much.

   If after a few attempts you still cannot find the right position, you can ask your client to lift her head a little for just long enough to let you arrange your hands properly and comfortably behind her occiput (see points 1–3).

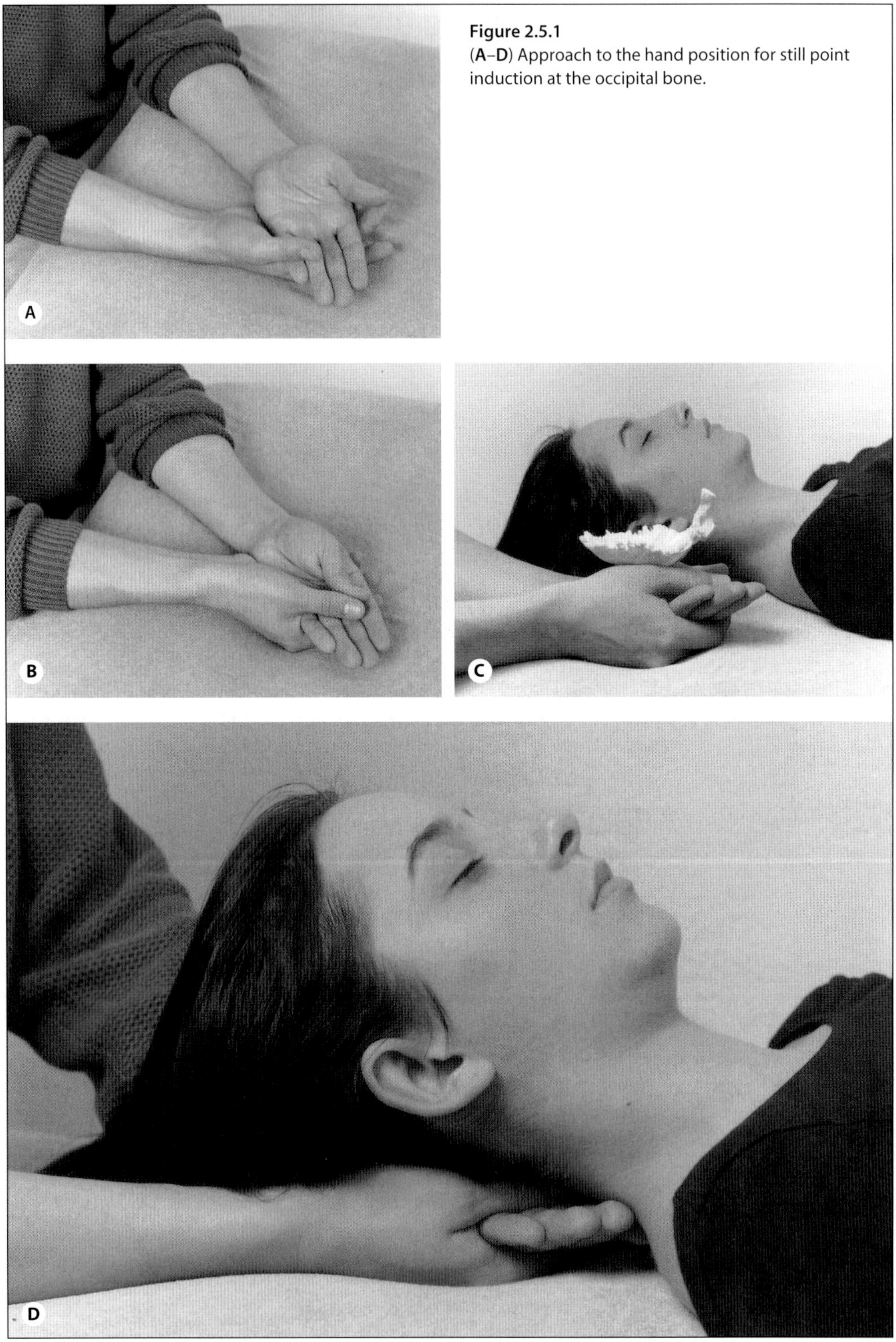

Figure 2.5.1
(**A–D**) Approach to the hand position for still point induction at the occipital bone.

Check the position of your thenar eminences to left and right, and make sure that you are the *right distance* from the treatment table, i.e. from the client's head, and that you are *seated at the right height*. Just as importantly, you need to ensure that your thenar eminences under the occiput are as soft as possible. With arms and shoulders relaxed and your torso grounded, consciously let the weight of your hands and of your client's head be absorbed into the padded surface of the table.

Important points

Take care that the points of contact of your thenar eminences are close enough to the middle of the occipital bone (at/to left and right of the *external occipital protuberance*. You can then avoid the area of the cranial sutures (transition to the parietal and temporal bones). Any prolonged compression on the cranial *sutures* can feel unpleasant for the client, or might cause slight pressure in the head, and you need to avoid this.

5. Let the correct position take effect on you. Your two soft thenar eminences should 'blend' with your client's occipital bone and the cranial membranes behind it, working through the hair and skin of the client's head. Expand your field of perception to include the fluctuation and the motion of the CSF. At the occiput, flexion feels like a process of becoming fuller and wider; extension like contracting and becoming smaller.
   Follow the flexion phase. At the occiput, this is sensed as a downward motion, in the direction of your hands and the table, at the same time becoming slightly broader laterally. Follow the extension phase. This is sensed as an upward motion, in the direction of the cranium, at the same time becoming slightly narrower. Follow the flexion phase again.
6. *When the next extension phase comes, follow this motion* inward and upward *with your thenar eminences*. With your thenar eminences, hold the occipital bone in position at its innermost point of extension, *so that you do not allow it to move into the opposite motion of flexion.* Do not apply any additional pressure to the occipital bone. This brings about the still point after a few moments or a few minutes.
7. Wait until you sense the stillness that marks the still point; then (with your hand, and in particular your thenar eminences) you once more *release the hold restraining the motion at the innermost point of extension (inward and upward)*. You do not perform any movement; you just completely relax your hands, arms and shoulders again.
8. Maintain the link within your palpatory awareness with the structures concerned, and wait for the moment when the slow motion of the craniosacral rhythm resumes. Follow and listen

in a differentiated manner to observe the strength, amplitude, symmetry and rate that appear now, after the still point. Are there any differences? What are the qualities of the rhythm if you compare them before and after the still point?

If it is still difficult to sense the craniosacral rhythm (either because you are a novice in the art of palpation or because the craniosacral rhythm at the client's occipital bone is considerably restricted), you can use the following directive, mechanical approach to induce a still point. (This version replaces the steps in points 6 and 7 above):

If after about 12–14 cycles you (still) cannot detect a craniosacral rhythm, then *without following the extension motion* you can simultaneously draw your thenar eminences slightly *inward and upward* and apply slight pressure there for about 3 min (in the direction of the fourth ventricle). Continue to be sensitive and to listen to what you can sense as you do this. Then palpate as in point 8.

These two techniques for the induction of a still point can help give you an initial theoretical and practical understanding of what is involved. However, both can be invasive in their effect, depending on how they are carried out; it is therefore advisable to begin by performing them with feedback, on a healthy subject, preferably by a group of craniosacral students during a course of training. Both versions are unsuitable for use on children or anyone who has recently suffered extreme force in the head, neck and shoulder region.

In addition, some gentler alternative methods of inducing the still point are described below. However, these assume that you are able to palpate the craniosacral rhythm for several cycles.

Alternative 1 (Hand position: thenar eminences under the person's occiput)

Follow the craniosacral rhythm in flexion and extension for a few cycles to familiarize yourself with the way it moves at each moment and so that you will be able to compare its motion after the still point with that before it.

Instead of stopping the occipital bone at its innermost point of extension, as described in point 6 above, follow the craniosacral rhythm, accompanying and slowly reducing its motion: use the ball of your thumbs under the occipital bone to *slow down and shorten the flexion motion each time*, and then follow the entire extent of the extension motion to the innermost point of IR. This automatically leads to a still point after about 15 cycles, if the wisdom of the body is willing.

Alternative 2 (Hand position: cradle hold)

In the cradle hold, follow the craniosacral rhythm at the occipital bone for a few cycles. Listen to the craniosacral rhythm, then reduce its motion slowly over several cycles: use the palms and edges of your hands that form roughly the middle of the 'cradle' to *slow down and shorten the flexion motion each time*; follow the entire extension motion each time. This automatically leads to a still point after about 15 cycles, if the wisdom of the body is willing.

Inviting or inducing the still point at the sacrum

Take up a position at the side of the treatment table

1. Sit facing the table, with the hand nearer the person's feet under the sacrum, as for the release of the pelvic region or sacroiliac joints. Place your cranial hand in the pelvic region, the abdominal region or another of the locations already mentioned, as you prefer.
2. Ensure that your position is comfortable to allow you to listen to the craniosacral rhythm at the sacrum for a few minutes, in a spacious, present and relaxed manner. With the upward-facing hand under the person's sacrum, sense through the skin and tissue to the bone. Remain relaxed, passive and attentive and listen to the rhythm. If you sense the region of the sacrum and pelvis *in 3-dimensional space*, you will be better able to perceive the craniosacral rhythm and the processes en route to release.
3. Follow the *flexion phase* at the sacrum. As the dural tube becomes fuller, the inferior apex of the sacrum moves 'upward' (in the direction of the ceiling). This flexion motion can be palpated particularly in the middle of your hand and on toward the thenar eminence.

   Be aware of the axis of this motion: as the apex of the sacrum moves, so the superior part of the sacrum, where your fingers are resting, pointing toward the person's lumbar spine, swings slightly downward, in the direction of the table.
4. Next, follow the *extension motion*; this time the inferior, caudad part of the sacrum moves downward, toward the table, meaning that the part resting in the middle of your hand (extending toward the thenar eminence) moves slightly downward.

   Be aware of the axis of this motion: as the apex of the sacrum moves, so the superior part of the sacrum, where your fingers are resting, pointing toward the person's lumbar spine, swings slightly upward.
5. With your fingers resting on the superior part of the sacrum, follow this tipping motion as it swings upward *into extension* (toward the ceiling) as far as you can. When you have clearly palpated a couple of cycles, you should also support this motion and hold the sacrum at its furthermost point of extension, not allowing it to move in the opposite direction into flexion. After a while, this will cause the still point to occur.
6. When you detect the stillness that indicates the still point, let your hands become soft and so cease to hold the bone in position at its innermost point of extension. You do not perform any movement; you just continue to relax your hands, arms and shoulders.
7. Then wait and listen for the motions of the craniosacral rhythm to resume. Follow these motions and listen in a differentiated manner for several cycles to observe the strength, amplitude, symmetry and rate. Are there any differences? What are the differences if you compare the qualities before and after the still point?

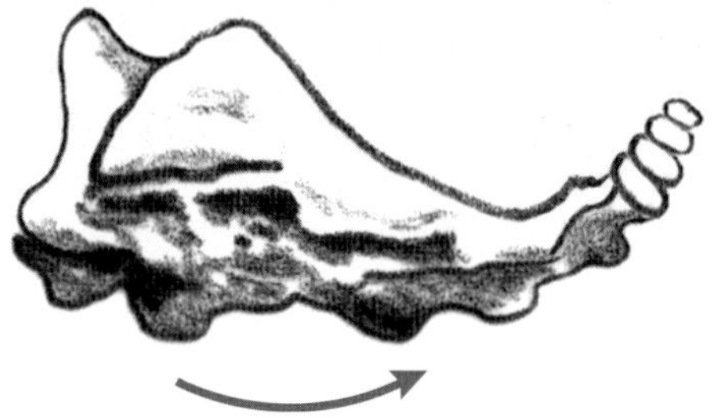

Figure 2.5.2
The sacrum in flexion.

Alternative

Instead of stopping the craniosacral rhythm at its innermost point of extension as described under point 5, you can *listen to the craniosacral rhythm* at the sacrum and slowly reduce the motions: *slow down and shorten the motion of flexion at the sacrum each time, and follow the full extent of each extension motion*. This automatically leads to a still point after about 15 cycles, if the wisdom of the body is willing (Fig. 2.5.2).

- A still point at the occipital bone or sacrum is a very effective longitudinal fluctuation technique. It is used, for example, for states of exhaustion, because on the one hand, it has a balancing and centering effect, and on the other it stimulates the cranial nerve nuclei in the region of the fourth ventricle, bringing about a vitalizing and strengthening effect.

Self-treatment techniques for the head

2.6

During a craniosacral therapy session, the client can passively lie there and enjoy the experience. However, there are also self-treatment techniques in which you can listen to your own craniosacral system and support its functions. An important by-product of such self-treatment is that, as a practitioner of this gentle therapy, you will be able to sense in your own body that little (if any) pressure is needed. This teaches you subtly to vary your quality of touch so that later you can more skillfully adapt to your client's wishes.

This chapter will focus on some preliminaries to treating the head, on still point induction at the occiput, and on the gentle ear pull technique – all presented as self-treatments. These may be used on a daily basis, ideally in a peaceful setting. In other chapters, you will read about additional treatments you can perform on yourself. Start with the exercises outlined here before graduating to the advanced self-treatment techniques.

Every head has its own unique individual shape. You may well be astonished how these self-treatments help you to 'rediscover' your own head.

Scalp massage

1. Feel your scalp with all 10 fingers. Try to move it gently, as far as possible *without your fingertips slipping*. Is your scalp resistant or can it be moved easily? Massage it using slow, circular movements. Vary the intensity, but always stay within the range that feels pleasantly comfortable. From time to time, move to a new position on your head. While performing this gentle scalp massage, simultaneously direct your attention through your finger pads to the different cranial sutures. Avoiding any deep pressure, continue to massage using circular movements over the surface.
2. Afterwards use all 10 fingers to feel for the muscles at the sides of your head, also those with attachments to the occipital ridge at the back, and gently massage using circular movements. If your touch feels unpleasant, adjust its intensity as appropriate.
3. Your hair also has continuity with your scalp and the muscles of your head. Experiment on yourself using the following simple technique from Gerda Boyesen's biodynamic body psychotherapy: take hold of a few tufts of hair between your fingers. As you *very lightly* pull your hair away from your head, this gently stretches your scalp and head muscles, which will slowly relax. Sometimes you will be able to hear sounds of

activated digestion – a kind of biofeedback signal of relaxation and tension release – and these are a good indication that self-regulatory processes are unfolding.

Using your fingers, hold your hair over a period of 5–10 seconds while pulling gently and evenly; or slowly pull your hair increasingly away from your head before deliberately slackening your hold at the end so that your hair is 'stroked outwards' as it runs through your fingers.

This can feel extremely pleasant, almost as if the mental ballast in your head due to the non-stop build-up of thoughts has found an escape route through your hair.

Massaging the masticatory muscles

Massage of the muscles used in chewing (see p. 192) can also be performed as self-treatment. This will relax the muscles involved and your temporomandibular joints (TMJs). At the same time, you will be supporting the natural craniosacral motion of the paired temporal bones and parietal bones that is reduced when your masticatory muscles are tense.

Using broad contact palpate your own TMJs on your face just in front of the auditory canal on each side. Then palpate your masticatory muscles, perhaps making slight chewing movements as you do so. You may sense your own TMJ tension and feel free to yawn. Now slowly massage the muscles under your TMJs using a downward stroking action.

Stroking your muscles at the occipital ridge

1. While seated or lying down, bring your hands from each side up against the back of your head and slide them down your occiput towards your neck, as far as the occipital ridge. Without applying pressure, *palpate your occipital ridge*, beginning at the middle and moving outwards:
   What shape is it? In particular, how are the muscle attachments at the lower edge of the occiput? How precisely do your muscles here feel? Is one side more relaxed than the other?
2. Using your index, middle and ring fingers in *broad contact*, touch the middle of the occipital ridge on your occiput. As you stroke the muscle attachments at the occiput and the muscles at the occipital ridge, make sure that you *never* exert pressure on the cervical vertebrae: the cervical vertebrae in this region are extremely sensitive. The purpose of this self-treatment is to stroke the muscles along the occipital ridge *sideways, not to exert deep pressure*! Now use your fingers to stroke the muscles sideways out from the middle of the occipital ridge (fingertips of left hand along the left side of the ridge, and fingertips of right hand along the right side) as far as the mastoid process of the temporal bone to which the powerful sternocleidomastoid muscle is attached. *You can repeat this lateral stroking several times and, if pleasant, intensify slightly.*

3. As an accompaniment to this exercise, allow your lower jaw to drop. This can be done with your mouth open or closed and it supports the relaxation process.

Still point induction at the occiput

Find two tennis balls (soft or well-used ones feel more comfortable) or, even better, two juggling balls. Take a sock that is sufficiently wide and flexible and push the two juggling balls as far forward as possible into the foot of the sock. Knot the sock so that the two balls are touching each other; they should lie firmly and compactly side by side and should not be pushed apart later by the weight of your head.

Lie down on a soft mat in a peaceful, undisturbed setting. Instead of a pillow, now place the two balls tied in the sock under your head at the level of your occiput (Fig. 2.6.1). The balls should be positioned 2 or 3 cm above your occipital ridge. Make sure that the balls are not too low (i.e. not on the occipital ridge) or too high (i.e. not on the sutures with the parietal bones). If the balls are correctly positioned, your head can rest relaxed on them for about 4–6 min.

The weight of your head exerts a constant, even pressure via the occiput on to the fourth cerebral ventricle, where a still point is generally established spontaneously after a few minutes. After a deep sigh or as you feel you need to, you can set the balls aside. Afterward turn on to your side and stand up again from that position.

Gentle ear pull technique

You can self-administer the gentle ear pull (cf. p. 189) in the seated, lying or standing position. As well as easing tension in a number of cranial sutures, this technique also helps the meninges, which are often taut or adherent, to become stretched and more flexible. In the same way

Figure 2.6.1
Still point induction at the occiput.

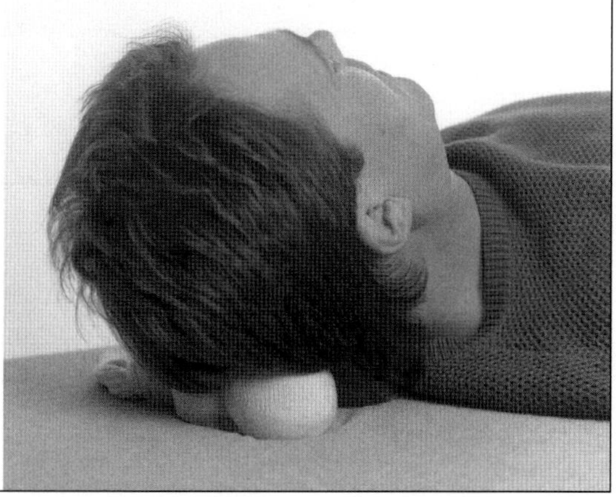

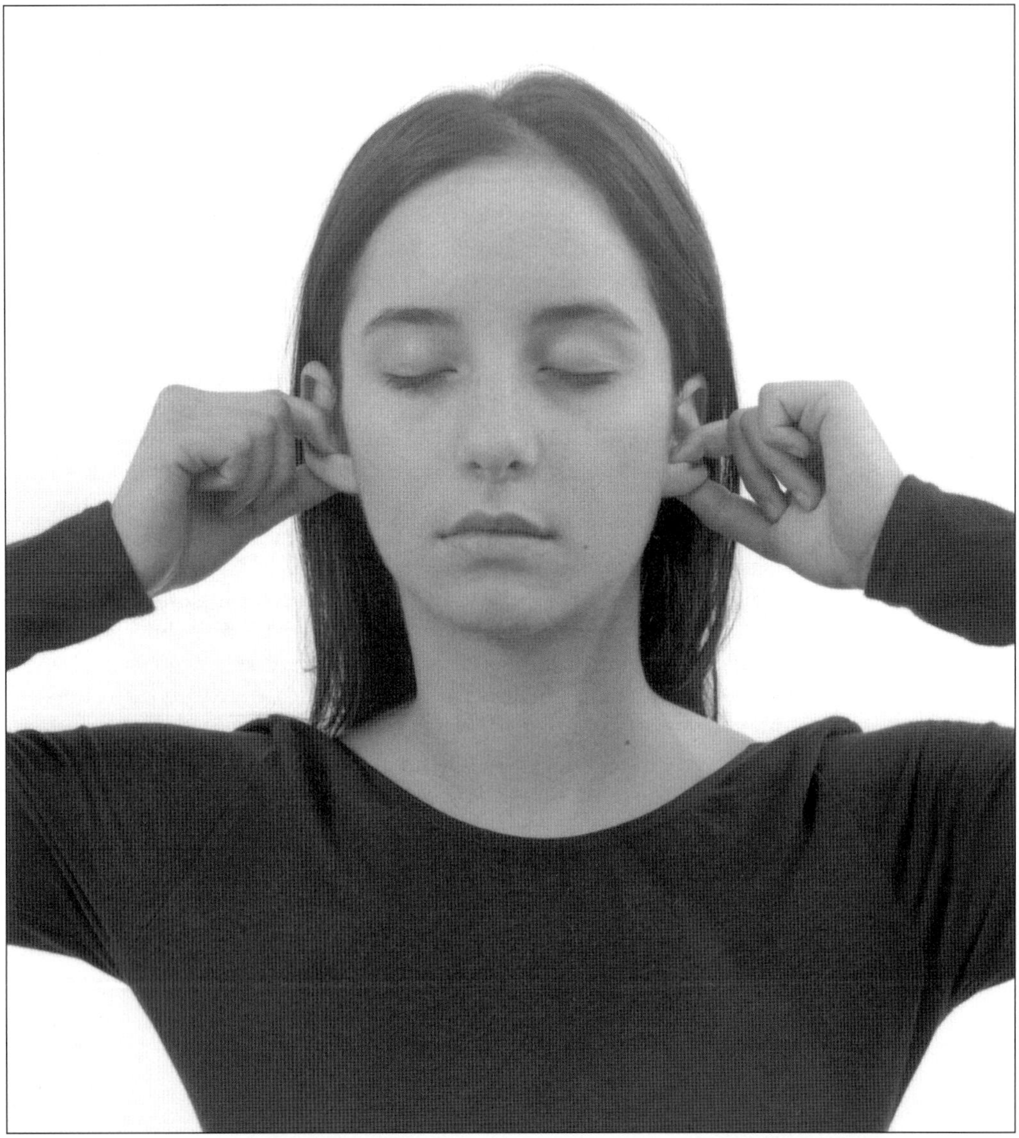

Figure 2.6.2
Gentle ear pull.

tension patterns are released in the tentorium cerebelli (the horizontal component in the intracranial membrane system), and at its points of contact with the falx cerebri and falx cerebelli (the vertical components in the intracranial membrane system). This also has a positive effect on the drainage of blood from the brain and can reduce the sensation of pressure.

Place each index finger inside the cartilage of your external ear diagonally behind and below your auditory canal: do not insert your finger into the auditory canal. With your thumbs behind your ear lobes, take a perceptible hold but without exerting pressure (Fig. 2.6.2). Slowly and gently offer just a suggestion of posterolateral traction, i.e. sideways and backward. At the same time listen to the innate motion of the structure. You might try occasionally closing your eyes and letting your lower jaw drop. While doing this remain within the breathing flow.

2.7 Treating the head

The combined effect of whole-body assessment, of releasing transverse layers of connective tissue from pelvis to cranial base, and of inviting still points is to relax the craniosacral system from the sacrum up the spine as far as the cranial base and to comprehensively prepare the way for treating the head. Now you can encourage release of the cranial bones and sutures and the meninges.

Earlier you learned that craniosacral therapy *involves clear contact rather than pressure*. Before starting, it is important that you treat yourself to a few craniosacral sessions with experienced practitioners. In general, I also recommend that you attend a basic course followed by supervised training before you practice these treatments and techniques on healthy adults. Move on to treating the head once you feel fairly familiar with the treatment outlined so far.

Asking open questions will generate feedback on how your client is feeling and on the quality of your touch, which you can then adjust appropriately, if necessary. Regulate your distance from the client, and make sure you are grounded and centered.

Touching someone's head demands that you show respect, an ability to empathize, and attentiveness. Establish touch contact slowly, carefully and with clarity. Here, on the head and close to the face, you come into particular proximity with an individual's personality, what makes her unique. Respectful appreciation and occasional reality-check questioning will help you go with your client in the best way possible – and will also minimize any tendency for you to project your own ideas or have a different agenda.

Preparing to treat the head

The preparations outlined here are useful as an initial introduction to your client's head and they pave the way for the subsequent release of individual cranial bones. Before you start treating your client's head, first carefully palpate and gently massage her scalp. Is it very resistant or does it move easily? Massage using slow, circular movements. Ask your client on the treatment table whether your touch feels pleasant or is too heavy.

When treating the head, begin with the cradle hold (cf. p. 112) and/or the cranial vault hold (cf. p. 196) and listen to the motion of the craniosacral rhythm. This will give you an initial overall impression of the head and the craniosacral rhythm.

As already mentioned with the cradle hold, *you should ensure a sufficient resting surface for your forearms in the various holds and treatment positions involving the head.* By establishing a fulcrum in this way, for example, you reduce the likelihood of slight breathing movements or any tension in your own torso being transmitted to your client on the treatment table. It is especially important to eliminate such effects when treating the head.

For most head positions it is recommended that at least half the length of your forearm should be resting on the treatment table. It may be that as she lies down, your client can shift down a little toward the foot-end of the table, although her heels should still be resting on the table. Otherwise a blanket or a table extension may help you to create a larger resting surface so that you can be stable and relaxed as you palpate and treat.

Before starting to treat the head, it is important that you perform a whole-body assessment and release any tension patterns in the transverse connective tissue layers, cranial base, sacroiliac joints and sacrum.

After all, how can the cranial bones move freely in time with the subtle craniosacral rhythm if the muscle and ligament attachments to the cranium, especially to the cranial base, are acting to restrict the craniosacral system?

Releasing the cranial bones and intracranial membranes

Basic principles

Craniosacral therapy of the head encourages the natural free motion of the cranial bones at their sutural articulations. This also promotes the release of tension in the intracranial membranes (*dura mater, arachnoid, pia mater*) and other intracranial structures (falx cerebri, falx cerebelli, tentorium cerebelli). The release of tension in one structure increases its motility as well as the mobility of the craniosacral system as a whole.

Do not start releasing the cranial bones until you have a sufficiently large resting surface for your forearms and you are seated at the correct height.

If you are a beginner, I recommend that before using any release techniques on your client's head, you should first have palpated and thoroughly familiarized yourself with the cranial regions on your own head. This self-palpation will bolster your confidence regarding the shape and location of the cranial bones before you use your fingers to palpate the structure of your client's head and will help you then to position your fingers accurately.

Detailed anatomical knowledge of the position of the individual cranial bones and an ability to locate them exactly is a prerequisite for properly informed treatment of the head. Illustrations depicting the most important cranial bones, the cranial sutures and the intracranial membrane system, together with details of nomenclature, can be found under The anatomy – an illustrated account, p. 15 and in any anatomy atlas. The figures in this chapter highlight the particular zone being treated in each case when releasing the cranial bones. The motion and qualities of the craniosacral rhythm are described on p. 49.

When releasing cranial tension, it is important that you as the practitioner should remain relaxed, as should your hands as they palpate and treat. Empty your mind of all thoughts, and enter increasingly into a state of stillness. Without exerting any pressure, allow your hands to blend with the cranial region being palpated and to listen passively so that they can sense the motion that is the expression of the Breath of Life.

The following sections presuppose an understanding of the theoretical and practical concepts outlined earlier in this book. References to 'treatment', 'lifting' or 'compression' should not be construed as firm manipulation but rather as a subtle invitation to the areas in question to let go, to relax. And even during these times of clear, gentle touch to release structures in your client's head, keep listening simultaneously for signals from the structure in response to your invitation indicating whether or when it wishes spontaneously to let go.

In between individual tension release techniques for the head and at the end of the session, use the cradle hold to listen to motion at the occiput and use the cranial vault hold to listen to the motion of individual or multiple structures at the same time. While doing this, make a before-and-after comparison.

In a structural basic treatment, release of cranial bones is often performed in the following sequence:

- frontal bone
- parietal bones
- sphenoid
- temporal bones.

Achieving the right quality of touch or 'Less is more'

- The 'traction' applied for cranial release is generally just 1–3 g, and *never* more than 5 g.

While the direction of release or compression is almost merely hinted at, it should nevertheless be felt subtly at the structural level while being hardly or only minimally perceived by the client. *Always remain below the treatment intensity* that would be classified as intrusive by the cranial suture receptors and the autonomic nervous system. This will avoid the situation in which the tissues seek to protect themselves – a natural defensive response – and consequently contract.

Also, by adopting the correct position at the treatment table, by purposefully checking your physical and emotional distance, and by allowing sufficient space, you will determine to a major degree whether or not your touch (and any subsequent structural release) is perceived as being harmonious. Brief enquiry will help you to correct your touch and to adapt to your client's wishes.

Listening to the body's self-corrective process and inviting release

Once your fingers are positioned accurately and the quality of your touch feels appropriate and pleasant, *listen* at these points without seeking to achieve anything. As you are patiently present and without any personal agenda, listen to the craniosacral rhythm and to the subtle changes that reveal themselves in the stillness. For the moment, listen to the body's own self-corrective process.

If the body's self-corrective mechanisms are impaired (e.g. due to a fall), compressions and adhesions at the sites in question can be released using specific techniques.

Release the individual cranial bones slowly and using constant, gentle, sustained traction or compression. In all this, remember that your clear, yet subtle impulse transmission as an 'invitation to let go' requires time until the cranial sutures begin to expand and widen slightly. Consequently, less 'traction' is often more effective and – to make up for this – it is usually performed for longer, i.e. from about 20 seconds up to about 1–2 min.

Via the cranial bones, you are encouraging two levels of release: the cranial bone level and the membrane/meningeal level. This automatically supports the *third level – that of the cerebrospinal fluid (CSF)*. The CSF carries a highly intelligent healing and self-regulating potency that is able to express

Tips for beginners

At the same time, beginners should be careful not to perform the following release techniques for too long. After each individual release, you can listen again for a few cycles at the site in question in order to sense whether any change has occurred and to encourage its integration. Afterward you can switch at any time to the cradle hold and/or the cranial vault hold and listen – What is your overall impression now? How is the craniosacral rhythm now? How is it now compared with before? A session is rarely concluded at the client's head but is rounded off, for example, by listening at the sacrum and feet.

You do not need to perform all the techniques at all positions in a single session – the priority is for treatment to be stress-free and attentive. However, in order to achieve more comprehensive release throughout the craniosacral system as a whole, you should not limit yourself exclusively to individual treatment techniques. Make the most of the wide range of possibilities to enhance your structural skills in all positions of this full basic treatment.

itself more freely if release occurs not only at the bone level but also particularly at the membrane level. It is therefore vitally important to allow sufficient time for the careful release of the cranial bones. Through the connective tissue collagen and elastin fibers that unite the sutures, your unhurried, light lifting impulse facilitates gentle release at the bone level. And it is not just the cranial sutures that become freer as a result. At the same time, via the meninges underneath, the intracranial membrane system – a reciprocal tension membrane – is gently stretched and relaxed. For all the reasons stated, it is important to perform release techniques continuously.

Releasing the frontal bone

Take up a position at the top end of the treatment table (near your client's head)

Using both ring fingers, palpate left and right at the outer end of your client's eyebrows for the small (rounded, hump-like) prominences at the lateral edges of the frontal bone and place your ring fingers immediately behind them. As you do this, make sure that you are touching the frontal bone and not the sphenoid wings. Then without pressure, establish broad contact over the frontal bone with your middle and index fingers. Your thumbs may touch in the middle of the frontal bone and, in energetic terms, create a connection between the left and right halves of the frontal bone. However, position your thumbs in such a way that they do not project into the coronal suture. Your two little fingers may rest against your ring fingers or may be slightly raised and play no part.

If you do not position your ring fingers accurately, you may touch a suture without meaning to. To avoid this happening, palpate with meticulous exactness or position both ring fingers more toward the middle of the frontal bone.

Make sure that *your fingers are positioned gently and with as broad a contact as possible and that they mold to the shape of the frontal bone*. In this process your palms should be angled slightly and not in contact with the cranium so as to prevent unintentional compression on the nearby coronal suture.

Through your broad finger contact, make a connection with your client's scalp, with the underlying tissues and then with the frontal bone underneath: without any pressure increase, use part of your attention to drop down gently, via the different receptors on your finger surfaces, and 'blend' with the osseous tissue of the frontal bone. Your hands, arms, shoulders and all their joints will probably become even softer.

Then use your palpatory awareness to establish contact with the meninges attached behind the frontal bone and with the inherent CSF fluctuation. You may need to reduce your weight of touch slightly, but without losing clear contact. As this happens, stay passive and relaxed. This makes it easier for the craniosacral rhythm to communicate with you in slow motion via the frontal bone.

Listen to the subtle and natural dynamics of the craniosacral rhythm. At the frontal bone, in simplified form, motion is as follows: in flexion/ER the supine client's frontal bone moves in slow motion up toward your hands, toward the ceiling. At the same time, the lateral parts of the frontal bone become broader while the central part – due to tension exerted by the falx cerebri at the front – shows a tendency to move slightly posteriorly, down toward the treatment table. After flexion/ER, as the direction of motion changes, there is sometimes a brief pause followed by the start of extension/IR. The lateral parts of the frontal bone slowly move back again toward the treatment table, perhaps halting briefly at the innermost point of extension/IR before going again into flexion/ER, and so on. Go with the craniosacral rhythm for several cycles (Fig. 2.7.1 and Fig. 2.7.2A, B).

Listen at the frontal bone and palpate:

- Overall, is the motion clear or almost imperceptible?
- Does this rhythm tend to be slow or fast?
- Do you tend to sense more flexion/ER or more extension/IR?
- Can you sense differences between the left side and the right side?
- Is one lateral part of the frontal bone freer than the other?
- Do the sutures with the nasal bone and orbits or the coronal suture have a freer feel to them?

Go with the next extension/IR motion, during which the lateral parts of the frontal bone slowly move down toward the treatment table (client supine). During subsequent flexion/ER, during which the lateral parts of the frontal bone slowly rise toward your hands, toward the ceiling, attentively support this motion using your ring, middle and index fingers on the frontal bone. Via these fingers you already have a good connection with the bony structure and your ring fingers are located over the

Figure 2.7.1
Direction of motion in flexion (simplified).

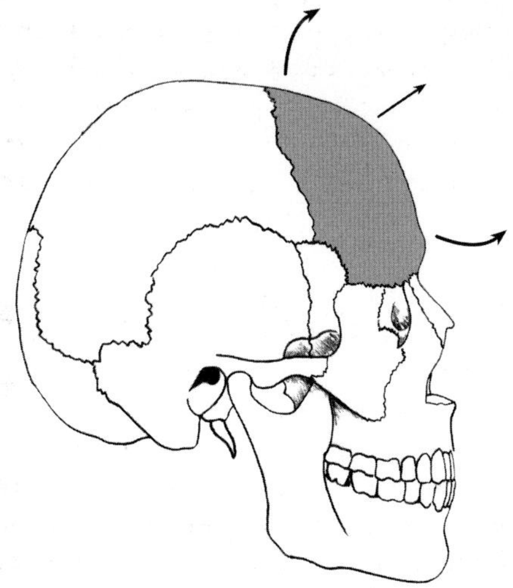

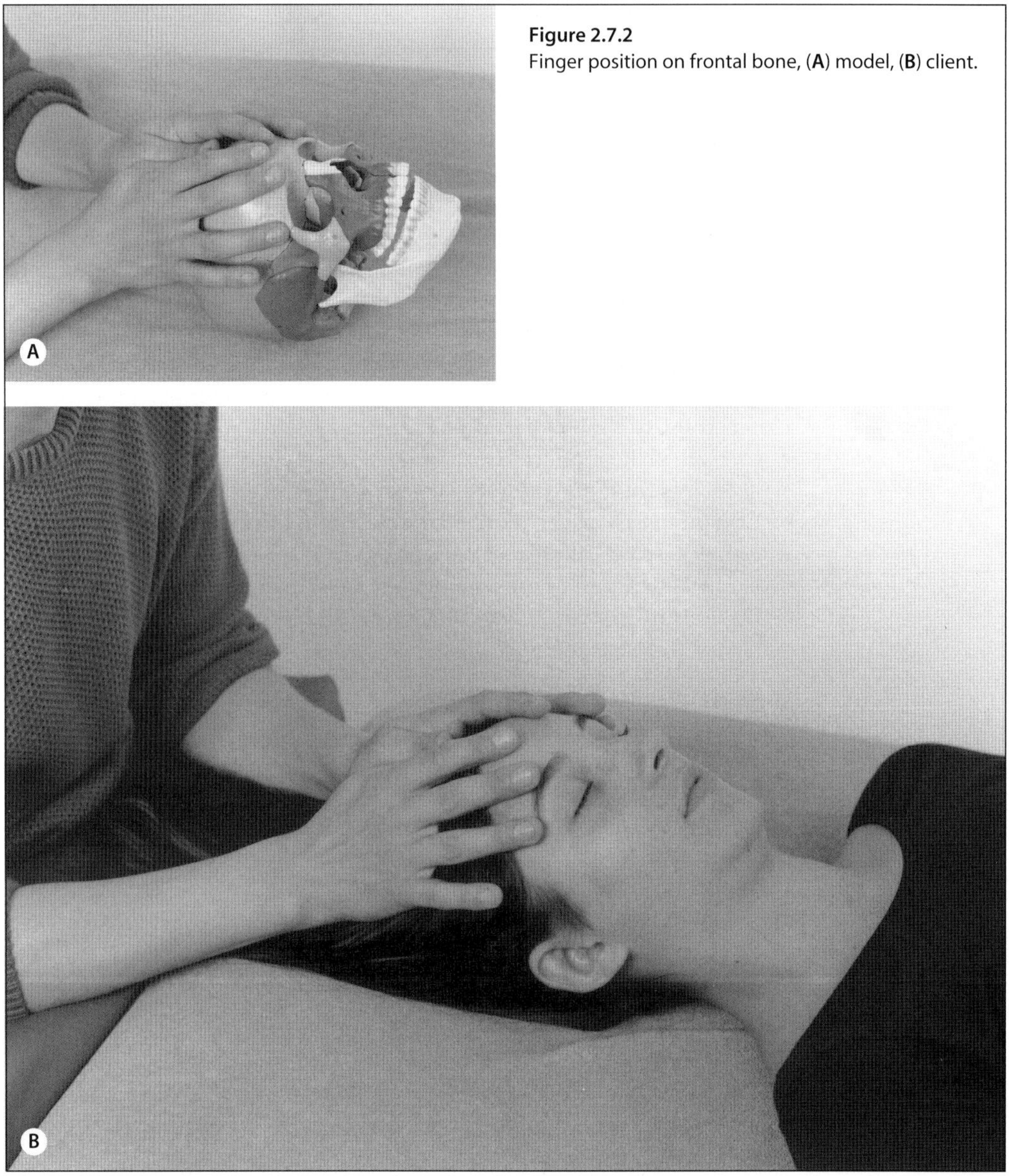

Figure 2.7.2
Finger position on frontal bone, (**A**) model, (**B**) client.

depression at the outer end of the client's eyebrows (or further in toward the middle).

Now, ideally during flexion/ER, slowly, gently and continuously start to lift the frontal bone slightly for about 1–3 min. Do not slacken your lift during the extension/IR phase that resumes afterwards. Maintain your continuous light traction diagonally at about 45° away from the sutures, i.e. simultaneously up toward you and the ceiling. To do this, use a gentle lifting force not greater than 1–3 g. Instead of diagonally at 45° away from the sutures, your light traction on the frontal bone can also be performed anteriorly/up toward the ceiling.

Stay receptive during this continuous light frontal bone lift, and simultaneously listen for release movements of the frontal bone – i.e. for whether, how and where the cranial sutures and meninges start to relax. You will be able to sense these movements more clearly if you continue to regulate your distance vis-à-vis your client and remain relaxed.

With the passage of time it may happen that your index and middle fingers come off from the frontal bone, leaving only your ring fingers (positioned over the small depression at the lateral borders of the frontal bone) to exert light traction. Maintain contact until your ring fingers also slip off upward by themselves. If it has still not been possible to sufficiently and comprehensively release the expansive area of the frontal bone (thus also bringing release to the meninges as well as to the bony structure), reposition your fingers and continue with this release technique. While lifting the frontal bone, you may also find it helpful to imagine your fingers with small suction pads on them.

When the gentle minimal expansion encounters the bony structure of the cranial sutures, this may sometimes feel relatively 'boggy' and inflexible. The more this level is released – perhaps over a period of several craniosacral therapy sessions – the more directly the treatment will act at the membrane level, i.e. at the level of the meninges. By comparison with the bone level, this feels supple and more stretchable, rather similar to a rubber band or an air mattress.

Once you have arrived at the membrane level with your frontal lift, reduce your lifting traction by half. At this level too try not to provoke any resistance. Instead, using sustained continuous traction, subtly stretch the meninges and parts of the falx cerebri. Now listen to the craniosacral rhythm and make a before-and-after comparison.

In general, a sequence of listening and treatment for the frontal bone and the other cranial bones lasts for between 2 and 5 min, depending on how well the sutures and meninges are released or whether they still require more time and treatment sessions, and on the client's response and wishes. A fixed time cannot be specified because the individual process has to be followed and the whole person treated.

Releasing the parietal bones

Take up a position at the top end of the treatment table (near your client's head)

Like the temporal bones with which they articulate at the squamoparietal suture, the two parietal bones are paired plates of cranial bone. They are capable of different types of motion in time with the craniosacral rhythm. In ER, the two parietal bones move outward. The head becomes broader, fuller and more rounded. During IR, the two parietal bones rotate slowly inward, and the head becomes narrower and rather more oval in shape (Fig. 2.7.3).

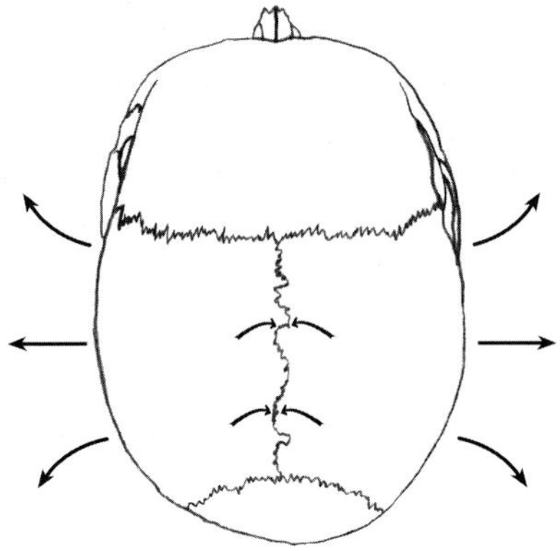

Figure 2.7.3
Direction of motion in flexion (simplified).

Among other things, supporting ER/IR releases the squamoparietal suture between the parietal and temporal bones from adhesions and thus also contributes to the more balanced craniosacral rhythm of all the cranial bones treated here. The superior sagittal sinus beneath the sagittal suture is drained and this brings a decisive improvement in CSF drainage.

Parietal bone release is achieved in several steps

1. Palpate and massage the squamoparietal sutures

With your fingers gently palpate the *squamoparietal sutures* between the parietal and temporal bones; located at the sides of the head, these sutures travel in a semi-circle around the ears, a few centimeters above them. Using circular movements, gently massage these sutures up the sides of the head (in a cranial direction, and avoiding deep pressure). Ask your client for feedback.

2. Locate the exact position

Now place your hands to the left and right of your client's head (with the outer edge of your little fingers resting on the soft covering of the treatment table) and slide them up toward you at the head of the table. Make sure that your terminal phalanges are located *2 cm above (cranial to) the previously massaged squamoparietal sutures.*

To do this, feel at the sides of your client's head for that area where the paired parietal bones begin to arch over markedly (toward the sagittal suture). *Just before they arch over*, find an area where you can palpate the parietal bones on their lateral surfaces. It may be that the terminal phalanges of your index, middle and ring fingers will need to work their way through the client's hair so that as far as possible they are *in clear contact with her scalp.*

3. Accurate, clear and spacious touch

Rest your *index and ring fingers* against your *middle finger* so that the *three together form a compact surface*. The terminal phalanges of your fingers should now be taking up the broadest possible contact with the two parietal bones. As you sense the client's scalp, blend with the *bony structure* through the contact surfaces of your fingers. Your two thumbs are angled slightly and may be touching each other or crossing over. They thus form a fulcrum and so provide stability. Your thumbs should be at a sufficient distance from the client's head; never compress this sometimes sensitive area (Fig. 2.7.4A, B).

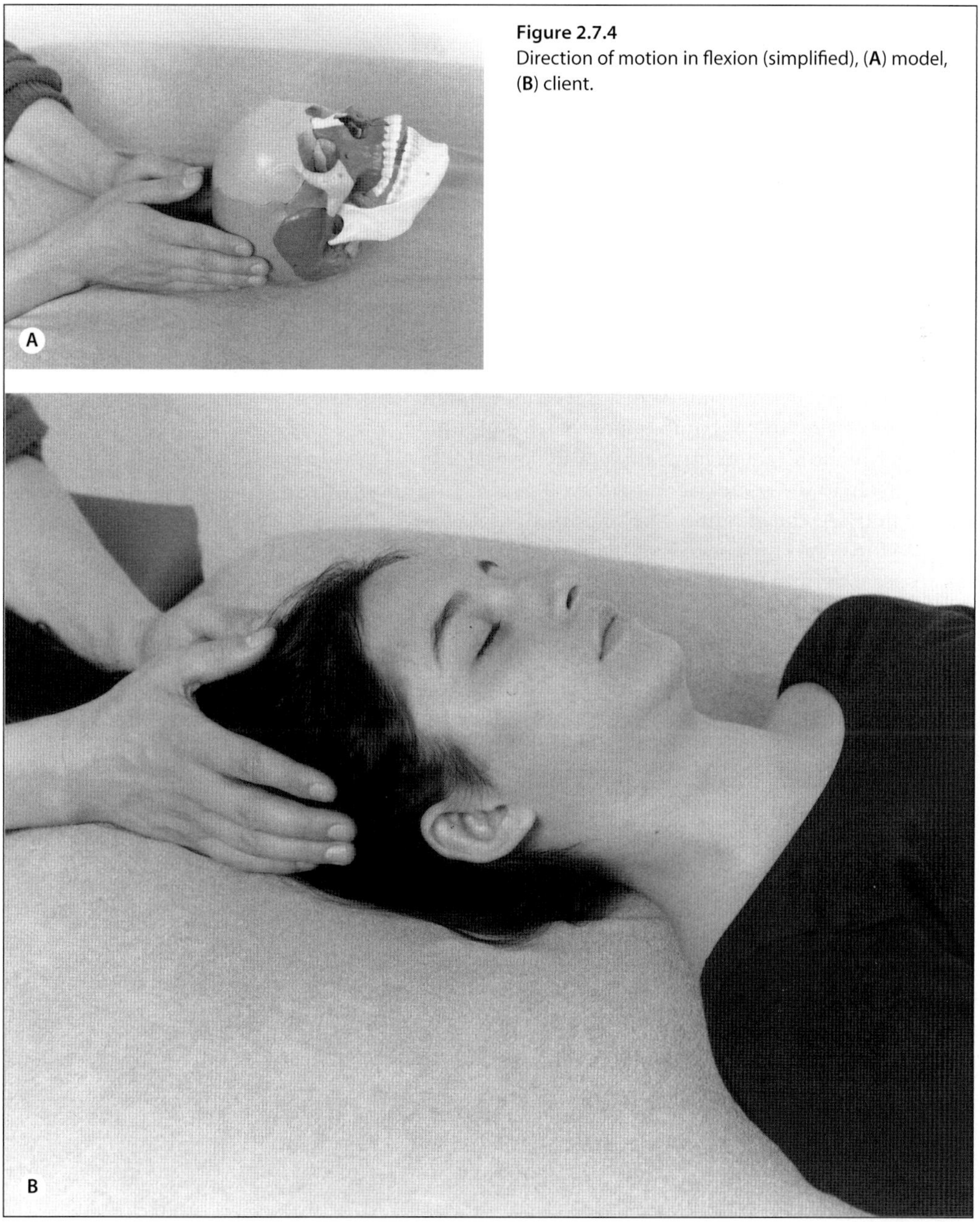

Figure 2.7.4
Direction of motion in flexion (simplified), (**A**) model, (**B**) client.

4. *Listen to the craniosacral rhythm*

Your fingers, hands, wrists, arms and shoulders should be free from tension – in fact, your whole body should stay relaxed. Are you sufficiently grounded and centered? Have you regulated your distance sufficiently?

Now listen to the motion of the craniosacral rhythm at the parietal bones. You may sense this more clearly if your level of perception remains clearly in contact with the bone level, while your sensory and intuitive awareness simultaneously also *extends to the level of the meninges and of CSF fluctuation*. If you listen to the stillness, then the slow craniosacral rhythm becomes more clearly perceptible. What are its qualities? How does external/internal rotation (ER/IR) reveal itself on the left side, and on the right side?

5. *Supporting internal rotation (IR)*

Follow ER and IR several times and then decide to support the next IR motion using your finger contact. Go with IR and *gently exaggerate this motion*. This may feel like a gentle compression of the two parietal bones (during IR, medially). When ER occurs, go with it but do not apply any compression at all. When IR recurs, go with it again using clear compression that is barely more than a suggestion. You can repeat this support and slight exaggeration of IR several times. However, always listen to the craniosacral rhythm and actively support its motion in IR. At the innermost point of IR do not use compression either to force the craniosacral system further into IR or to prevent the craniosacral rhythm from going into ER. Always go with the craniosacral rhythm.

6. *Gentle cranial lift on the parietal bones*

Re-establish broad contact with your index, middle and ring fingers at the same location, as described above under 2. Your thumbs may be touching or crossing over again, providing stability, but are not in contact with the client's cranium or hair.

Again go with ER/IR. Can you sense approximately the midpoint or neutral position of these two physiological motions?

Now using both sets of finger surfaces simultaneously (if possible in the neutral position or ER), start *gently lifting the two parietal bones cranially, i.e. toward the top of the client's head*, toward you. Maintain this almost imperceptible, evenly light decompression for about 1–2 min. At the same time, keep listening attentively: Are the structures on both sides releasing evenly? Or is one side releasing more easily, better, more smoothly?

With the resultant release of their cranial sutures (coronal, squamoparietal and lambdoid sutures), the parietal bones together with the meninges and in particular the falx cerebri will be subtly stretched and mobilized.

7. Listening to ER/IR motion, before-and-after comparison
Now listen again to ER/IR for several cycles. Has the motion altered? If so, how? Is the craniosacral rhythm stronger, more balanced? Is the release of the paired parietal bones (which cover a large area of the cranium) also affecting the neighboring cranial bones, e.g. the frontal bone treated previously? If so, how?

At any time you may specifically palpate individual bones, switch to the cradle hold or cranial vault hold and make a *before-and-after comparison*.

Going with the motion of the sphenoid

The sphenoid occupies the most central position of all 22 cranial bones. All the components of the cranium and intracranial structures are in direct or indirect continuity with the sphenoid and are influenced by its position and motion, and vice versa.

Together with the occiput (and the petrous bones), the sphenoid bone forms the main part of the cranial base. The articulation that connects the two is known as the sphenobasilar joint or sphenobasilar synchondrosis (SBS). It possesses no interdigitating articulated connections and is a long, cartilaginous structure that does not become ossified until the age of about 18–25 years. The definitions of flexion and extension relate to the motion of the pterygoid (or winged) processes of the sphenoid and of the occipital condyles, viewed from the (external) inferior cranial base:

- The pterygoid processes and occipital condyles move toward each other = flexion, flexion motion, bending.
- The pterygoid processes and occipital condyles move away from each other = extension, extension motion, stretching.

Shaped rather like a butterfly, the sphenoid bone traverses the cranium horizontally and can be palpated externally at its two greater wings in the temporal region (Fig. 2.7.5).

Figure 2.7.5
Sphenoid motion in flexion, simplified.

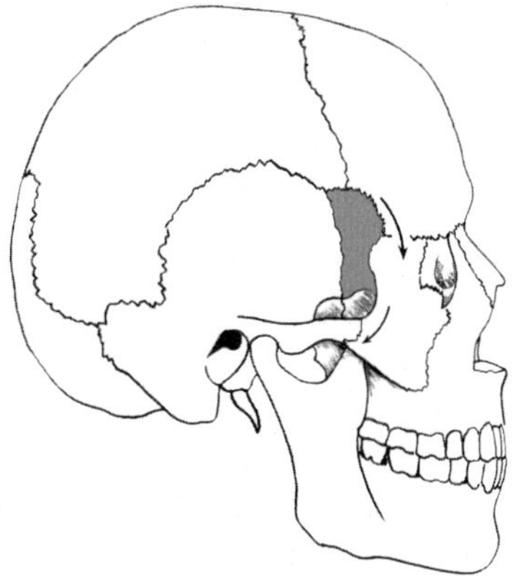

Experience suggests that a balancing and integrating effect on the sphenoid can already be achieved by gently touching the two sphenoid wings, then tuning in to its subtle motion in flexion and extension, and going with the craniosacral motion in a relaxed manner.

Because the illustrated release of multiple cranial bones creates altogether more space for all cranial components, this also benefits the sphenoid in its central location. Any attentive treatment will therefore improve its balance and motion.

Important points

For the moment be careful not to perform any manipulation on the sphenoid and do not treat it in isolation. The sphenoid and temporal region may be sensitive to pressure. The following general rules therefore apply:

Contact should be without pressure; touch that is gentle yet clear is sufficient (ask for feedback).

Deliberate correction of sphenoid dysfunctions should be undertaken only by practitioners with sufficient course experience (including supervised work), and should never be attempted if the craniosacral rhythm cannot be palpated clearly over several cycles.

Take up a position at the top end of the treatment table (near your client's head)

With open palms upward, place your hands on the treatment table, one on each side of the client's head. Leading with your little fingers, slip your hands in sideways toward the middle, toward the occiput.

Now carefully feel at the sides of the client's head for the two greater wings of the sphenoid: locate an area with a softer feel in the temporal region, roughly level with her eyes and at the outer edge of the eyebrows. The sphenoid wings are located there in a tiny depression, and are lightly covered over with muscles and other tissues.

Carefully position your thumbs to establish as broad a contact as possible with the left and right sphenoid wings. Do not apply firm pressure and keep your fingers, hands, wrists, elbows, shoulders and torso relaxed (Fig. 2.7.6A, B). Sense your pelvis, legs and feet and become grounded. Ask for feedback about how your touch feels – e.g. your client can rate your touch intensity on a scale from 1 (= wonderfully light) to 5 (= highly unpleasant, release contact).

Motion/terminology

Now listen to and go with the motion of the sphenoid. Use the contact surfaces of your thumbs to go with the *motion into flexion*, signaled by a slow, fine tilting movement away from you, toward your client's

Figure 2.7.6
Finger position on the sphenoid, (**A**) model, (**B**) client.

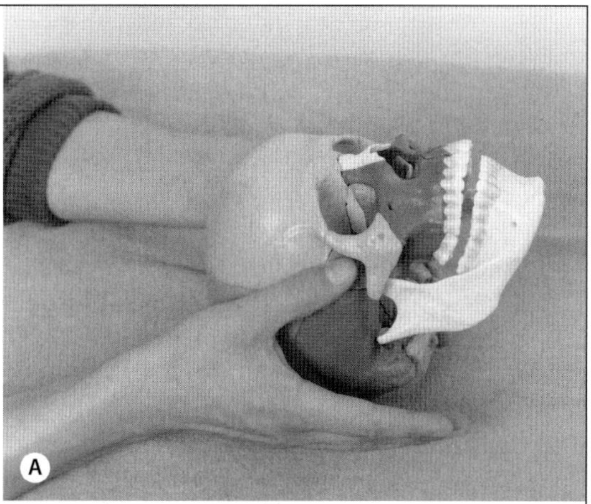

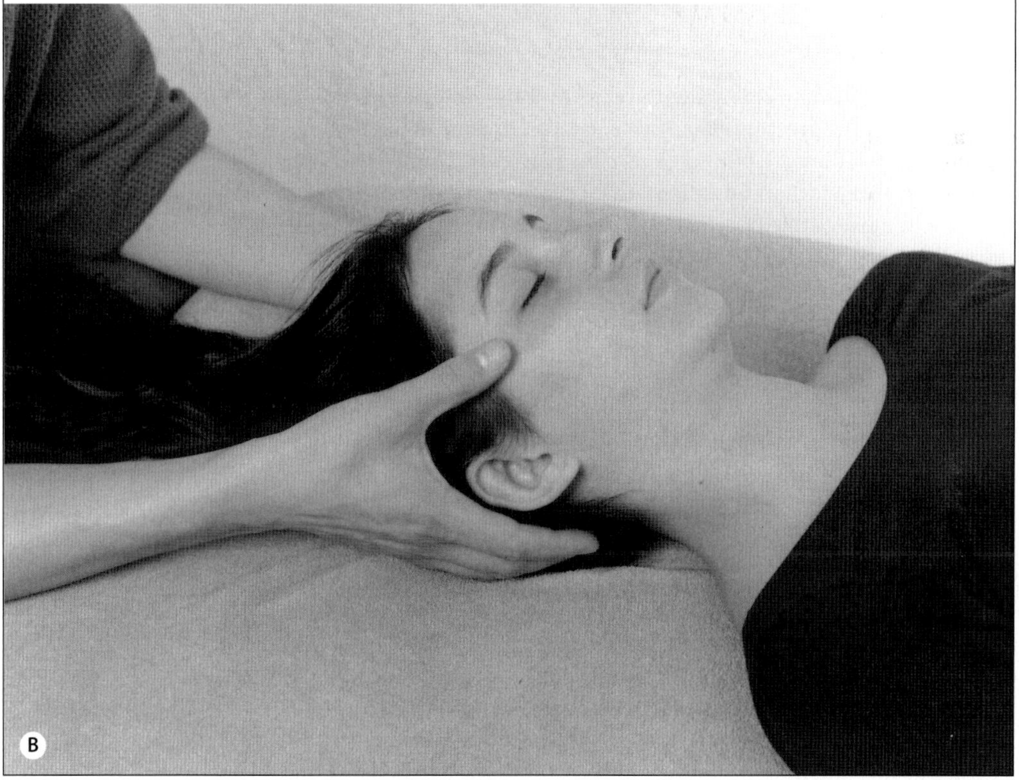

feet. Similarly, go with the *motion into extension* marked by a fine tilting movement toward you, toward the top of your client's head. With your little fingers at the occiput, you may also sense its motion into flexion and extension. If your hands are too small or your client's head is too large for you to place your little fingers on the occiput without straining, leave it. Listen attentively and go with the physiological motion that you sense in your thumbs.

These movements are extremely subtle and it requires considerable practice, centeredness and patience to clearly sense motion into flexion and extension. Use this listening station simply as a further opportunity to hone your palpation skills.

Once you can clearly sense these tilting movements toward your client's body and head, try as you palpate to form an idea of the location of the midpoint of the motion – and hence the *neutral position*. Do not perform *any manipulation on the sphenoid*, but go with the motion that reveals itself. You may also be able to palpate whether the sphenoid moves more into flexion or more into extension, or whether other motion patterns become apparent; make a mental note of this.

Listen for several cycles to establish whether and how the craniosacral rhythm balances itself. If you are able to perceive this motion, then release the broad contact of your thumbs and little fingers by taking your hands away to the sides, ideally during neutral.

Alternative

Instead of establishing contact with your thumbs, you can position *your index fingers* at the greater wings of the sphenoid. Your hands will not be overstretched if they are placed *more to the side* of the client's head (instead of snug up against it). In this alternative option, your loose finger and wrist joints facilitate accurate positioning. Locate your little fingers laterally on the occiput. (For further details, see Cranial vault hold, p. 196.)

Releasing the temporal bones

Take up a position at the top end of the treatment table (near your client's head)

The two temporal bones are also very interesting because of their anatomy and physiological motion. In the region of the cranial base, the petrous parts of the temporal bones housing the auditory canal communicate medially with the sphenoid and occiput. In addition, the *temporomandibular joints (TMJs)* articulate with the temporal bones close to the ears and are principally responsible for the movement of the mandible (lower jaw) and for occlusion (bite).

Due to broadening of the skull in ER, the temporal bones rotate toward the facial bones, and simultaneously *outward*, especially in the vicinity of the squamoparietal suture (Fig. 2.7.7). In IR, the temporal bones rotate toward the occiput and simultaneously *inward* in the vicinity of the squamoparietal suture. In the following sections, three methods are explained in detail for releasing the paired temporal bones. *They may be combined at will. In each case, take up a position at the top end of the treatment table (near your client's head).*

Finger-in-ear position: going with the motion of the two temporal bones

Place the outer edge of your hands vertically on the treatment table to the left and right of the client's head. Bring your left middle finger up to

Figure 2.7.7
Direction of temporal bone motion in flexion (simplified).

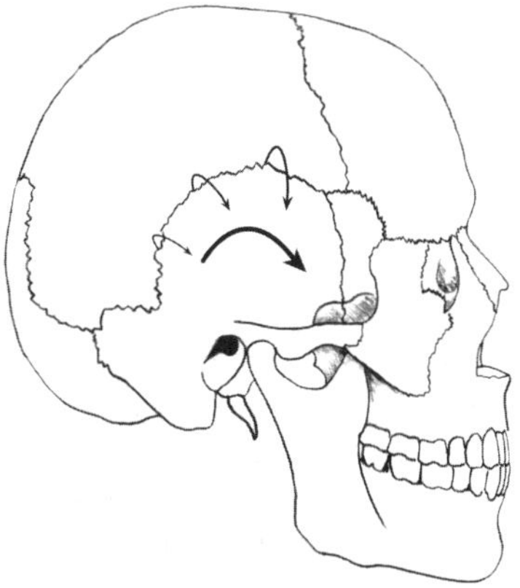

your client's left auditory canal, and your right middle finger up to her right auditory canal. Make sure you do not exert any pressure because your middle fingers in the client's ears are intended merely as rotational axes. With your index fingers now feel for the zygomatic arches. One part of the zygomatic arch belongs to the temporal bone, and the other to the zygomatic bone. It is therefore important that you position your index fingers on the part of the zygomatic arch that belongs to the temporal bone, i.e. about 1–2 cm away from the auditory canal. Place your index fingers there with their terminal phalanges achieving as broad a contact as possible. Position your ring fingers directly behind the ear/ear lobe on the mastoid process on each side. Without tension in your hands and fingers direct your attention then to these sites where your index and ring fingers are listening to the slow rhythm of the temporal bones. While doing this keep your middle fingers in the auditory canal without pressure (Fig. 2.7.8A–C).

Palpate the motion of the temporal bones and go with it. Is the tilting movement outward in ER and toward the facial bones greater than the opposite motion in IR, toward the occiput? If you sense motion: where is its midpoint, the neutral position? How does the left side move compared with the right side: are they synchronous or different?

Releasing the mastoid processes

The mastoid process is located immediately behind the ear and is a conical projection downward (toward the feet/caudally) from the posterior part of the temporal bone, roughly behind the ear lobes. Feel for the bony mastoid processes on the left and right side (Fig. 2.7.9A, B on p. 188).

Place your hands to the right and left of your client's head, close to her shoulders and neck. Move your fingers under her neck so that they overlap: to do this, press your fingers and hands lightly into the padded surface of the treatment table, then slip your loose fingers under the middle of the client's neck so that they overlap. Now carefully move your hands to the left and right of her spine cranially and position your *thenar eminences* on each side immediately behind her ears at the mastoid processes. If you cannot quite get this positioning right, even after some

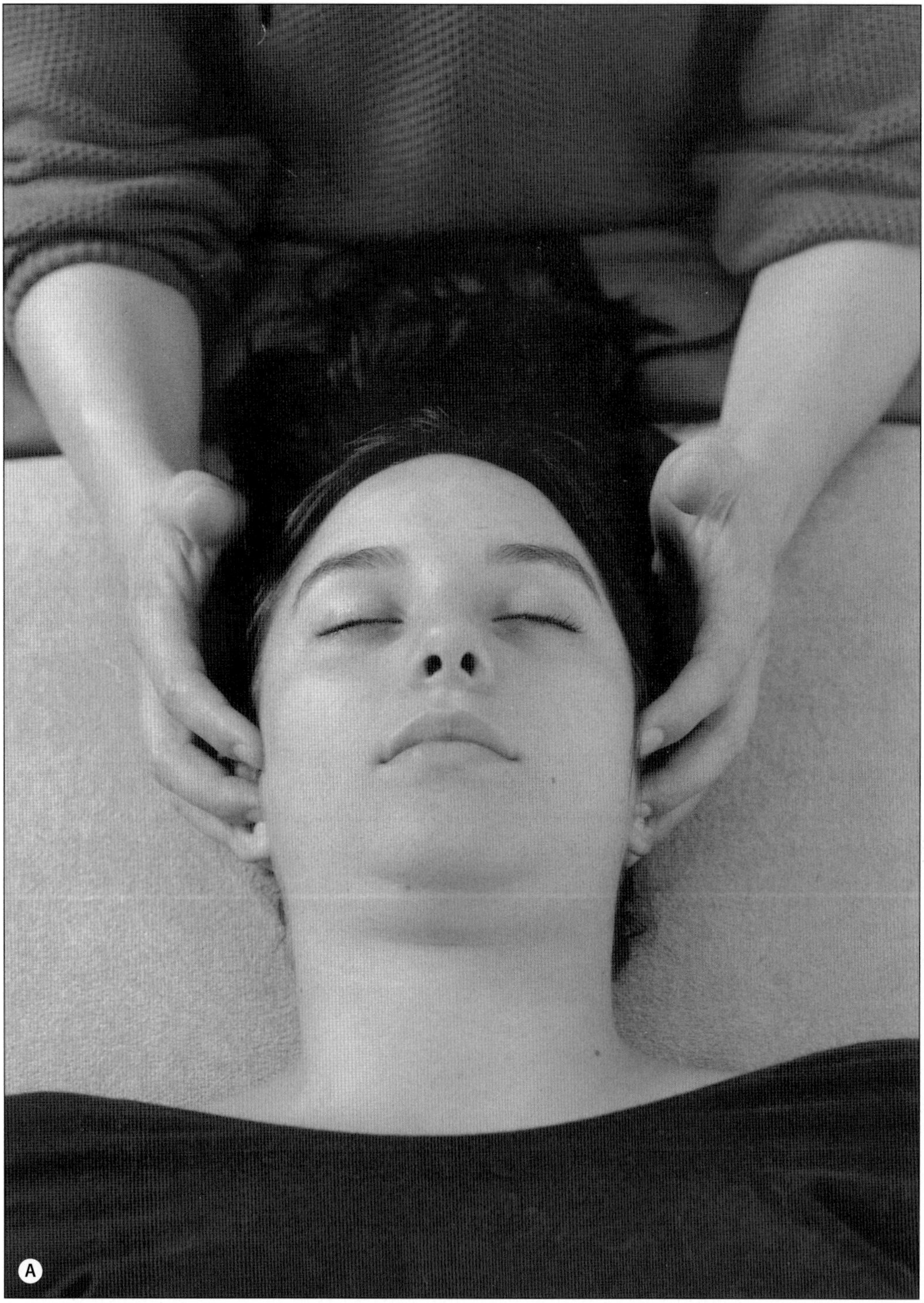

Figure 2.7.8
(**A–C**) Finger-in-ear position (*Continued on next page*).

Figure 2.7.8 *(Continued)*

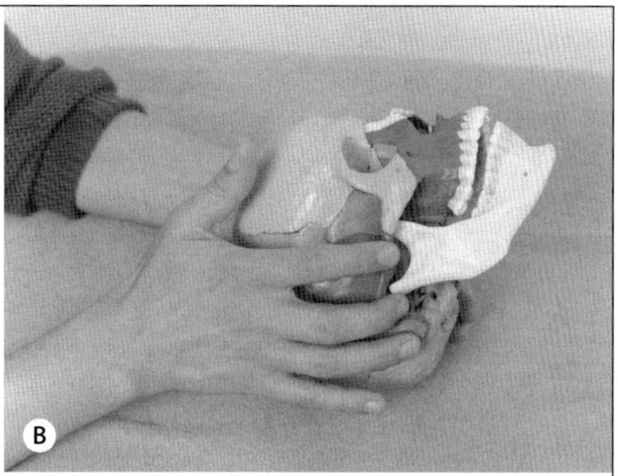

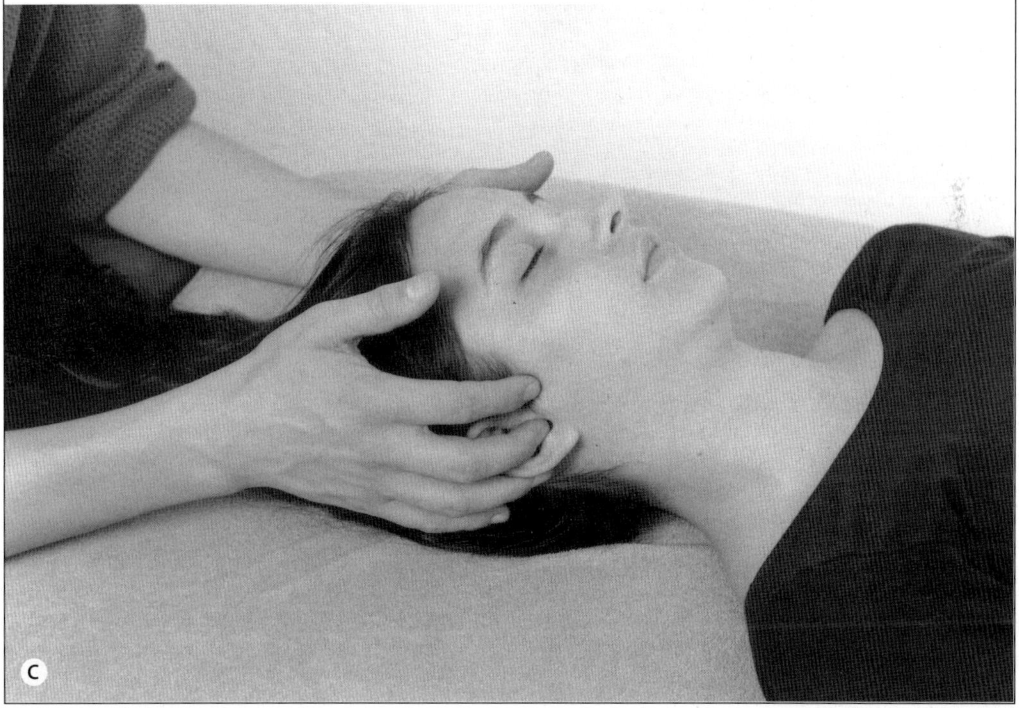

practice, your client may also gently raise her head so that you can adjust your thenar eminences accurately and comfortably. To keep your client's head as horizontal as possible, allow the weight of your hands to sink into the padded surface.

Your fingers are now slightly overlapping under your client's neck muscles, and your hands and both thenar eminences should stay relaxed. Make sure that you do not exert any pressure toward the torso of your supine client, but instead, via the contact between your thenar eminences and her mastoid processes, *slowly* perform very fine traction in a cranial

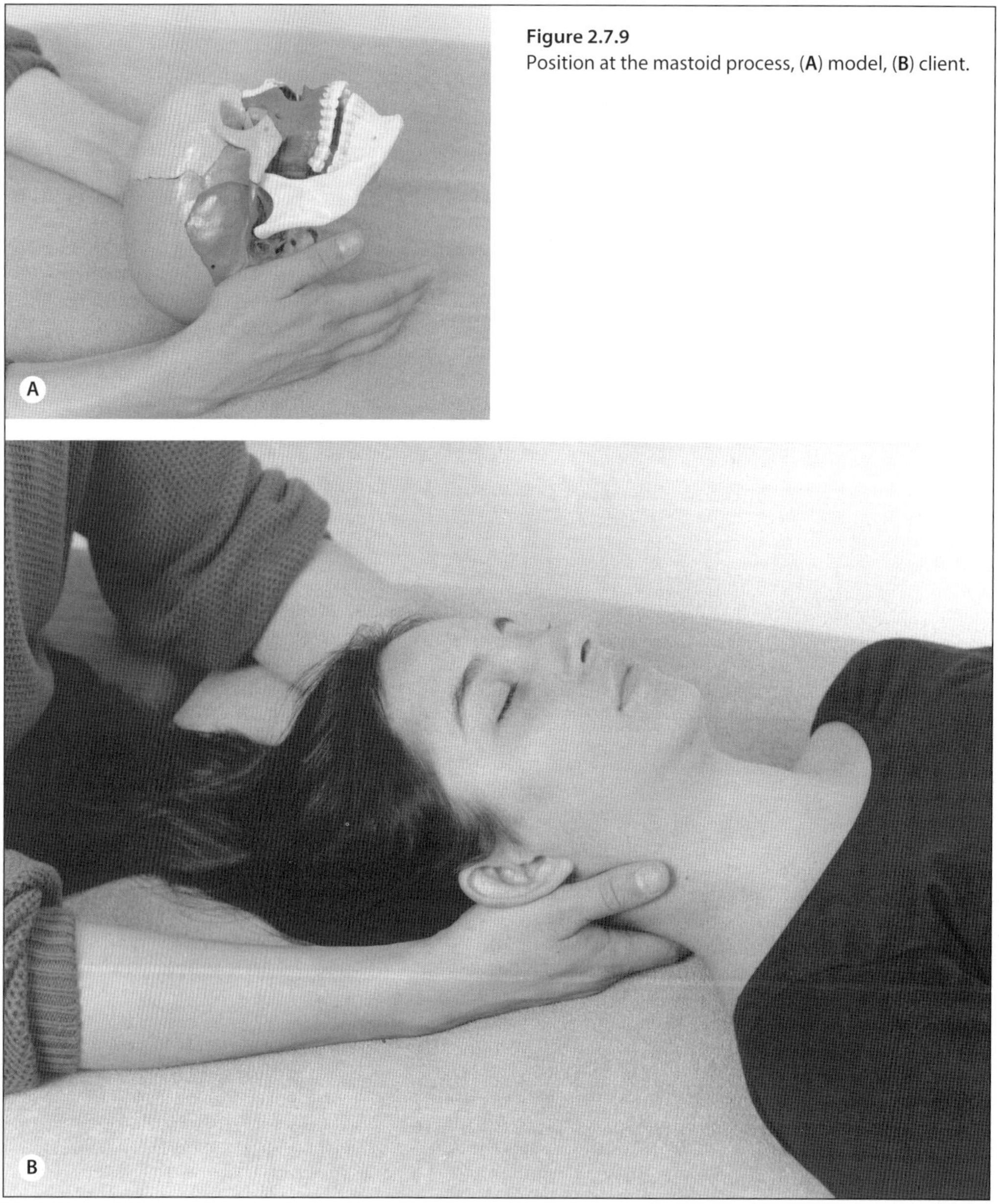

Figure 2.7.9
Position at the mastoid process, (**A**) model, (**B**) client.

direction. This often acts to release tension in the neck muscles and cervical spine.

With both thenar eminences now contact and feel consciously for the bony substance of the two mastoid processes, as if you were blending with them. During motion of the temporal bones in ER the mastoid processes move inward (medially). During IR of the temporal bones the mastoid processes move outward (laterally). Palpate this fine motion with your thenar eminences. How does it feel? Is it evenly expressed or different on the left and right sides?

Go with this medial–lateral motion of the mastoid processes for a few cycles. Lightly support this motion during the next inward (medial) rotation so as to gently amplify *the IR of the two mastoid processes*. As above, when supporting ER/IR of the two temporal bones, also make certain at the mastoid processes that you always go with the craniosacral rhythm, i.e. that you are not working against it. You can support and amplify IR of the mastoid processes, but at the innermost point of IR do not exert any compression; instead go with it again into ER. Afterwards, listen to ER/IR for several cycles: Is the craniosacral rhythm now balanced? Perhaps you need to repeat the gentle, mere hint of compression at the mastoid processes during IR several times – but always with the craniosacral rhythm. In this way you will encourage the motion of the paired temporal bones overall and help them and the entire region – including the cranial base and the now slightly expanded squamoparietal suture – to experience greater release.

Gentle ear pull (ear pull technique)

Via the connective tissues and the bony substance of the temporal bones, the auricle (or external ear) and the auditory canal are continuous with the dura mater and thus indirectly with the entire intracranial membrane system. The tentorium cerebelli covers the cerebellum like a tent and has attachments left and right to the petrous parts of the two temporal bones.

Gentle pulling on the auricle directly releases the temporal bones, but also indirectly causes subtle stretching of the dura mater and, in particular, of the tentorium cerebelli. With this procedure, it is again important to calculate the intensity of pull extremely finely so as not to provoke the tissues into contraction, but instead to invite release.

With your hands relaxed, place them on the treatment table next to your client's ears. Position each thumb in the bottom third of the cartilage of her external ear (not in her auditory canal). With your index and middle fingers take hold of the back of the ear cartilage, without excessive pressure (Fig. 2.7.10).

Relax and deliberately ground yourself. Then with both hands very gently offer just a suggestion of steady and continuous traction sideways, away from your client's head. At the same time listen and simply be open to any possible direction of motion that you perceive in your left or right hand: go with it in the direction of ease that is revealed, both outward (laterally) as well as up and down (cranially/caudally). If you sense resistance, stop but maintain the steady gentle ear pull. Go with it into the new free direction only if further release is evident. This is similar to gentle 'unwinding' in which the direction of free motion is always supported and any limit of motion is accepted.

After you have supported the temporal bones, and through them indirectly the tentorium cerebelli, in their spontaneous free motion via the external ear, you may additionally define a clear direction in order to

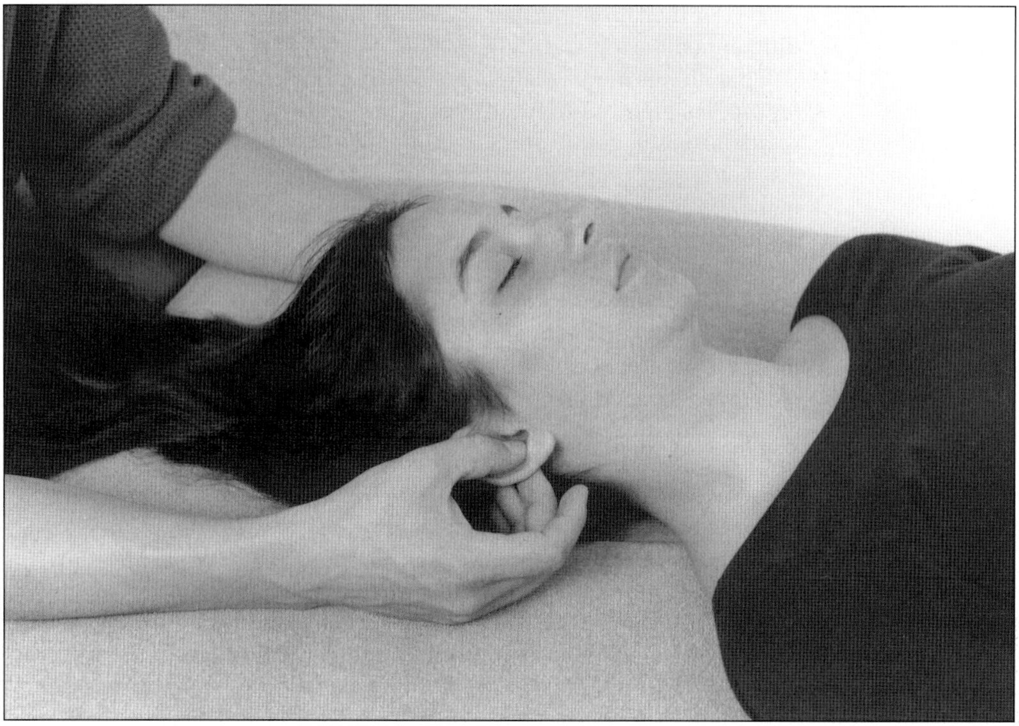

Figure 2.7.10
Finger position for gentle ear pull.

release these structures more specifically. For this, place gentle traction on both external ears simultaneously along an oblique, posterolateral line that would roughly be an extension of the petrous part of the temporal bone, i.e. slightly to the side and toward the client's occiput. Then release the gentle ear pull and let go of the external ear. Now use the finger-in-ear position at the mastoid process, the cradle hold or the cranial vault hold to listen to the craniosacral rhythm. Has anything changed, and if so, what? Is the craniosacral rhythm clearer, more balanced, and if so, how?

The finger-in-ear position, mastoid process release and gentle ear pull technique may be performed individually or may be combined in whatever sequence you wish. The gentle ear pull is also suitable as an integrative technique to conclude the three temporal bone release techniques.

The following positions and techniques can be used in any combination following cranial bone release:

- still point invitation/induction
- dural tube release
- cranial vault hold.

Releasing the temporomandibular joints

2.8

The temporomandibular joints (TMJs) are frequently under considerable tension or found to be restricted. Some of the muscles involved in chewing are among the most powerful in the human body, enabling trapeze artists, for example, to suspend their whole body weight by hanging from their teeth. Concepts such as food utilization, aggression, combativeness, anger, and 'gritting your teeth', not to mention laughter and pleasure, have resonant associations with the TMJ region and lower jaw. If the lower jaw is relaxed, then experience from the fields of biodynamics and bioenergetics suggests that half the body is relaxed.

The position of the temporal bones, with which the TMJs articulate, exerts a decisive influence on the position of the lower jaw and hence also on tooth alignment and correct bite (Fig. 2.8.1).

Never treat the lower jaw in isolation or using powerful manipulation.

Treatment of the TMJs via the lower jaw should be preceded by release techniques at the sacrum, thoracic inlet, hyoid bone, cranial base (atlanto-occipital release) and both temporal bones.

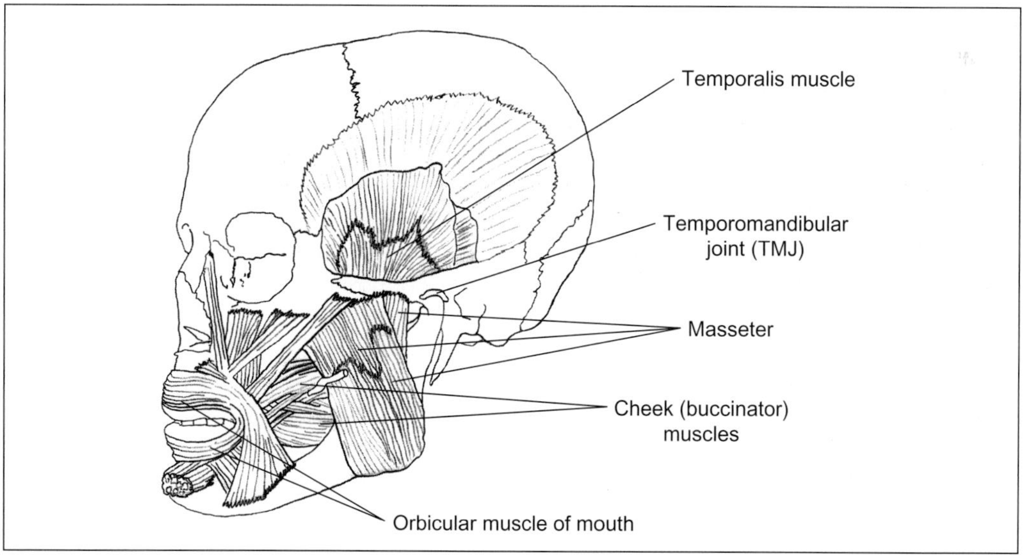

Figure 2.8.1
Masticatory muscles (*temporalis, masseter*), cheek muscles and the circular muscle (*orbicularis oris*) that closes the mouth.

Massaging the masticatory muscles

Together with the large temporalis muscle and the temporal fascia, the muscles involved in chewing extend well up into the territory of the frontal and parietal bones, with some even reaching the greater wing of the sphenoid. The powerful masseter muscles and the lateral pterygoid muscles extend laterally and below the TMJ on each side.

Release your own masticatory muscles, for example, by not clenching your teeth or by deliberately allowing your lower jaw to drop. At this point, refer back to the self-treatment section on *massaging your own masticatory muscles* (p. 166).

Employing circular movements, massage your client's masticatory muscles, establishing as broad a contact as possible using the terminal phalanges of your fingers, but without touching the TMJ itself. Pressure sensitivity is highly individual, especially in the vicinity of the TMJ muscles. Ask your supine client about the intensity of pressure she finds acceptable.

Start above the auditory canal and TMJ by massaging the temporalis muscle upward toward the cranial vault, and then continue below the auditory canal and TMJ by massaging the masseter downward as far as the lower jaw. Then remove your hands and allow your client time to enjoy the ongoing effects.

Releasing the lower jaw

This should never be done in isolation from the treatment techniques described above. Your touch should be clear and light and should allow the entire TMJ region ample time to let go. As is usual in craniosacral therapy, never force anything here; instead, issue an invitation to the connective tissues and muscles in this region (and via the lower jaw to the TMJ) to become widened and softened, to permit themselves to relax.

Perform the additional option of compression–decompression using the indirect–direct technique: first go a short way into the range of tension to identify the existing usual direction of pull – offer light compression into the abnormal restriction pattern, but do not go beyond the limit of motion in the process. Then slowly go in the opposite direction (= decompression) to invite release carefully, patiently and steadily. As soon as you sense the least tissue resistance, pause and wait for the restriction to resolve. Then use gentle decompression to go again with the further subtle releases of the lower jaw.

Take up a position at the top end of the treatment table (near your client's head)

After gently massaging the masticatory muscles, rest the outer edges of your hands vertically at either side of your client's head. Broadly and carefully feel for her mandible on both sides using your index, middle and ring fingers. Now take up *broad finger contact* with the mandible, at an angle of about 45° to the padded surface.

Using as much of your finger surfaces as possible, establish clear contact via the skin and connective tissues with the bony element of the lower jaw and 'blend' with it. While doing this, make sure that your hands leave some space either side of your client's head, and under no circumstances compress this with your hands (Fig. 2.8.2A, B).

Once your finger surfaces have blended well with the bone of the lower jaw, slowly offer just a suggestion of compression for a few moments, *directed toward the TMJ*. Can you sense whether one side is more resistant than the other?

Next allow about 2–3 min for the longer decompression in the opposite direction. Again, perform this slowly using uniform, steady and very gentle traction. While doing this listen attentively and accept any 'stop' indicated by the tissues/muscles or TMJ. As soon as you sense the least resistance, pause and wait until the resistance/restriction is resolved. Then continue with decompression or go with the TMJ in the direction of ease.

During this gentle decompression, again performed with as broad a finger contact as possible and at an angle of 45°, try to discriminate the directions of motion you can sense. Does the lower jaw show greater motion up toward the ceiling or down toward your client's feet? During this decompression, can you sense any differences between the left and right side of the lower jaw? Is one side freer than the other? Pause at each 'stop' indicated by the tissues and allow the structure concerned to relax. Then continue with the decompression. Slowly take your hands away upward in the direction of release and allow your client time to enjoy the ongoing effects.

Figure 2.8.2
Finger position on the lower jaw, (**A**) model, (**B**) client (*Continued overleaf*).

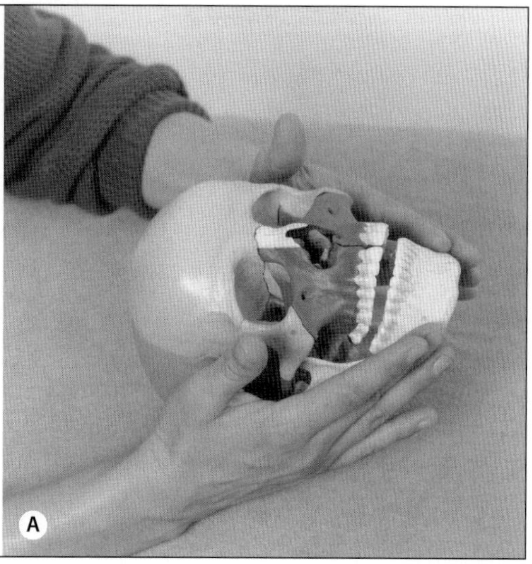

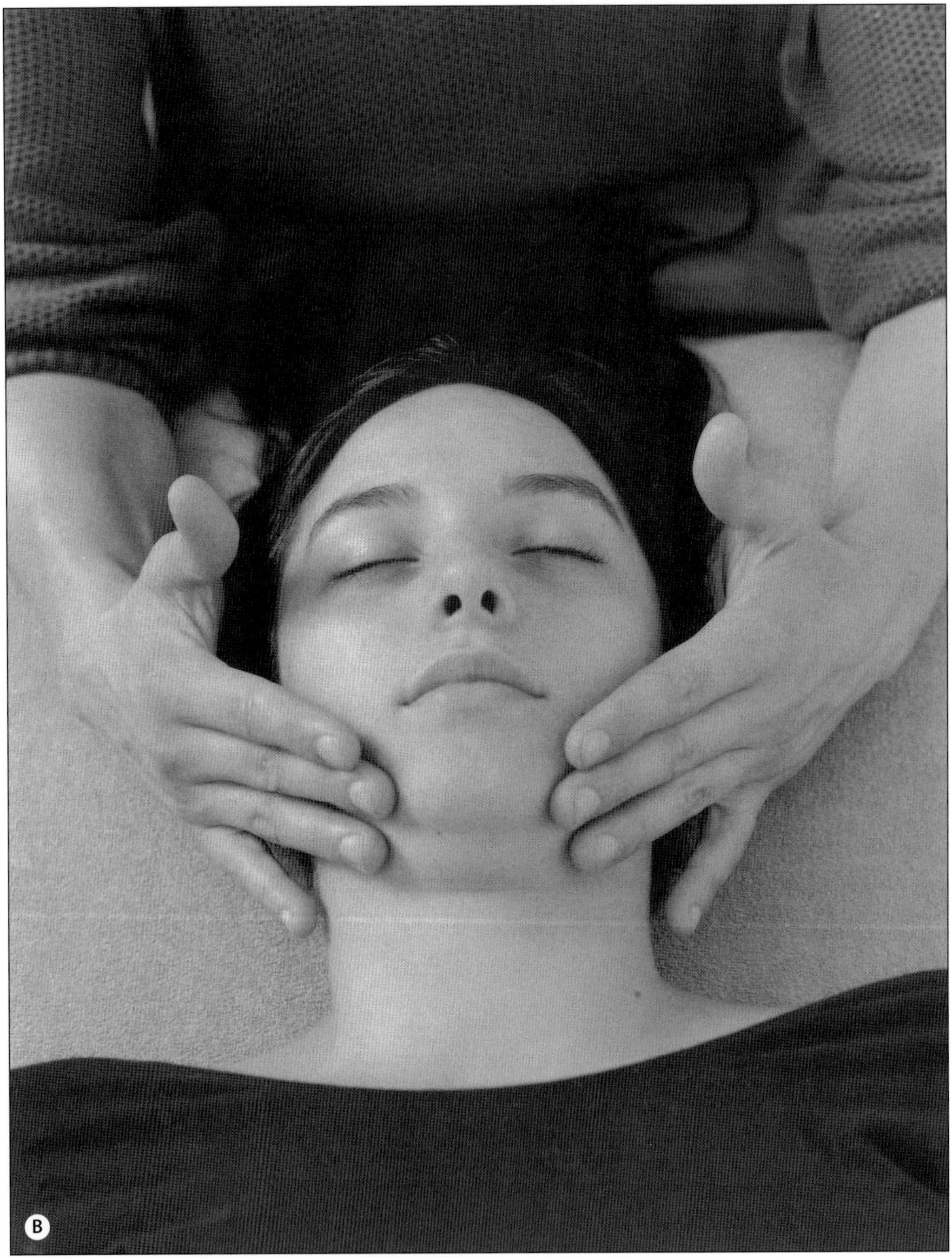

Figure 2.8.2 (*Continued*)

Functional treatment

Instead of performing light compression–decompression on the lower jaw using the indirect–direct technique, as an alternative you may support the lower jaw 3-dimensionally in the directions toward which it moves with ease. In so doing, *never apply testing for motion restriction* or indirect–direct release techniques, but continuously go with the inherent motion and tissue stops.

If you as the practitioner regulate the distance and are yourself relaxed, your clear, spacious touch will often help the lower jaw and TMJ to release spontaneously and find a better balance. Listen attentively to these spontaneous corrections.

Tips

Before performing release on the lower jaw, it is essential that you as the practitioner should optimally adjust your seat height (lower = better) and distance from the treatment table. Before you take up contact, rest your elbows on the table, *ideally one at either side of your client's head.* This enables you to create a stable fulcrum, which prevents your own body posture (or agitation) from being transmitted to the client. Pay attention to your own posture and breathing. Let your own lower jaw relax and again deliberately regulate the distance before you take up touch contact. Exhale slightly to one side so as not to breathe into your client's face.

After releasing the lower jaw, it is recommended that you listen to the craniosacral rhythm at the following stations:

- temporal bones, possibly using the gentle ear pull
- cranial vault hold
- cradle hold.

In normal circumstances, you will not conclude the craniosacral therapy session with the lower jaw; instead observe at the head, torso and feet and thus deepen the integration of treatment in the body as a whole.

2.9 The cranial vault hold: 'Listening to the cranial orchestra'

The cranial vault hold enables you to *listen* to the motion of the craniosacral rhythm both *specifically for individual cranial bones* and *for the cranium as a whole*. All finger positions should be as accurate as possible: this is made easier by precise observation and feeling for the structure using supple hands and fingers.

The cranial vault hold can be used as the sole listening station at the head. It can be readily combined with the cradle hold. The cranial vault hold is useful in particular before and after every release technique at the head for making before-and-after comparisons and for establishing whether and how local release of individual cranial bones has improved overall cranial mobility.

Get yourself ready by loosening your hands and wrists; one way you can do this is to let your arms hang and then wiggle and shake all your fingers. Next, spread your hands and fingers and stretch them a little but without over-tensing them. Then let all tension go again, perhaps loosening your hands once more. Stretching and spreading the muscles of your hands occasionally or a luxurious relaxing hand massage can also help; this will stretch your joints and muscles and so enable your hands to adapt ever more subtly to the shape and size of individual heads without exerting tension.

Before establishing touch contact, re-check your height and distance from the table, regulate the physical and emotional space, and make sure you are grounded and centered. Sit up straight and relaxed and let your breathing flow.

The cranial vault hold lets you palpate the varied motion of the cranial bones using all fingers simultaneously.

Method

With thumbs upward, place your hands vertically on the treatment table either side of your client's head. Spread your fingers, especially your middle and ring fingers. Now bring both hands up against your client's head in such a way that her ears are located between your middle and ring fingers. In this position, your middle finger is precisely over the zygomatic arch close to the ear, and your ring finger behind the ear over the mastoid process. Your middle and ring fingers can now palpate the motion of the temporal bones. Slowly and lightly place your index fingers precisely at the two greater wings of the sphenoid. Use your two little fingers to listen at the occiput. Make sure that your touch is clear, but not firm, just very gentle. Then check the quality of your touch with the client (Fig. 2.9.1A–C).

In this position, with your individual fingers on the respective cranial bones, you can now follow their inherent, *intrinsic capacity* for motion (motility). As you stay flexible and relaxed in your fingers, with some practice and patience you will also be able to distinguish increasingly between lateral fluctuation and longitudinal fluctuation.

As you focus attention on the motion perceived by all your fingers together, you will with some practice and patience be able to palpate the

Figure 2.9.1
(**A–C**) Finger position for the cranial vault hold (*Continued overleaf*).

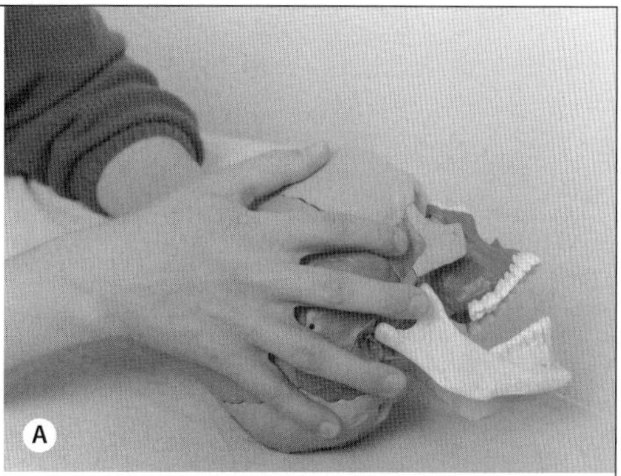

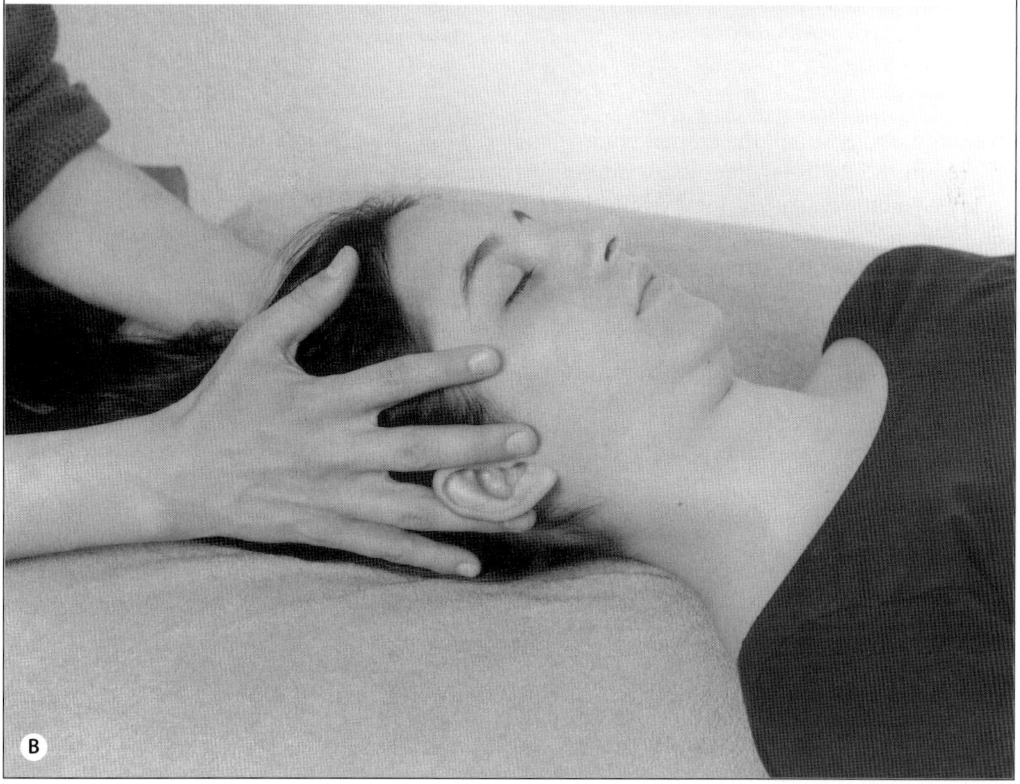

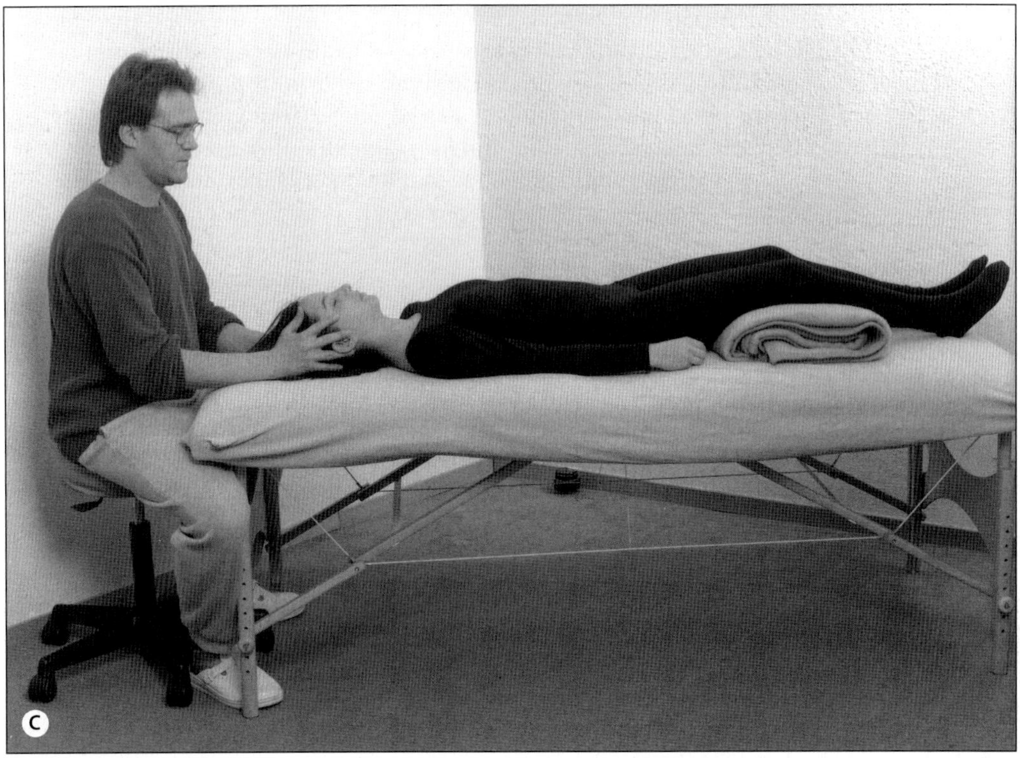

Figure 2.9.1 (*Continued*)

motion (mobility) of all the cranial bones *simultaneously*. Then you will be able to appreciate the ensemble playing of this cranial orchestra.

After you have listened for a while, make a before-and-after comparison.

It is also recommended that you do not merely listen to the 'cranial respiration', but that you broaden your perceptual field to include the entire craniosacral system and the whole body as a unit.

Harmonization and integration of head and torso 2.10

After releasing restrictions in the head, use the cranial vault hold or cradle hold – without any accompanying technique at all – to listen to how the entire cranial system is harmonizing the motion of the cranial bones overall.

You can invite a still point by cooperating deliberately with the stillness. However, do not use further techniques or pressure to force the craniosacral system to do anything – trust the inner healer and the expression of the Breath of Life that is re-organizing the body outward from the midline.

As already recommended following the release of transverse layers of connective tissue in the torso and spinal region, you should now follow release techniques involving the head by encouraging the *harmonization of head and torso and the integration of the session as a whole.*

In this final part of the treatment session, your intention is less to 'release and relax' but rather to round off the treatment as a whole – that means: 'connecting', 'integrating' or consciously 'listening to the whole body as a unit'.

At the same time, this final integration step again gives you the opportunity quietly and sensitively to sense any changes that have taken place compared with the start of the session. This session review is important – not least because it enables you to make a clearer evaluation of the treatment and its direct benefits. This inner reflection helps both the documentation process and the follow-up dialog with the client at the end of the session to become easier, clearer and more precise.

Examples of structure-connecting hand positions for head and torso integration after treating the head include:

- Head–neck balance (take up a position at the client's head). Place one hand transversely at the occiput, and the other transversely in the cervical region C2–C6/7.
- Head–shoulder balance (take up a position at the client's head). Place one hand transversely at the occiput, and the other transversely in the cervical-upper thoracic region C3–T2. Place one hand transversely at the occiput, with the other touching the sternum and clavicles.
- Palpate both shoulders with your hands.
- Shoulder–neck balance (take up a position on one side, roughly level with client's head). Invite 3-dimensional body awareness in the shoulder-neck region. As for the arm bridge at both sides of the pelvis, exert light pressure into the padded surface of the table, inserting your 'more cranial' hand under the client's shoulder region (ca. C4–T3). Position your other arm over the client's shoulder girdle in such a way that your fingers are

touching the shoulder on the far side, and your forearm the shoulder on the side closer to you. Make sure that your position at the table is comfortable and relaxed.

Do not exert any traction on the shoulders but connect and listen to the tissue and its motion in time with the respiratory and craniosacral cycle. What can you sense with your fingers and forearm in the anterior shoulder region, and what can you sense with your other hand underneath your client in the middle of the shoulder region? How do you perceive this region in 3-dimensional terms?

These and the following positions can also be combined with supplementary treatment elements (p. 202).

As you take up a position on one side, roughly level with client's head, here are some examples of general hand positions for head and torso integration:

- Place one hand transversely under the occiput (or slightly lower), and the other simultaneously:
  - — on the costal arch/solar plexus
  - — on/under the abdominal or pelvic region
  - — under the sacrum.

Now take note of the sensations, releases and slow movements:

- first with one hand
- then with the other hand
- and finally with both hands simultaneously.

Then listen to the structure *between your hands*, 3-dimensionally. Listen to the whole: how is the entire body moving together, as a unity?

If you can sense the craniosacral rhythm:

- Is it now more balanced overall?
- Is the rhythm at the occiput and sacrum about equally strong, and harmonious overall?
- Or can you now sense how the craniosacral rhythm in the torso is also starting to balance?

In just the same way, it can be useful to remove your contact for a short time; at a sufficient distance from the table now reflect:

- What is your overall impression compared with the start of the session?
- Is there any visible evidence to indicate any changes in the client?
- How is the atmosphere in the room now?
- How does the client feel?
- Where in the client's body does she have a pleasant feeling?
- Where in her body has there been some – perhaps particularly marked – change?

The integration of release in the head, both with immediately neighboring structures and with the body as a whole, is also encouraged by touching and listening at the following stations:

- Mid-torso: inferior thoracic inlet/solar plexus.
- Upper and lower torso simultaneously: double arm bridge.

- Base of torso/pelvis: 3-dimensional pelvis awareness phase or at both sides of the pelvis.
- Thighs, knees or feet: listen to the craniosacral rhythm, what is the difference between the start of the session and now?

What is your overall assessment now? How is the craniosacral rhythm now compared with before? Does your client show any evidence not only of palpable but also of visible change compared with the start of treatment? Ask your client how she feels and whether anything has changed compared with the start of treatment. If so: what, where and how? Where do things now feel most pleasant?

2.11 Supplementary treatment elements

While the following treatment steps may stand alone, they may also be used to conclude a craniosacral therapy session or to aid integration following severe physical or psychological processes.

Supporting the craniosacral rhythm with the client lying on her side

Instruct the client to lie down, preferably on her left side, with her cervical spine supported, for example, with a pillow, towel or thinly-folded blanket placed under her head. Ask her whether she feels more comfortable with some padding or a cushion between her knees and covered over with a blanket.

Take up your position behind the client at the side of the treatment table. Place one hand on her occiput and the other on her sacrum (Fig. 2.11.1). Allow your hands to blend with these two bones, stay passive for the time

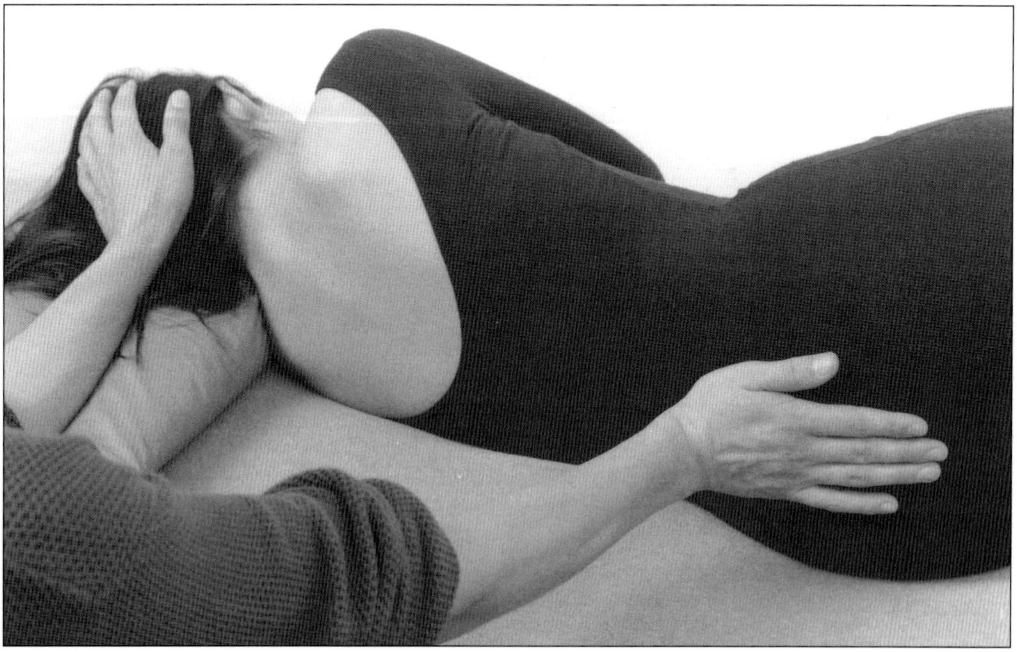

Figure 2.11.1
Hand position on occiput and sacrum with client lying on her side.

being and palpate the craniosacral rhythm. Go with the motion. You may exaggerate this slightly, but always go *with* the craniosacral rhythm, never against it. Alternate by using your hand at the sacrum to gently stretch this caudally during flexion, and your hand at the occiput to gently support this in a cranial direction during extension. In this process do not exert any pressure on the bones; instead what is happening is *a lateral widening and gliding*.

Support the craniosacral motion with your hands as they go cranially and caudally in this fine rocking movement, perhaps amplifying it slightly and thus also gently stretching and widening the dural tube. This has the effect of helping the craniosacral rhythm to become stronger, clearer and more balanced.

Make a *before-and-after comparison*: Can you clearly sense the bone level here at the sacrum and occiput? If so, what is it like? And beyond this bone level can you sense the dural tube between your hands? If so, what is it like?

To conclude, listen to the craniosacral rhythm for a few cycles: is there any change compared with the start of treatment? If so, what and how?

Supporting and harmonizing energy flow with the client lying on her side

In energetic terms, ascending energy often gets stuck in the neck region, whereas descending energy can be held up around the respiratory diaphragm/abdomen or umbilicus. The hand position illustrated in Fig. 2.11.2 is derived from Gerda Boyesen's biodynamics method and

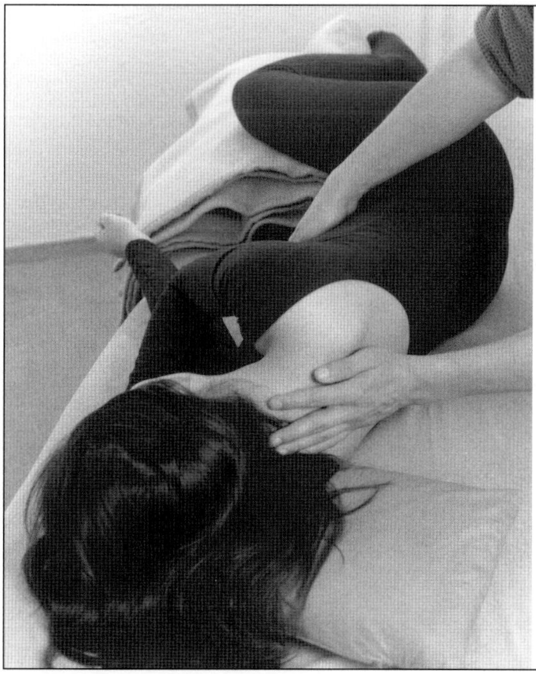

Figure 2.11.2
Hand position for neck and abdomen.

can be employed either on its own or as an add-on to the previous supporting technique.

With your client lying preferably on her left side, position her head horizontally using a small pillow or folded blanket. Sit or stand relaxed beside the treatment table behind the client. Place your 'more cranial' hand at the back of her neck. Pass your 'more caudal' hand over her torso and place it gently and without pressure to establish broad contact just below your client's navel, at the hara. Ask the client about the quality of your touch and adjust this, as necessary.

Remain in this position for about 2–5 min.

Releasing the dural tube

The dural tube is the continuation of the meninges and extends down the spinal cord as far as the coccyx. In its free state, it has attachments at just three points: at the foramen magnum in the occiput, in the vicinity of the second and third cervical vertebrae, and at the upper part of the sacrum (S2). Over the remainder of its course along the spinal cord, it should be flexible and freely mobile so that it can adapt to all the movements of the body. During flexion, for example, the posterior aspect of the dural tube is stretched.

The following simple release technique can be used to free the dural tube from adhesions and slight torsion. Lesions of this type may occur along the whole length of the spinal column down as far as the sacrum and are often caused by sedentary lifestyle, incorrect posture, falls, stress and trauma.

In preparation for this treatment, restrictions in transverse layers of connective tissue should be released, especially the top and bottom ends of the spinal column. This encourages preparatory release of the dural tube from peripheral structures and in the midline areas. If this is achieved to a sufficient degree, you will encounter fewer tensions, adhesions or torsions in the dural tube, and this will improve the effectiveness of the following short supplementary treatment.

Recall that the dural tube consists of the spinal dura mater, inside which are the arachnoid and the spinal pia mater where the cerebrospinal fluid (CSF) flows which, in turn, protects and nourishes the spinal cord.

When it is free and flexible, the dural tube promotes CSF flow and is better able to protect the spinal cord: moreover, the cleansing of the many exit points for spinal nerves is improved, as is their supply of fresh CSF.

Method

Start at the top of the spinal column with the client's occiput in the *cradle hold* or at the bottom end of the spine by placing one hand under the client's *sacrum*.

Once your hands are relaxed and positioned in the *cradle hold*, slowly shift your own body weight backward a little. As your hands glide toward you, this will automatically exert gentle traction via the occiput on to the dural tube attached there, stretching it minimally.

Down the length of the dural tube, sense how flexible and free it feels. Along its length are there areas of slight resistance where the tube feels 'snagged'? Some practitioners can *sense* the sites of restriction, while others have a more sensory visual gift and 'see' the restriction; during gentle traction, practitioners with mental training are able to count down the individual vertebrae and in this way, obtain information about possible restrictions. Where the dural tube seems to be caught, pause without reducing or increasing the gentle traction on the occiput, and wait. In this way, the bound region is slowly and minimally invited to let go. Once this happens, maintain steady traction and continue to sense your way down the dural tube until you come to the next 'snag' point or restriction, and so on. When you sense the sacrum at the occiput along the dural tube, this indicates that the dural tube is now largely free. Depending on motion type and structural restriction, it may take several basic treatments, specific advanced techniques or, depending on the client, a modified treatment approach to free the dural tube.

If slight resistance or restriction is not released, then remove your hands from underneath the occiput and position yourself slightly to the side of your client. Place one hand transversely under her occiput and the other hand on the torso area affected by the restriction (either at the back or front of the body). With your hand underneath the occiput, again offer gentle cranial traction and with your other hand release the connective tissues, possibly combined with a light fascial glide. Once this site is released, position yourself at the client's head for the cradle hold again (or at the sacrum) and listen.

Now how is the motion of the craniosacral rhythm in the head? How free is the dural tube now?

Next, position one relaxed hand *at the client's sacrum*. Shift your body weight slightly toward the client's feet, thus stretching the dural tube via the sacrum from the bottom up. While doing this place your other hand in support at any location you wish or at precisely the point reached by your light traction on the dural tube. If this site is not released, treat the connective tissues, possibly combined with a light fascial glide.

Once you have released restrictions in the dural tube working *down* from the occiput, you can then *switch to the sacrum*, listen there and start to release the dural tube from the bottom up.

Once you have released restrictions in the dural tube working *up* from the sacrum, you can then *switch to the occiput*, listen there and start to release the dural tube from the top down.

To finish off, move to one side of the treatment table. Place one hand transversely under the client's occiput and the other hand transversely under her sacrum. Without making any effort, move your arms and hands apart: this simultaneously coaxes gentle stretching and widening for the top and bottom ends of the spinal column and consequently also for the entire length of the dural tube. As an alternative to being in the supine position, the client may also lie on her side for this.

Stroking the sternocleidomastoid and trapezius muscles

Take up a position at the top end of the treatment table (near your client's head)

Rest your hands loosely on the treatment table to the left and right of your client's head. Allow your shoulders to droop and perhaps let your lower jaw drop a few millimeters. Once you are centered and relaxed, start by gently stroking the client's neck muscles, especially the trapezius muscles, on the left and right sides over her shoulders and toward her upper arms.

Method

Angle both wrists and place the surface of the backs of your hands directly at the end of the mastoid processes *on the sternocleidomastoid muscles*. Listen as the client breathes in and out a few times. When you are ready, use the finger surfaces of both hands to gently stroke along the muscle surface down toward the neck and from there outward, over the shoulders toward the upper arms (Fig. 2.11.3A–D). When stroking, make sure that you do this using minimal pressure. *This technique does not involve deep pressure but entails lateral stretching and stroking along the course of the sternocleidomastoid and trapezius muscles*. Do not apply traction or pressure on bones and joints (especially the shoulder). After all, your objective is for the tension in the client's neck and shoulders to be stroked away and diverted through her shoulders.

You may repeat this stroking several times. Ask the client for feedback about rate and intensity so that you can vary these, as appropriate.

Releasing the shoulder blades

Take up a position at the top end of the treatment table (near your client's head)

Many throat, neck and shoulder muscles are also attached to – or pass close to – the shoulder blades. To encourage the release of restrictions in this area it is helpful to touch your supine client's shoulder blades with the palms of both hands for a few minutes.

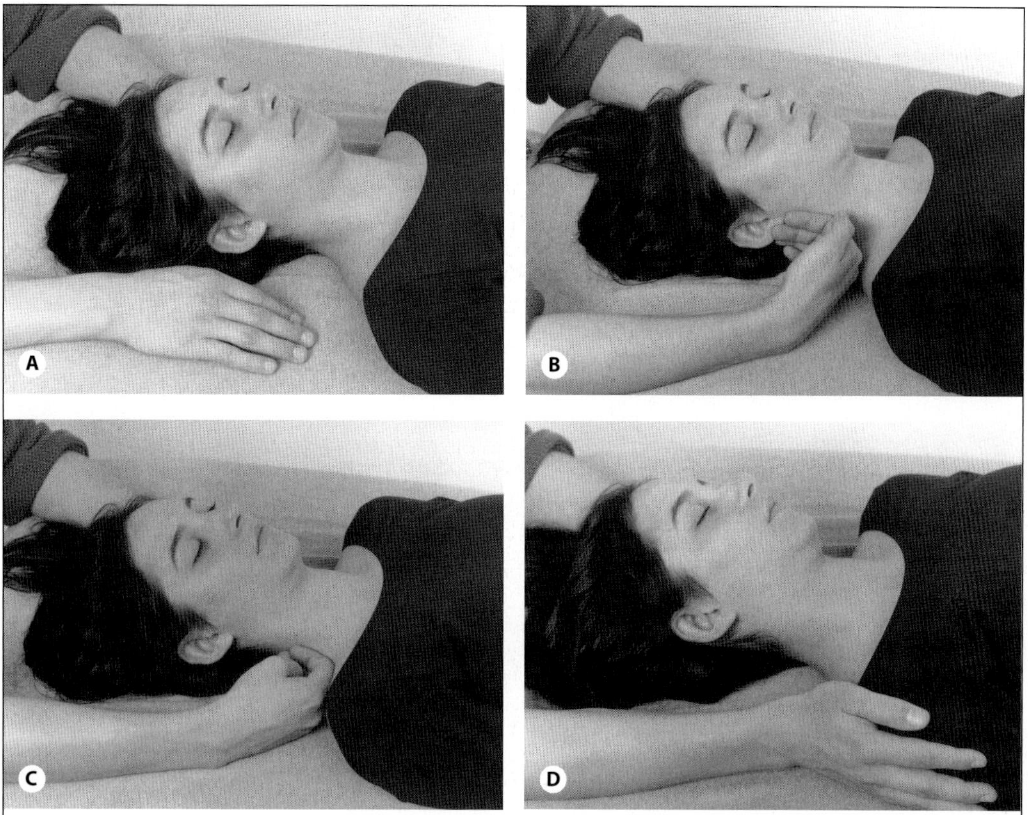

Figure 2.11.3
(**A–D**) Stroking the muscles of the throat and neck.

You can also explore the wide range of motion of the two shoulder blades. While doing so, it is advisable to pause occasionally. This sends a signal to the muscles, tendons, ligaments and fasciae and to the shoulder blade that it is possible to let go in different directions – and the different tissue structures are allowed time for the spontaneous re-integration of any release that has already occurred.

Method

Approaching from the top of the shoulders, push your hands into the padded surface of the table and down toward your client's shoulder blades. As you do this, stretch your fingers out toward her shoulder blades. Position your hands (open palm upward) precisely under the two shoulder blades. Your left hand is now under the client's left shoulder blade, and your right hand under her right shoulder blade (Fig. 2.11.4). Your fingers, hands, arms, and shoulders should remain relaxed.

Using the palpatory awareness that you have developed, take note of the tone of the individual shoulder blades: Are there differences?

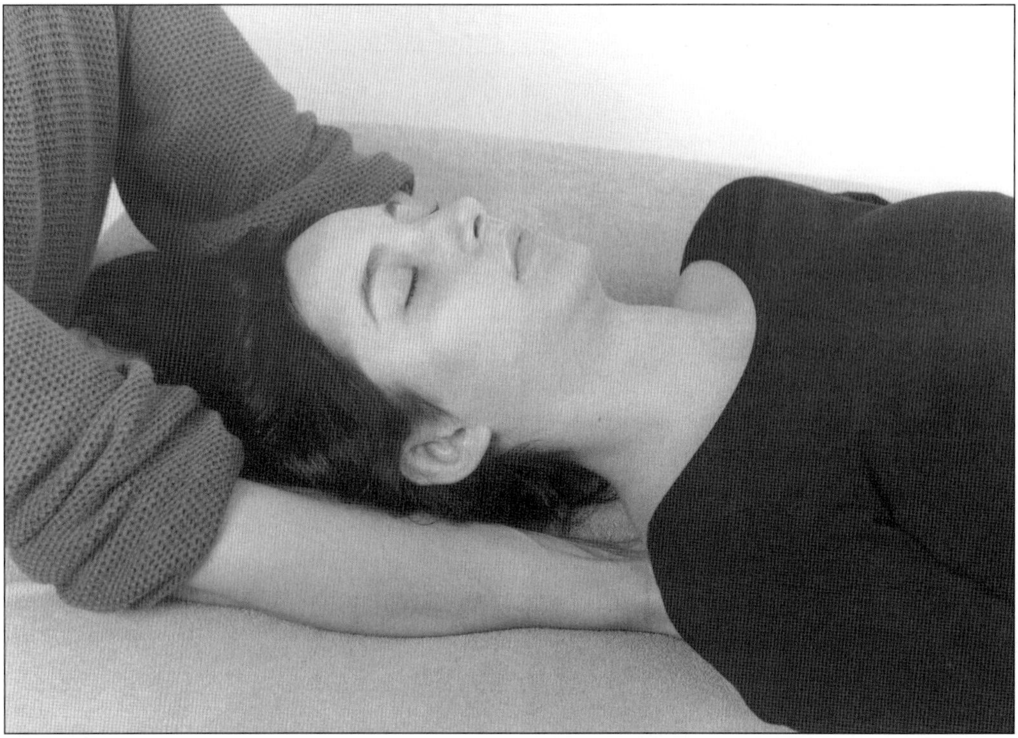

Figure 2.11.4
Hands positioned under the left and right shoulder blades.

Can you feel the client breathing, and if so, how? Is anything changing, possibly as a result of your spacious and finely-tuned touch? Now tune in to the first palpable tension level of connective tissue, fascia or muscle. Support the shoulder blades and their immediate area using the same technique as for the release of transverse layers of connective tissue. You do this, for example, as your hands slowly take over this same tension level, create space and wait for release or as you use a light fascial glide.

Then offer just a hint of movement to the two shoulder blades by allowing both your hands to go a few millimeters in the direction of ease. If your hands are stopped in the direction of ease, pause there with the option later of perhaps going even further into the newly created direction of ease. You may then also slowly move the two shoulder blades into the direction of restriction, in which case you should stop at the first palpable restriction, with the option later of perhaps going even further into the direction of restriction.

Afterwards, consciously relax both your hands and hold the client's shoulder blades in your hands without doing anything. Can you already sense how this zone is starting to relax without your further active intervention? Listen to and go with all the directions of motion into which both shoulder blades are now spontaneously released.

If the client's own spontaneous release mechanism and your spacious presence still do not enable any local release of restrictions, you may use supple hands to *lift her shoulder blades slightly*. Again this occurs in slow motion and is hardly perceptible: very gently (and listening at the same time) lift her two shoulder blades together a little toward the ceiling, wait and return to the starting position, wait and then take her shoulder blades in the opposite direction, more toward the treatment table, by allowing the weight of your own two hands to sink a little into the padded surface. Here, too, wait for a few moments so that the tissue in question can register this invitation to release. As you do this, if you sense the direction of greater ease for the individual shoulder blades, you may slightly amplify this direction of ease and later perhaps guide the structure slowly and lightly into the direction of restriction.

As a supplementary technique, you may also gently move the client's shoulder blades *alternately*, one up toward the ceiling and the other simultaneously down toward the table: i.e. left shoulder blade up (by lifting your left hand), and right shoulder blade down (by lightly pressing your right hand into the padded surface), and vice versa. While you are doing this, pause occasionally for a few moments and listen to the inherent motion. This helps the client and you to sense any changes occurring.

While your hands invite the client's shoulder blades to become heavier/lighter and to let go of any muscle tension, you may also use both your hands to deliver one or two gentle vibrations. This additionally supports the loosening of the muscles.

All these different techniques are performed very delicately, almost merely as a suggestion. These minuscule movements that can be spontaneously integrated coax the area in question toward a release that also continues after local therapy at this site has ended. As you build up experience, you will be able to freely combine the various methods for the comprehensive release of the shoulder blades.

Supporting release in the shoulder region (arm bridge)

To release restrictions in the shoulder–neck region you can also practice the same arm bridge as used in the pelvis awareness phase during sacroiliac joint release: Take up a position at one side of the treatment table, level with your client's head. Place your 'more cranial' hand under her torso, in the middle of her back in the region of the upper thoracic vertebrae, with your fingers between her shoulder blades. Position this hand as for the release of restrictions at the upper thoracic inlet. With your free hand, touch the shoulder on the opposite side in such a way that you are able simultaneously to touch the shoulder closer to you with your forearm. Your hand and forearm thus form an arm bridge at the client's shoulders (Fig. 2.11.5A, B).

Then use this contact to sense your way into the connective tissues of this region without tensing yourself or your own shoulders in the

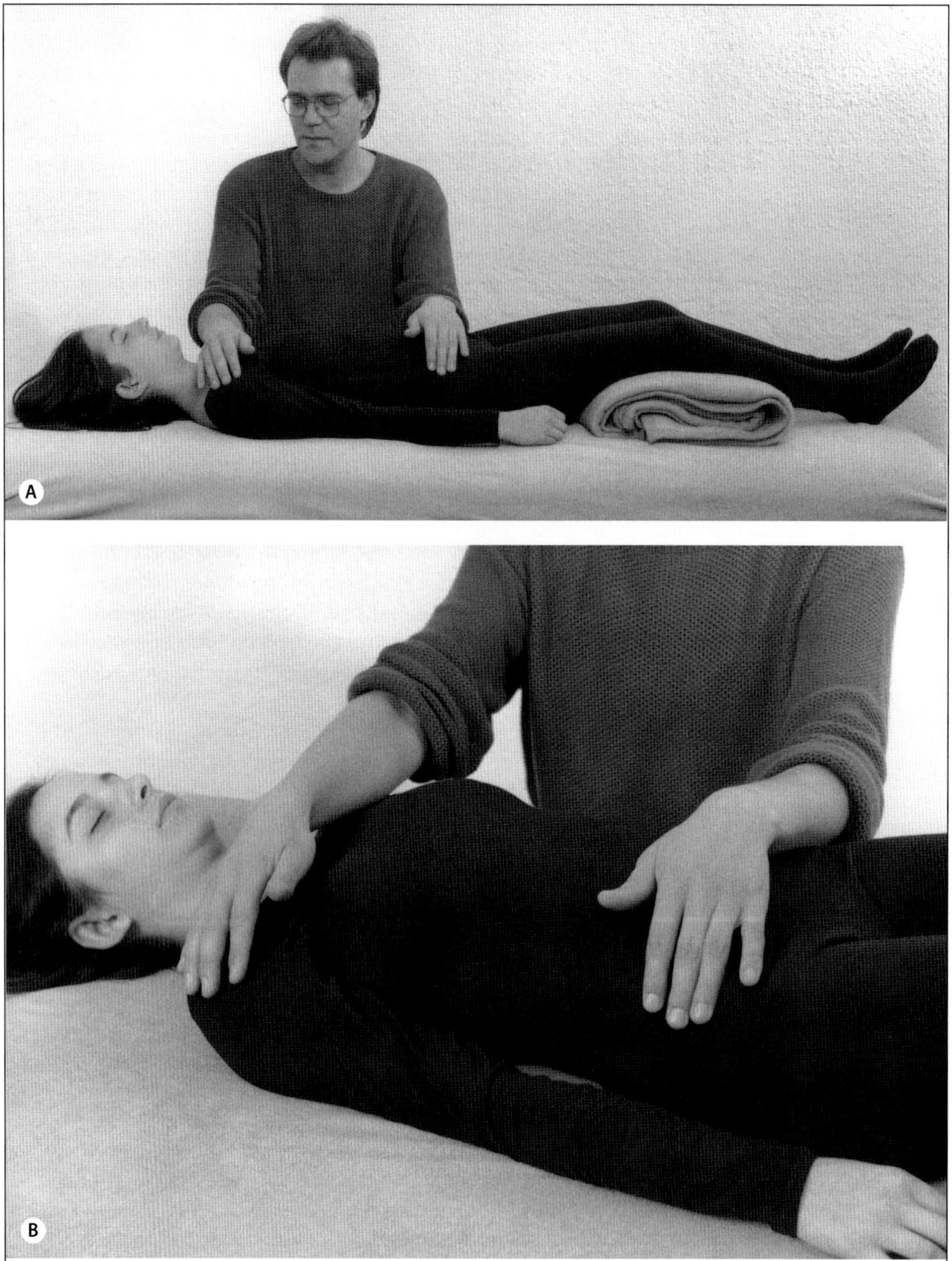

Figure 2.11.5
(**A, B**) Double arm bridge at the shoulders and anterior superior iliac spines.

process. The two contact points at the shoulders together with your hand placed underneath the client should form a relaxing, awareness-enhancing, 3-dimensional 'feel' that helps the shoulder-neck region to let go and to relax.

If the pelvic region has already been released, you may also use a *double arm bridge* after the arm bridge at the shoulders: to do this, take up a position at one side of the table, level with the middle of the client's torso. With the hand and forearm of one arm, establish contact with the two anterior superior iliac spines, while simultaneously touching the client's two shoulders with the hand and forearm of your other arm. Your touch should be clear, empathic, spacious, and listening. Take note of what you sense in the pelvic region on the one hand and in the shoulder–neck region on the other. Now broaden your perceptual field to include also the entire torso *between* your two contacts. After a while include the *whole body* in your sensitive listening, from the client's feet to the crown of her head and back again.

Connecting body regions and segments

From my experience with Gerda Boyesen's biodynamic massage, I already knew as a newcomer to the craniosacral method about the importance of *body segments as defined by Wilhelm Reich*. Therefore, when releasing transverse layers of connective tissue using the craniosacral concept, it seemed self-evident to me that as a simultaneous result the body segments would be better connected at their transitions.

Experience gained from my own practice and self-treatment indicates that the connection of body regions/segments is beneficial for:

- the overall mechanical forces acting on the body
- communication between abdomen, heart and head
- holistic body awareness, awareness of unity
- improving the flow of all body fluids
- energy flow in the body
- sensation and expressive ability.

Evaluation of body regions and segments can be performed using criteria such as 'too little' – 'too much' – 'balanced' as well as 'free'/'relaxed' – 'restricted'/'tense', along with aforementioned criteria such as the quality of motion of the craniosacral rhythm and the mobility of the dural tube in this area.

Version 1

Instead of releasing the connective tissues from the pelvis up to the cranial base, you can start by treating the segment that is most free. Right from the outset, therefore, the focus is resource-oriented on what is vital and healthy, and this aspect is correspondingly encouraged.

If a degree of symmetry or further tension release is found there, change position and continue at the transition with the next segment. Your intention/invitation here is for the transition from this segment to

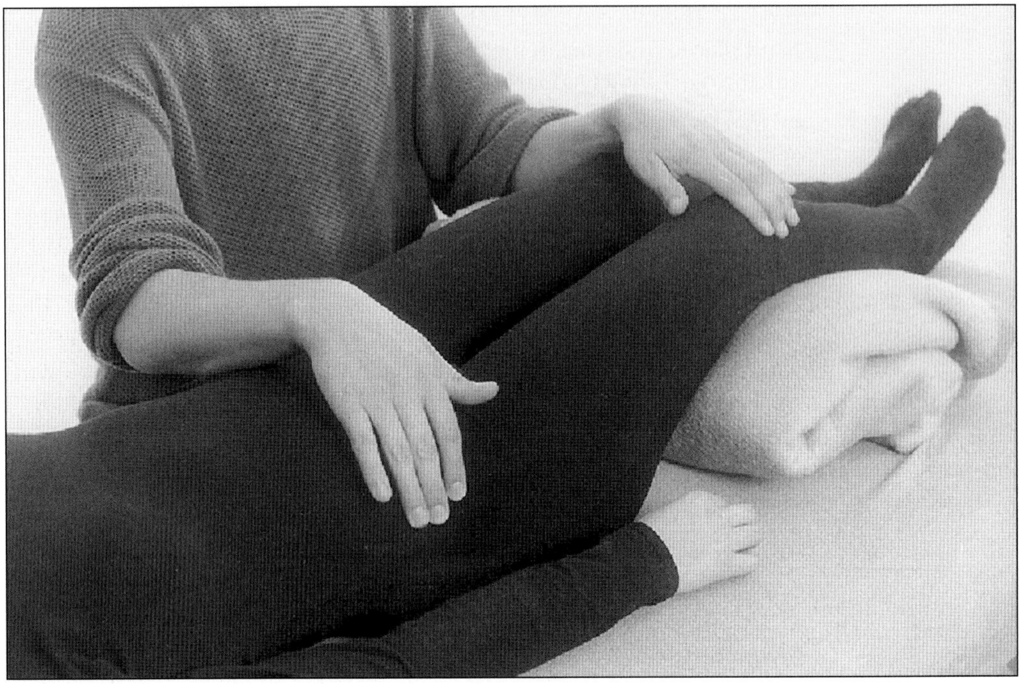

Figure 2.11.6
Connecting body region pelvis with thigh and knee.

the next to start to release, in response to pleasant touch, spontaneous physiological motion, and the energy in the segment that is most free (Fig. 2.11.6). Once this segment transition is released, establish touch contact in the territory of the 'new' segment or continue at another neighboring segment transition. After each segmental release or to conclude, you can listen to the craniosacral rhythm at the occiput and sacrum and evaluate the dural tube.

Version 2

Another supplementary treatment sequence consists of using broad contact with the surfaces of your arms and hands *to connect multiple body regions and segments simultaneously*. The body as a whole is harmonized through the agency of finely-tuned touch, the potency of the intrinsic rhythms and the energy in the free segments. Even the extremities, together with their articulated transitions, can be included here. This relieves strain there and they are described, for example, as 'increasingly belonging to the whole'.

If you take up broad contact using both arms and hands, you can comfortably connect several body regions and segments. Figure 2.11.7 illustrates how to make a connection from below the left knee with the thigh, pelvis and abdominal segment, with the liver, with the diaphragm/costal arch on the right side and with the thoracic segment.

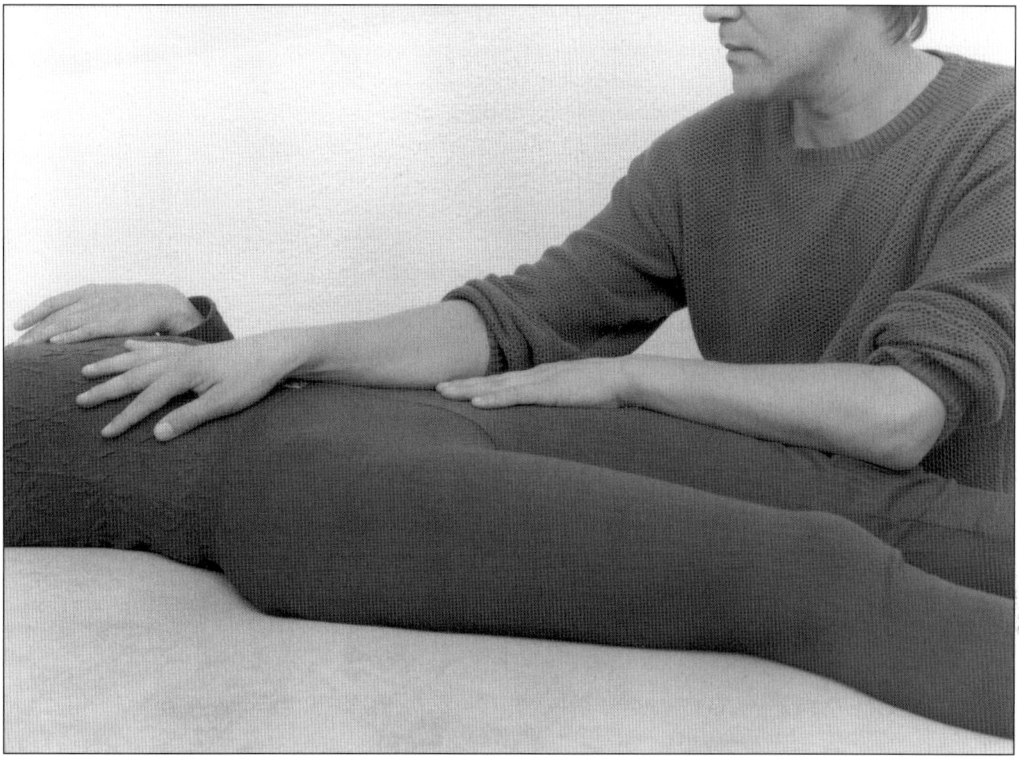

Figure 2.11.7
Connecting body regions and segments.

Energy is therefore not retained in segments but is available to the body as a whole. The flowing current of energy or the balancing of polarities or chakras can be sensed particularly well in the relaxed state.

Directing energy with fingers and hands

Everything in the universe has an energy form, and therefore even energy processes that cannot yet be measured may also be effective and successful. The mere thermal reaction produced by your hand placement when palpating the craniosacral rhythm supports relaxation and the freeing of restrictions.

As a further treatment technique, you can intentionally try 'directing energy' with your fingers. This can help restrictions to start to let go or resolve more swiftly. Place a fingertip, finger or hand diagonally to cranial sutures or to body sites that require healing or are painful. In your mind's eye imagine that this contact is sending a releasing and healing energy that widens and relaxes the tissues increasingly. This treatment method was already described by William Garner Sutherland who called it 'directing the tide'. Some of his pupils, and decades later John E. Upledger and thousands of craniosacral therapists, have also subsequently performed successful treatments using this technique.

As craniosacral therapy has become more widely used in the past 20 years, 'directing the tide' and the 'V-spread' have been taught and performed differently by teachers and practitioners – depending on treatment approach and the individual needs of the client.

Directing energy can be applied at different levels (musculoskeletal apparatus, bones, membranes, CSF, fluid body) and in different ways. Practice extensively on yourself and fellow students of craniosacral therapy first before you use it on clients.

During treatment, make sure that your hands and fingers are held loosely.

At points where restrictions of any kind are present, proceed as follows:

1. Place your index and middle fingers, spread into a V-shape, on the site affected by the restriction.
2. Place the extended index finger of your other hand at the corresponding location on the opposite side of the body. Point it diagonally at the restriction and direct releasing energy transversely through the tissues to the restricted, V-spread site. This serves as the target and collecting point for the releasing energy. The procedure is often followed by the production of warmth, a therapeutic process, and then by noticeable relaxation (Fig. 2.11.8A, B).

There are different versions depending on the energy that is utilized/employed

Version 1: The practitioner directs his personal energy (active).

Version 2: The practitioner does not direct his personal energy into the client's body, but remains grounded, centered and connected with the universal life force, which makes the releasing energy available.

Version 3: The practitioner utilizes the fluctuations of the CSF/ craniosacral rhythm (passive).

Version 4: The practitioner utilizes the fluctuations of the fluid body.

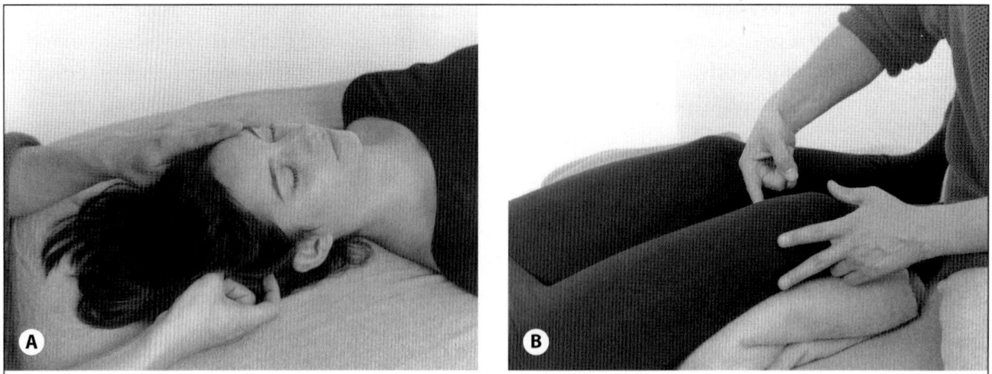

Figure 2.11.8
Directing energy to the (**A**) head and (**B**) knee.

Directing energy may take place with a varied range of intentions:

- The practitioner delivers *one* energy impulse into the system and waits for the spontaneous reaction of the client. This impulse can be repeated once or several times.
- Over several seconds or for a minute the practitioner continuously directs energy toward the restriction and it emerges through the V-spread site.
- The practitioner directs relaxing energy diagonally to the restriction; from there it is sent back again and finally it is directed yet again to the restriction, where it emerges through the V-spread site.
- The practitioner directs energy once or several times; it flows back and forth several times until the restriction starts to resolve or has resolved. This may be repeated once or several times.
- The energy has an ordering, releasing, balancing, harmonizing quality/ purpose and is used by the inner healer at the place where it is needed.

Alternatively, instead of spreading your two fingers into a V-shape, place one hand at the site of the restriction, and the other hand diagonally opposite. Your hands should be free from tension, they should be transparent and supple or 'like water'.

Visceral therapy: perceiving and releasing organs

You can broaden your perceptual field at any time and, once contact is established, you can direct your attention to organs in general or specifically to individual organs. Particularly while releasing transverse layers of connective tissue, it is an obvious step to take up contact not only with connective tissues and muscles, but also with the membranes covering the organs and with the organs themselves. Listen to the intrinsic motion of individual organs and to their movement in the overall setting. Organ function can be supported in this way.

You can encourage organ release and function by your gentle touch and attentive contact (exactly as described already in Releasing transverse layers of connective tissue, p. 120), by your listening and by your invitation of space and increased widening.

Visceral release may be combined with a gentle fascial glide. Palpate:

- in the pelvic region, for example, the bladder, uterus, Fallopian tubes or prostate
- in the abdominal region, the liver, gallbladder, spleen, kidneys, stomach, large intestine or small intestine
- in the thorax, the lungs and heart.

This may help the client – perhaps for the first time – to experience individual organs consciously or in a deeper way. The organs also reflect an individual's history and current state of health, as well as vitality and emotional state.

Any craniosacral therapy can be supplemented by or include elements of visceral therapy. The mechanical forces generated by the organs act on the musculoskeletal system and indirectly on the craniosacral system with its rhythmic activity – and vice versa – because the body is a functional unit.

Naturally, visceral therapy *can also be performed as self-treatment* by experienced practitioners. Regular use will deepen your palpatory awareness. At the same time, organ functions will be improved and become more balanced overall.

2.12 Suggestions for short treatment sessions

The suggestions in Table 2.12.1 for short treatment sessions are recommended only after you have scrupulously checked for any contraindications.

Before you apply individual treatment options, study the topics addressed in this book, e.g. 'Your inner attitude', 'Regulating the distance', 'The neutral point and stillness'. A pleasant and effective short treatment session also depends on extensive practical experience with the techniques presented so far, both in an instructional setting and in a practice group.

Important points

The stated time required may vary. Among other factors, this will depend greatly on the skill and experience of the practitioner. It may be that an experienced practitioner will achieve greater release in a far shorter time.

Table 2.12.1 ● Short treatment session suggestions

	Time required (approx.)
Listen to the craniosacral rhythm and spontaneous still points	≥10 min
Induce/invite still point	5–10 min
Treat client lying on her side	15–20 min
Release torso and neck, including integration	20 min
Followed immediately, for example, by:	
Release of upper spine (atlanto-occipital joint) (never do this on its own/ in isolation)	10 min
Release of lowest lumbar vertebrae (lumbosacral joint, L5/S1)	5–10 min
Release of sacrum	2–5 min
Encouraging sacroiliac joint release (arm bridge)	5 min
Release of head–shoulder–neck region	5 min
Using one position at the head, e.g. cranial vault hold	5 min
All the supplementary treatment elements described in the previous chapter may be used individually or in combination.	
To conclude the treatment (see 'Integration of release in torso', p. 153, 'Harmonization and integration of head and torso', p. 199):	
Invite still point	10 min
Whole-body assessment (before-and-after comparison)	5–10 min
Touch feet to ground yourself, before-and-after comparison of CSR	2–3 min

2.13 Basic treatment for beginners

The basic craniosacral treatment outlined in Table 2.13.1 supports release as a whole and the experience of 'body-mind-soul' unity, while serving to integrate the various self-regulatory mechanisms of the body. Among other things, the immune system is strengthened as a result. This basic craniosacral treatment promotes health in general; at the same time, it provides (body) perception and awareness training for the practitioner and for the client being treated.

Review the chapter on 'Indications and contraindications', on p. 63. Please note that patients suffering from health problems/illnesses must not be treated by people without professional training. Such cases require allopathic medical investigation and therapeutic management by specialists qualified to do so.

In individual cases, following medical diagnosis and in consultation with trained craniosacral therapists, people requiring care may also be treated. To be eligible to give treatment in such circumstances, you should have attended a number of craniosacral courses and one-to-one supervision sessions. In addition to possessing thorough familiarity with the basic techniques, it is recommended that you should have personal experience of craniosacral treatment at the hands of other practitioners, and be regularly treating yourself.

This basic treatment gently releases tension and restrictions in the body, e.g. in connective tissues, muscles, and joints. At the head, your weight of touch should be about 1–3 g.

The duration of treatment depends on regular practice, the experience of the practitioner, and the harmoniousness of treatment overall. A decisive factor here is *also the reaction of the client's body*, its capacity for self-regulation. On the one hand, it is important to support release of the craniosacral system at various points. At the same time, you should treat in a manner that is stress-free. As a beginner, it is better if you opt to perform fewer positions so as not to interfere with the self-regulatory mechanisms because of your own nervousness or uncertainty. Regulate your physical and emotional space and do not treat for too long. About 50–60 min is sufficient because the craniosacral system should never be over-stimulated. Sometimes a 45-min session is quite sufficient. Divide the treatment period up wisely.

Only embark on the overall structural basic treatment once you have carried out a few short sessions using the simpler treatment suggestions listed earlier and have received positive feedback.

Table 2.13.1 ● Basic treatment for beginners

Whole-body assessment, palpation of:

Feet
Knees, possibly thighs
Anterior superior iliac spines/both sides of pelvis
Costal arch
Shoulders
Head/cranium

Connective tissue release at:

Pelvic region
Costal arch
Thoracic inlet
Hyoid bone region
Occiput/cranial base (atlanto-occipital joint)
Lumbosacral junction (L5/S1)
Sacrum
Sacroiliac joint

Treating the head:

The following release techniques involving the head are very gentle, using a maximum weight of 3 g. Terms such as 'lifting' or 'decompression' should be construed more as a hint, a subtle invitation to release and *not as firm manipulation*.

Start with the cradle hold, and invite a still point.

Support the craniosacral rhythm at the:	***Release technique:***
Occiput	Cradle hold
Occiput	Still point invitation
Frontal bone	Frontal lift
Parietal bones	Go with IR, support, perhaps amplifying slightly in time with the craniosacral rhythm; cranial lift
Sphenoid	Listen to and go with tilting motion (no pressure, no manipulation)
Temporal bones	Finger-in-ear position
	Gentle ear pull
	Go with mastoid process motion, perhaps amplifying slightly in time with the craniosacral rhythm
	Massage masticatory muscles: upward above the auditory canal, and downward below the TMJ
Lower jaw	Gentle compression-decompression or go with inherent motion

Use the cranial vault hold or cradle hold to conclude your treatment of the head.

Integration/finishing off the session:

At least one position on torso	Invite still point
Listen to craniosacral rhythm, touch client's feet, 'grounding'	Before-and-after comparison
Overall impression	Before-and-after comparison

As is usual in basic craniosacral therapy, place your hands gently. Rather than manipulating with excessive pressure, you are instead inviting natural release.

Wherever possible, also use touch to encourage release in the head. Resistance patterns in the torso also have repercussions at the cranial base and on other structures in the head. Conclude your treatment of the client's head in plenty of time to allow for integration in the cradle hold and induction of a still point, for example. Finally, palpate the craniosacral rhythm at a few listening stations. Allow sufficient time for the integration of the treatment and then make a before-and-after comparison. Touch the client's feet briefly to ground yourself. To conclude the session, the client can rest on her side if she wishes and have time to enjoy the ongoing effects of treatment.

With regular practice, you will become familiar with craniosacral rhythm palpation and with the treatment sequence, and you will need only a few minutes for whole-body assessment at the listening stations. This will leave you with more time for releasing restrictions in the torso and cranium and for integration at the end of the session. As you grow in experience, your listening and treatment will no longer be separate activities, but will be performed together in immediate conjunction.

After the session, your client should sit up *from the side-lying position*, taking care to support her back. As she takes a few slow steps around the treatment table, she will be able to sense the new feeling in her body while standing and to communicate vital feedback about this.

Instruct your client to drink plenty of water afterwards.

Section 3

Experiences from craniosacral therapy practice

3.1 Practice and experience

It is important to practice the described techniques continuously, always operating from a fundamental position of respect. Regular practice, for example, in a training group or practice group, will help you become more attentive to the qualities of the craniosacral rhythm and whole-body interrelationships, and in particular will give you the assured confidence you need as you negotiate the treatment sequence. You will find that you will be guided increasingly by your intuition and become freer in structuring the treatment sequence, while still preserving the basic techniques and a cautious approach in the process.

Make sure that you always adopt a comfortable body posture in which you can rest for a few minutes before positioning your hands exactly. Relax your body by consciously grounding yourself. Perhaps you can sense your own points of tension; take note of these without changing anything and resolve to direct them downward through your pelvis, legs and feet. Allow your shoulders to droop as far as they will go and let your arms and hands become even looser.

Allow yourself to enter a natural state of relaxation, stillness and passivity. This state should not be confused with daydreaming or mental absence; instead, it is characterized by an alert presence and a heightened yet relaxed attentiveness.

- It is the messages communicated by the client's body that help to determine the course of the session; these messages draw our attention to the body's inner healing potential and the path to healing.

Resting in a place of stillness, you will be better able to palpate the various types of extremely fine motion in the body, both in yourself and others. It is at this point that craniosacral therapy becomes awareness training for both parties involved. During treatment, your underlying attitude should be as open as possible and your perception should be without judgment or expectation. Inner reflection before, during and after each session is valuable for your own learning, for the client and for the quality of your sessions. Sometimes you will be palpating and find yourself wondering: 'Is that the client's pulse or my own that I can now feel so strongly in my hand?'

The more practice, feedback, craniosacral course experience and personal experience you have, the better equipped you will be to differentiate between sensations that come from you and those that reflect fine motion in the client. And you do not always need to attribute and explain everything;

simply be present and listen to the flow of the slow rhythms and to the body's spontaneous self-regulation. Without having to cling tightly to individual 'sensations', you can trust the process.

While it is advisable and important to acquire essential specialist knowledge of structure and function, your experience in craniosacral therapy will grow as the number of your treatment sessions increases.

3.2 Stories from craniosacral therapy practice

Marlene had fallen on her left knee while hiking in the mountains. After the accident, she experienced stabbing pains in her right hip. The medication prescribed by her doctor relieved the pain for a few hours only. On palpation, the craniosacral rhythm in her pelvic and sacral regions was very weak and faltering. As a result of craniosacral therapy, the tension referred to her torso by the fall on to her knee was released as if in a chain reaction: the restriction in her pelvis disappeared and subsequently tissue restrictions were released as far up as her sternum and shoulders. The cramps she experienced occasionally in her left calf also disappeared completely after the second session.

Hans is a successful businessman. Because of the high stress levels associated with his job, he sometimes had the feeling of being 'full and empty inside at the same time'. He had also complained for months of disturbed sleep and chronic gastritis and constipation due, so he surmised, to all the business dinners he had to attend. Although Hans did not want to close his eyes during the entire session, he felt a noticeable sense of letting go after restriction release in his torso and at the top and bottom of his spine, and after his body entered a spontaneous still point. Gurgling sounds were evident in his gastrointestinal tract. Hans had diarrhea for hours after this first treatment session and was able to sleep through the following nights. Over the next two sessions, he gained the feeling of being inwardly centered of having rediscovered his center. At the start of the fourth session, he closed his eyes after a short time and enjoyed the treatment, which again was accompanied by prolonged and loud digestive noises – especially after the top and bottom of his spine (atlanto-occipital and lumbosacral joints) had been released even further; his chronic gastric pressure had disappeared. Craniosacral therapy also resolved the diffuse pressure in his esophagus and harmonized his central nervous system. Together with a change in diet, it helped him to live and work free from symptoms and to enjoy refreshing sleep at night.

Simona, a 16-year-old girl, complained of severe back and neck problems caused by high stress levels brought on by school. She also often suffered from cystitis and very painful menstruation. Her craniosacral rhythm was restricted throughout her torso, particularly at the shoulders. After two basic craniosacral treatment sessions, there was a marked improvement in the overall tone of her musculoskeletal system, and her back and neck tension had disappeared – not least because the two craniosacral sessions had enabled Simona to develop a different attitude towards her learning-related stress. There were only rare recurrences of cystitis, usually due to negligence on Simona's part; her menstrual pain was reduced to a tolerable minimum.

Gerda S. was diagnosed with a 4-cm uterine cyst that disappeared after just one basic treatment session. If the cyst had remained the same size, it would have necessitated surgical excision a few weeks later.

For **Christine,** a lively woman with rare back problems but no pathological findings, her very first craniosacral treatment session was a watershed experience. During craniosacral rhythm palpation, she experienced the onset of a pleasant sense of calm. The release of restrictions in the transverse connective tissue layers in her pelvic and abdominal regions was felt as a liberating widening in all directions. Her respiratory rhythm slowed when my hand was placed on her costal arch and hence on her diaphragm. My hand placed on her costal arch established contact without pressure. After a short time, Christine's solar plexus region started to vibrate slightly. When I asked what was happening at that moment, she replied tersely: 'I don't know exactly – I can't see anything.' Her eyes were a bit screwed up and her left eyelid began to twitch irregularly. When I repeated the question, it was met with the same response as on the first occasion. Her costal arch region between my hands became increasingly warm and finally hot. Because the client wanted my touch to remain exactly as it was, treatment at the costal arch was continued for a further 10 min without further techniques, simply and exclusively using spacious presence and trust. Christine then sighed deeply and fell asleep for a while afterwards. Meanwhile, I continued attentively with the session. At the precise moment when the still point at her head was past and her craniosacral rhythm resumed more powerfully than before, Christine breathed deeply a few times and was then wide awake. She was able to recall precisely how, several years previously while on holiday, she had been violently struck by a tent pole on her left eyelid. All the tension that had still been palpably present at the start of the session had disappeared. The dull sensation in her lumbar spine at the start of the session, at those sites where Christine occasionally felt back pain, came and went over the period up to the next session. Since her second session, Christine has been free of problems and occasionally comes along for a craniosacral session to help her cope better with day-to-day life and work.

Agnes, a 40-year-old mother and part-time office worker, presented for craniosacral therapy because of bladder problems and transient symptoms of paralysis in her left arm, her physician's prescription suggesting that these might be of psychosomatic origin. At the age of 9 years, she had sustained a riding accident, and in the same year, she had another accident on an escalator; the resulting patellar operations were extremely painful. After I had palpated her craniosacral rhythm, and once points of attention had manifested themselves and I was cradling her head at the end of the whole-body assessment, I had a clear picture of the tension state in her body: her entire left side was characterized by markedly increased muscle tone, and her head also had a definite tendency to turn to the left. Her whole neck region was restricted. Above her left iliac crest, my hands sensed a mildly stabbing area of densification, a compensatory inertial fulcrum. During transverse connective tissue layer release, starting at the costal arch/respiratory diaphragm, Agnes also sensed this site above her left iliac crest. In the course of the slow unwinding motion of her left leg and the simultaneous involvement of the region around the inertial fulcrum, tensions at varying depths were released (over the next 20 min). At the end of the session, the client felt pleasantly relaxed and 'whole'. Now, after a long period, she felt that all the parts of her body belonged to her again. She felt that her vertebral column was hugely reinforced and strengthened. Afterward this client sought out a female craniosacral practitioner so that the possible psychosomatic background to her bladder and abdomen problems could be worked through with a woman.

Roman, a masseur whom I had got to know years before at a training course, wanted to discover practically how craniosacral therapy works. He had read an article about it and felt that it promised relief for his persistent neck problems and the latent tension in his thoracic spine. Because Roman's craniosacral rhythm was restricted at the pelvis and sacrum, I left one hand under his sacrum for a relatively long time and began applying various relaxation and release techniques in his pelvic region. After only the first 5 min the client was better able to feel his legs and feet and experienced general relief. I treated the connective tissues in his pelvic and abdominal region, used the sacroiliac joint release technique, and finished off with L5/S1 decompression and a still point at the sacrum in the pelvic region. Because his solar plexus then started to vibrate powerfully, I intuitively placed one hand under his neck, and the other in the region of his solar plexus. The production of warmth – already sensed previously – became even more pronounced, his breathing grew faster, and beads of perspiration ran down Roman's face. Subsequent interactive support of the client's process in conjunction with attentive therapeutic dialog revealed that because of a previous road traffic accident, Roman had developed a habitual reflex: as soon as another vehicle approached within 2 m behind his own, he was overcome by a now subconscious, habitual fear that caused him to become rigidly tense in the regions of his neck, solar plexus and pelvis – this was his individual way of reacting instinctively to this trauma activation. Once I had finished treating his head the client became calm, and with the onset of slow unwinding in all his extremities as well as at the neck and head, he had returned to his normal respiratory rate and at the end of the session he kept on exhaling deeply with exhaustion. Roman telephoned me 1 week later and thanked me for the treatment. He had still felt very tired for a few days, but after the fourth day, he felt more energy than ever before. His fears about being rear-ended by another vehicle have since disappeared.

If they play frequently over a period of years, **musicians** whose instruments necessitate use of the head and neck may develop problems with tension in their shoulders and neck. It is not uncommon for their hearing also to become affected over time, especially if they play loud, sometimes shrill-sounding instruments held close to the ear, e.g. the violin or flute. This may result in annoying noises in the ear (tinnitus), as illustrated by the following case.

All her life, **Rita** had loved playing the piccolo, the archetypal Basel *Fasnacht* (carnival) instrument. Both eardrums became blocked due to chronic inflammation of the nasal mucosa and paranasal sinuses. As a result, playing the piccolo and piano became painful for her and produced severe bilateral tinnitus. During the first craniosacral therapy session, I found that the craniosacral rhythm in her whole body could be palpated only very weakly. At both temporal bones, there was minimal, curtailed motion into IR and hardly any motion into ER. The transverse connective tissue layers were very taut in all her body segments. It was there that I started treatment, after inviting a still point from the feet. I first treated Rita in the pelvic region because she had been suffering for months from severe low back pain. Slowly the restrictions in her body were released up as far as the costal arch where her solar plexus felt as if it was trembling but was slightly softer than at the start of the session. After I had treated her upper spine with atlanto-occipital release, her low back pain disappeared. After I had treated her head, especially in the temporal region, Rita felt that her head was released and broader. Her tinnitus had receded somewhat and was no longer as high-pitched as at the start of the session. In the second session, I treated her head more extensively. After initially treating her upper spine, I listened and treated at the sphenoid, temporal bones and TMJs, combined with intra-oral work and accompanied by spontaneous and externally induced still points. At the end of the third session, where the emphasis was on balancing the sphenoid and temporal bones, on going with unwinding at the neck and on release of maxillary restrictions, Rita felt completely free of problems for the first time in ages. Tinnitus was still present but had receded even further. Subsequently, it would become more problematic again if Rita did not allow herself the necessary rest. Rita maintains positive body awareness with weekly sessions of backstroke swimming. She occasionally still attends for a craniosacral therapy session. In the meantime, she now regularly uses still point induction and the ear pull technique to treat herself.

Mario came from the Italian-speaking part of Switzerland and was visiting relatives in Basel. He made the most of that opportunity to attend for some craniosacral treatment sessions with me. Following an eye operation under a general anesthetic, Mario had experienced initially mild and later severe whooshing sounds in his ears after taking antibiotics. A few weeks after eye surgery, the whooshing sounds grew into an annoying whistling; this was accompanied by hearing and balance problems and transiently by mild dizziness. Over the course of five sessions, I treated him intensively, on each occasion using more advanced intra-oral and head techniques. Mario combined these craniosacral treatment sessions with acupuncture therapy. Even after five craniosacral sessions and some acupuncture therapy, the ear noises did not abate entirely but they did lessen. The whistling noises disappeared and the client was only rarely aware of the whooshing sounds; these were sometimes louder and sometimes almost disappeared completely. I recommended Mario visit a fellow craniosacral practitioner in his home locality so that he could undergo further craniosacral treatment over a longer period in the hope that the improvement in his condition might stabilize and be consolidated further.

Katharina complained of daily headaches. Thanks to acupuncture she now suffered 'just' from headaches instead of daily migraines, as before. She reported back pain extending into her coccyx region; this was particularly severe in the mornings and after long periods of sitting or standing. Katharina had previously undergone surgery for an inguinal hernia; since then she experienced pain in both thighs after just a few hours of activity. Her craniosacral rhythm was more pronounced and still palpable on the left side of her body; the craniosacral rhythm on her right side showed delay and slight restriction. I treated her mainly in the pelvic region and using positions from the basic treatment outlined in this book. After the initial session, the client had no further thigh pain from the fourth morning onward. Her back pain was also reduced. In the second session, the treatment was focused primarily on the pelvic and lumbar regions. Release of restrictions in the upper spine and lower jaw brought the client considerable relief on a physical, mental and spiritual level. After the second session, Katharina claimed she no longer had any back pain or 'depressive lows'. During the third session, when I positioned one hand under her sacrum and the other at the pelvis–abdomen transition, I suddenly sensed a strong pounding and considerable heat. Katharina's face expressed pain, which she was able to pinpoint at the fourth lumbar vertebra, radiating to the right side, and at the point where my upper hand was positioned. I kept my hand on this point and repositioned my other hand under her sacrum to one side, obliquely above the iliac crest in the vicinity of L2–S1. This was followed by the release of connective tissue layers. The entrapped pain in her pelvis and abdomen diminished and resolved. After the three following sessions, which involved support of slow, spontaneous neck unwinding, and TMJ and intra-oral techniques, Katharina's back pain was noticeable only if she had overdone things. Also, the formerly daily headaches now occurred only very rarely.

As a company director, **Andrea** had a great deal of responsibility and stress. As well as hypertension, she also suffered from asthma attacks, particularly when she was lying down and resting. Years before she had also had a ruptured diaphragm. After seven single-practitioner sessions and two multiple hands-on sessions, the client was able to reach a state of greater inner calm. The craniosacral therapy sessions gave her a sense of greater spaciousness in her body, especially in the thoracic region. In particular, when lying down, Andrea was no longer afraid of having an asthma attack, allowing her rest phases to become times of refreshment again.

Anna-Marie complained of back and neck problems and wanted her first session to take place at the Institute. Her right side was relatively free, but on her left side, the craniosacral rhythm was irregular, faltering, and restricted. During release in the pelvic region, the client experienced powerful 'lightning flashes' emanating from her pelvis and traveling to her head. I observed twitching over her whole face, especially around her eyes and mouth. Anna-Marie reported that she was feeling slight pain at the weak points in her body, i.e. both knees and her ascending colon. She sensed how her body was becoming heavier and her left side was more restricted than her right. The lightning flashes and twitching resolved slowly and were suddenly gone. At the end of the session, the client was aware of a subtle flowing sensation in her head from her occiput forward to her frontal bone. When Anna-Marie sat up, all the symptoms that had occurred during the session had disappeared. She felt that the left and right sides of her body were now balanced. She felt light and had the feeling that she was floating.

Tina came to the practice with a susceptibility to allergy, asthma and a TMJ syndrome brought on by an accident she had sustained when she was 9 years old. In addition, her right ankle was chronically inflamed following a sprain; cortisone injections had provided no relief for the inflammation. Over the course of 10 sessions, I accompanied Tina through many physical and emotional experiences. After the first session, she experienced pronounced warmth in her TMJs. After the second session, so Tina told me, she had been aware of an enormous abundance of energy and great feelings of happiness over several days. The further course of therapy, including comprehensive release of the sphenoid, temporal bones, masticatory muscles and maxillae and support of spontaneous unwinding of the extremities, was accompanied by feelings such as tiredness, impulsiveness or even anger. Overall, however, Tina felt more balanced and relaxed session by session. Her breathing was deep and she sensed a bodily widening. The chronic inflammation subsided and had completely resolved within 12 weeks.

Two years previously **Susanne** had fallen on to her right shoulder while cycling. The pain in her right shoulder subsided after a few weeks but the pain in her sternum remained constant. A medical examination was inconclusive and 12 sessions of manual therapy helped only transiently. Susanne learned about craniosacral therapy through a magazine article and embarked on a course of treatments. Her neck muscles and head showed a marked tendency to the right, and no craniosacral rhythm could be palpated at either shoulder. During treatment, her left shoulder was painful, and her right shoulder felt 'stiff as a board'. Without any active motion testing, her sphenoid showed right torsion combined with left sidebending. I carefully supported the functional release of this motion pattern; Susanne already felt pleasantly relaxed after the first session. During the second session, I again treated her entire torso and head and supported the minimal spontaneous unwinding in her neck region. During release of the sphenobasilar synchondrosis via the sphenoid and occiput, mild pain radiated briefly from the client's left shoulder. After the second session, Susanne was again able to sleep right through the night: she had not been able to do this ever since the birth of her child 5 years previously, because at night she still subconsciously listened out for noises from the child's room. The pain in her sternum lessened for a time, but was still always present. During the third and fourth sessions, I treated her sternum, shoulder–neck region, the cranial bones – mainly the sphenoid and temporal bones – as well as peripheral sites. After the fourth session, her sternal pain had disappeared: Susanne had already forgotten all about it at the start of the fifth session. However, mild diffuse pain was noticeable in her left shoulder and in the lumbar region on her left side. Over the following three sessions, among other things, I supported the body's spontaneous unwinding; the renewed balance of the sphenoid, occiput and temporal bones noticeably reduced the tendency of her head to pull to the right. At the same time, the dull pain in her left shoulder and lumbar region resolved itself. During the following two sessions, my attention was drawn to a site above her left iliac crest and to Susanne's cesarean section scar. For her, the treatments were a journey through the most varied emotions, accompanied by pictures and feelings from the past. After the tenth session, Susanne had the feeling that the most significant traumatic events of her recent past had been dealt with. Since then she occasionally comes along for a session as a 'special treat'; this happens particularly at times when she senses a noticeable dip in her body's capacity for spontaneous self-regulation.

Patricia had had two road traffic accidents and suffered from chronic pain; in addition, she had scoliosis involving the thoracic spine. For 5 years previously, the pain had stopped her from sleeping more than a very little. All the allopathic and alternative medical therapies she tried brought hardly any relief. While cortisone achieved a temporary reduction in pain, it led to hair loss and other unpleasant side-effects. Throughout the treatment period (12 sessions at regular intervals of 1 to a maximum of 3 weeks), I treated her using the full range of craniosacral techniques that appeared reasonable to me, accompanied by regular pauses to listen. When Patricia appeared after 4 weeks for her third session, I was struck by her very clear gaze. She told me that she had been virtually pain-free since the second session. After the third session, she had the feeling of having been 'put back together again'. Patricia's feedback before the fourth session was that she was sleeping better and also generally feeling very much better. Moreover, her hearing improved significantly after the fifth session. During the ensuing treatments, I supported unwinding throughout her body as a whole, supplemented by release of the facial bones and by elements of visceral therapy. My attention was drawn mainly to the right side of Patricia's body, from her right shoulder blade (area of scoliosis) and right lumbar region to her right eye. Many sensations, including past pain, came to the surface and left her body again. From the start of the sixth session onward, Patricia's feedback comments included: 'I have the feeling I'm growing', 'At last I feel at ease again in my body', and 'A lot of things in my body are settling down'. Every session was intensive, both for Patricia and for me. Sometimes I would remain for 20 min with one hand at one site so that the structure could experience deep release and balance layer by layer. I treated her for between 60 min and a maximum of 75 min per session. Her whole personality changed over the 4 months. After 12 treatments, I said goodbye to a happy client who was 'upright again'.

(The names used in this Chapter are fictitious.)

After 16 years as a practitioner, I personally still feel tremendous gratitude for the craniosacral method and its enormous capacity for activating the self-healing forces in the body. The cases described here and thousands of others clearly illustrate the magnitude of the healing potential released by craniosacral therapy. The inner healer or the potency of the Breath of Life is supported so that healing can take place. This happens not only through precise techniques gently executed by the practitioner, but also because the ego is set aside. This means that neither the client nor the practitioner hinders the process of balance directed toward greater wholeness, i.e. they do not become obstacles to health.

The craniosacral practitioner encourages the body's spontaneous self-healing process using all the means at his disposal, such as knowledge, technical proficiency, experience, intuition, listening and resting in the stillness, resource-oriented therapeutic dialog, and support for the client's process, all of which are deployed with attentiveness and respect for the welfare of the client.

3.3 Frequently asked questions and tips

This chapter lists a number of questions **(Q)** that crop up repeatedly during training courses and practice sessions, together with possible answers **(A)**.

Q: What if I can't palpate the craniosacral rhythm at all or can palpate it only some of the time?

A1: When you take up your position at the treatment table, make sure that your inner attitude is right, and that you have prepared yourself properly and are inwardly 'tuned in'. Even minimal practitioner discomfort, e.g. a seat adjusted to the wrong height, can interfere with relaxed palpation.

A2: It may be that the craniosacral system has momentarily reached a still point or has suddenly shut down. Stay relaxed and keep listening. Fine readjustments of bones, joints, muscles, and connective tissues are often unfolding in the body during a still point. You may perhaps be able to sense these. Continue listening with a receptive attitude so that you can go with the motion of the craniosacral rhythm once it resumes after the still point is over.

A3: Do not be too fixated on wanting to palpate the craniosacral rhythm. The mere fact of exaggerated expectation can prevent you from feeling the rhythm. Listen with an attentively passive or meditative attitude. It is then more likely that the slow, subtle ebb-and-flow rhythm will communicate itself to you. Sometimes, the craniosacral rhythm only becomes palpable when the practitioner has stopped 'wanting' to feel it.

A4: It is almost as if there is an 'inner scale' on which you can change your palpatory perception setting. After you have trained your hands for a while, combined with your sensitive, spacious presence, you will sometimes feel the craniosacral rhythm as a large, slow impulse.

A5: Even if you cannot palpate the craniosacral rhythm, it can still be supported and become more balanced through your palpating presence. Listen for a while to the respiratory movements and then see later whether any slower rhythms become perceptible.

A6: It may be that the craniosacral rhythm at the palpated body site specifically, or in this particular client generally, can be palpated only very weakly, if at all. In most cases, it will become more readily palpable if you listen to the stillness in yourself, in the client and in the room, or after you have induced a still point.

A7: How is your touch? Is your finger/hand contact as broad as possible and have you reduced the intensity of your touch again by half *without losing clear contact with the structure?* If you are familiar with other manual therapies and are accustomed to the weight of pressure used there, your treatment pressure may be consistently too strong for craniosacral therapy. The lighter and softer your touch, the better you will be able to palpate and discriminate between respiratory and craniosacral motion, for example.

A8: Allow yourself and the client time to become slower and more sensitive. **Other tips**: Regulate the distance (physical, emotional, mental, energetic), wait, do not be fixated, and perhaps palpate your own back. *Listen* instead of doing; rest in the stillness instead of being active or feeling compelled to make something happen.

A9: It may be that your client's already very relaxed body is in the rhythm of the mid-tide; this is several times slower than the craniosacral rhythm and runs at 2–3 cycles/min.

A10: Accept the craniosacral rhythm as a gift that reveals itself when it wishes to. This gift will reveal itself to you if you yourself are at least as slow as the slow body rhythms, or even slower. Become totally attentive and still; listen into your own stillness. And once this inner stillness has deepened, listen to the stillness in the client.

Q: What if the client falls asleep during the session?

A1: Carry on attentively with the treatment. Falling asleep is a sign that the client is well, relaxed, and trusts you. Craniosacral therapy works even if the client is asleep. Often when this happens, brain activity is 'turned down' to a deeply relaxing frequency and the body rests in its center. The demanding stresses of everyday living can be erased or put into perspective. In most cases, the client wakes up centered and refreshed. Before or after the sleep, the body can often be perceived as a relaxed unity – not only at the physical level but also the immediate unity of body-mind-spirit.

A2: If the client attends for craniosacral therapy so that symptoms or diseases can be resolved, then – depending on the goal of treatment – it is recommended after a few 'sleeping' sessions that you ask the client to become more actively involved. Engagement in therapeutic dialog will help in this.

A3: Therapeutic dialog can be used so that the client does not fall asleep but is able to remain relaxed and present at the same time.

A4: Falling asleep may also reflect a protective or flight mechanism on the part of the subconscious.

A5: If the client falls asleep, her body and its organizing fluids are often better able to harmonize, to find a new inner balance, and simultaneously to start integrating changes. Our brain, our heart and our spirit know how to use this 'interruption of wakefulness' to best effect.

Q: What if the client's eyes are open?

A1: She may keep her eyes open. It may be that this external spatial orientation helps her to accept touch without any anxious connotations, and to relax physically. However, the client will benefit more from craniosacral therapy if she occasionally closes her eyes and directs her attention inward. It may take a few sessions before she is ready for this.

A2: Invite her to close her eyes and to become aware of her most pleasant bodily sensations, then perhaps also including those sites where your hands are currently positioned. Check whether the situation suits your client and ask for feedback on your quality of touch, which you should adjust accordingly.

Q: Should there be any talking during the session?

A: While some sessions are entirely silent, there will be others where verbal communication takes place occasionally. There is justification for both scenarios. It is useful now and again to enquire how your client is feeling – also to obtain feedback on the desired weight of manual contact. Avoid asking closed questions, i.e. those that can be answered with a simple 'yes' or 'no'. Brief dialogs during the session often help the client come to a deeper awareness. Things that are sensed at deeper levels can be anchored more effectively when they are expressed verbally; the subjects and feelings can sometimes be reflected and experienced more clearly in everyday reality. However, deep insight on a non-verbal level can also be equally powerful.

Q: What if the client talks non-stop?

A1: Listen closely for a while and pay attention to important keywords and physical changes where you can *make the connection to the bodily level* and ask the client *what she feels in her body* while she is saying this.

A2: You can inform your client about any pronounced physical changes that you, as the practitioner, clearly perceive, and in this way, you can draw your client's attention more concretely to *physical aspects and how she is feeling at that moment in time*. After a while, you can suggest that she tries to *become aware of how her body feels from the inside* and, for example, to focus attention on her 'inner healer'.

Q: Is it essential to keep to the sequence of treatment steps?

A1: It is recommended initially that you keep to the sequence of treatment steps. By following this sequence, you will learn a structural basic craniosacral treatment that will balance the craniosacral system as a whole. If you have omitted a particular treatment position, you can go back to it after completing the current position, but it is not essential to do so. Small subsets from the total treatment sequence tend to be more comprehensively effective in the hands of advanced practitioners. Once you are familiar with the basic treatment, you can modify or enlarge the treatment sequence, listen and treat more specifically. In particular, once you have gained in-depth practical experience after several hundred sessions with different people, you will know when it is advisable to depart from or shorten the treatment in specific ways.

A2: This depends on the knowledge and experience of the practitioner and on the treatment approach adopted. It is beneficial to carry out the structural treatment exactly, to engage interactively with the situation revealed at any given moment, and simultaneously to go with your intuition – and it is also important to involve the client to the full by occasionally asking open questions instead of 'fixing' her with techniques.

Q: How can I tell that tissue release is occurring?

A: There is a wide range of signs at every sensory level, and these are again dependent on the moment and on the individuality of practitioner and client. For example, tissue release may manifest itself as follows: gradual 'sinking in' of the practitioner's hand as the tissues become softer and softer; deep breathing in and out by the client; twitching, prickling or marked pounding (known as the 'therapeutic pulse'); the qualities of the craniosacral rhythm change and become more balanced; the practitioner senses tissue relaxation and 'letting go' in the client as well as in himself; broader/altered kinesthetic awareness; changes in skin quality; heat is produced when retained energy is released – cold may also be released from the tissues.

Q: How long should I stay at one location, e.g. when releasing transverse connective tissue layers?

A1: Once a release process gets under way at one location, stay there until this is more or less complete – provided this is what your client wishes.

A2: Some clients may require several craniosacral sessions before their trust grows sufficiently, their body accepts your gentle touch, or ingrained patterns of resistance become softened. Consequently, it is at the practitioner's discretion to remain at one location for longer (say 5, 10, or 15 min) to allow the tissues there sufficient time for appropriate release from the inside out. Where only a few areas on the body are treated, it might be beneficial also to involve the other end of the craniosacral system, e.g. bottom – top – bottom.

A3: If nothing changes at one site on the torso, you can ask the client if it is OK to continue at another position. Do not remain too long at any body site that is not yet ready for release. As you perform the next two or three positions you will probably find some sites that feel different and are more open to your touch and treatment. Remain there for slightly longer.

Q: What is happening when I can sense pronounced heat being released beneath my hands, or a strong pulsating, pounding and tingling?

A: It is a good sign that changes are occurring beneath your hands. Keep your hands on this site. Note whether the client's respiratory rhythm has altered. Ask how this body site feels. In all probability, what you are sensing is a 'therapeutic process', signaled by a 'therapeutic pulse'. This has nothing to do with the heartbeat or the craniosacral rhythm, but indicates that the tissues beneath your hands are working. It may be that retained energy is being released, after which a new point of balance will be established. Observe and go with it passively, i.e. as you remain attentive and allow space, *go with the process and trust it*. Ask the client from time to time what she senses.

Q: Why does the client say there is too much pressure even when I'm exerting no pressure?

A1: In most cases, the pressure is too great anyway, as is the intensity of the practitioner's attentiveness. Check for yourself whether the pressure might be coming from you or whether it should be interpreted as a therapeutic response emanating from the client. Have you regulated your distance?

A2: It may be that your touch is still too heavy. This may be due to actual physical pressure (1–3 g is sufficient when treating the head) or to the fact that – because of your inner attitude – you, the practitioner, are subconsciously trying to make something happen, wanting to achieve too much, or feeling that you have to be perfect, all of which may be perceived by the client in energetic terms as pressure/compression.

A3: Check whether the client can be positioned better. Also check your own sitting position.

A4: It is possible that certain sites on the body and head do not 'want' to be touched during a session or for a certain period of time (e.g. as self-protection because a major process is under way, the time is not right, or due to neuralgic discomfort). You should always accept this, and move on to the next treatment step or proceed to the body site that reveals itself currently as the most free or most pleasant for the client.

A5: And sometimes it is just the re-experiencing of old pressure from the past, e.g. 'birth pressure', and is part of the therapeutic process.

Q: At the start of a session, should I proceed directly to body locations that are particularly dysfunctional?

A1: Hardly ever. You could perhaps begin at a body location that is free from dysfunction but that corresponds to the dysfunctional part of the body.

A2: Wherever possible, begin at the feet, shoulders or a body location on the craniosacral system that the client feels to be pleasant.

Q: Is it the general rule for initial worsening or symptom intensification to occur during and after craniosacral therapy?

A1: This is not generally the case. However, part of the healing process may be for the body to start to resolve ingrained, chronic dysfunctions and for this territory to be activated first. When structures that have been 'stuck' start to flow again, it can take several minutes, hours, days, or weeks until a new balance is found at a freer level.

A2: In the pre-session dialog the client should be informed that you, as the practitioner, will do all you can to work carefully and to the best of your knowledge and ability. An individual session as well as a series of 6–12 sessions may be accompanied by a worsening of symptoms. These generally subside during or after the session. However, it is also possible that symptoms may persist for a while or migrate from place to place.

A3: People vary in their degree of body awareness. Sometimes they have a deeper awareness of their body only during or after release, with the result that not only released sites are sensed, but also those that are restricted or painful.

A4: Treatment will have varying effects in different individuals and from session to session. While release is happening, the cell memory may 'let go' of traumatic energy, giving rise to a whole range of reactions. When symptoms become intensified, the client may *simultaneously* be aware of those body sites that are most pleasant, while the practitioner interactively supports the process using a resource-oriented approach. The timely inclusion of integrating components at the end of the session will support overall integration.

A5: Do not be put off by symptoms that appear briefly and then disappear again or perhaps by symptoms that are constantly migrating from place to place. Listen to the craniosacral rhythm and release the craniosacral system as a whole, instead of just treating individual locally restricted sites exclusively. If the client wishes, continue with the treatment and encourage her to make inner contact with the symptoms or body sites and perhaps to enter into 'conversation' with them. If no change occurs there after the first part of the session, specific treatment can be given. If integrative treatment techniques are performed in the final third of the session, the symptoms often resolve just as quickly as they appeared or else they become fewer or subside.

A6: It may happen that the body temporarily produces fewer endorphins to combat pain. If there is a fall in current endorphin production (before settling at a new level), increased pain may be felt for a short time.

A7: At the end of the session, the client should always allow herself some time to enjoy the ongoing effects and to spontaneously do whatever seems appropriate, e.g. snuggle down and stretch or perform improvised movements on the floor. Remind the client to drink plenty of water after the session and to move around sufficiently but not too much, e.g. by taking a short walk. With sufficient activity followed by a sleep, the fine processes will be particularly well integrated.

A8: See also A9 below.

Q: Should I remove my hands if the client says that symptoms have become intensified?

A1: Ask the client whether you should leave your hands where they are or remove them.

A2: Make certain that the symptoms have not been provoked by the weight of your touch or by your fixation on this particular part of the body. Provided that the symptoms are not very severe or painful and are part of the therapeutic energetic process, it is generally advisable to leave your hands where they are.

A3: Is the body trying to use the symptom or the pain to say something? If so, what?

A4: Keep your hands at this location. Use therapeutic dialog to steer attention first to a body location/region that feels good or is less affected. If the client wants to, she can go back and forth once or twice between the symptomatic and the 'pleasant' location; describe the sensations there and perhaps explore the causes and background to this.

A5: If the symptoms or pain are too severe, place your hands on an adjacent or more remote body area that feels good for the client. You will thus enable the client to broaden her body awareness and not to be fixated solely on the body area that is currently 'working'. By doing this you will also support the better distribution and balance of free energies in the body.

A6: As the practitioner, you have the freedom to remove your hands at any time. Depending on the situation, however, it might perhaps be a pity not to stay with it if a therapeutic process is getting under way, and something is changing. Stay with it – it can be very impressive and interesting to observe what has changed and what is released once the therapeutic pulse dies away during the process.

A7: Why should the practitioner immediately do something if the change in the way the client is feeling is due to the onset of a therapeutic process at that moment? Ask what is happening and where/how this is perceived in the body.

To react immediately to such symptoms would mean acting in response to a momentary, perhaps unfavorable situation with the aim of avoiding or improving something. By doing this, however, you would already be 'boarding the train' that takes you into the realm of 'symptom–symptom management', an approach that is more akin to the cause-and-effect philosophy of allopathic medicine. Instead you can view and recognize the *therapeutic process during a craniosacral session overall* as treatment and so learn many valuable lessons about the forces and mechanisms of self-healing. By adopting this perspective, you will broaden your own perceptual field and locate yourself instead as an observer who supports the process. This means that any symptoms/painful sensations occurring during treatment should attract *only part of the practitioner's attention*. At the same time, another part of you should keep watch for what is causing the effect and in particular, over and above this, for what is healthy in the client – this also includes the slow body rhythms being palpated at that moment, which are a direct expression of the Breath of Life.

A8: Induce one or more still points.

A9: In-depth experience in craniosacral therapy is important. Have you attended an adequate number of specialist courses, including therapeutic dialog and how to support the client's process; have you received one-to-one supervision or undergone comprehensive further training in craniosacral therapy? Broaden your experience, e.g. practice regularly with other students/practitioners in your local geographical area; go along for individual treatment sessions with qualified craniosacral practitioners. Practical confidence in interactive process support and in therapeutic intervention (p. 95) is indispensable for treating clients with (persistent) symptoms.

Q: What can I do if too much routine has crept into the basic treatment?

A1: In asking this question you have already taken the first step toward changing things. Use your inquiring mind. Listen increasingly to the craniosacral rhythm or slower rhythms. Step out increasingly into the realm of intuition by allowing your *hands* to take charge of the session instead of your head or rigidly adhering to a set sequence – but do not lose sight of the structural context and inner reflection.

A2: Are you using all the positions and techniques in the basic treatment or are you leaving some out? You can combine these and the more advanced basic structural techniques with each other and by listening again to the craniosacral rhythm, you can go with the release of the craniosacral system. Introduce greater variation using additional treatment techniques with the aim of providing more specific support for your client. In foundation-level and advanced courses you will discover how to broaden and deepen treatment considerably.

Q: How regularly should craniosacral therapy sessions be scheduled?

A: This will differ from client to client and cannot be defined in general terms. It has been found that the first 3–4 sessions can be arranged at intervals of 1–2 weeks (or every 2–3 weeks if there is a strong reaction; this should be discussed individually with the client). After that, further sessions can also be scheduled at intervals of 2–4 weeks.

Tips

For the practitioner: Divide the time up properly

A treatment session lasting for about 1 hour often passes relatively quickly. Take care to divide the time up properly and leave the final 15 min for finishing off the session and for a short follow-up dialog.

For the practitioner: Change treatment sides

If you are performing more than one craniosacral therapy session, in the next session change sides for those positions taken up at the side of the treatment table: This will keep you flexible so that you are able to treat from both sides of the table and so that you continuously train the sensory and fine-motor skills of both hands. At the same time, you will be preventing unbalanced postural patterns.

For the client: Take time after the session

For a while after the session, clients should take time to enjoy and experience the ongoing effects of the deep relaxation that frequently occurs. Clients may react to a session very differently. In every case, to purify your body, it is advisable to drink plenty of water (e.g. energized, non-carbonated water). Before driving again afterwards, it is important for you to take a short stroll (e.g. in the park) to make absolutely sure you are not in a half-trance and that you will not be a danger to yourself and other road users.

Section 4

Waking the inner healer: The integration of body, mind and spirit

It is not all about activity and technique. Supremely, it is the open and attentive attitude of the practitioner and his palpatory skills that guide him to the free locations as well as to the restrictions in the client's body. In this way, the trained practitioner is escorted through the session by the *messages communicated by the client's body.*

The release of the client on a physical, emotional, and spiritual level supports and activates the inner healing forces. First-hand experience of the freedom of existence, awareness of body-mind-spirit unity, sensing the currents of flow in the body, recognizing yourself as a unit in a greater whole, feeling sensations of peace and happiness – all these factors have a healing action.

In craniosacral therapy, we learn to operate less and less by critical thought processes. Rather than merely finding and releasing restrictions and pain points, you instead also support the body in its natural 'letting go' and self-regulation. Do not get in the way of this process by using too many techniques or performing them too rapidly. Allow yourself as the practitioner, as well as your client, sufficient time so that the body's spontaneous self-corrective process can occur.

It is not only technical proficiency and your treatment that make for an effective session; just as much credit for this must go to the secure setting and your *respectful accompaniment of this natural process* of self-regulation. Also, learn to trust the inner healing force, which spontaneously operates at the right time and place to bring about health.

4.1 Neutral and stillness

As already mentioned on several occasions, the practitioner should be grounded and centered and regulate the physical and emotional distance. It is not a question of using inflexible techniques to invasively 'maltreat' the client's craniosacral system, but of creating a secure space within which self-regulation and self-healing can unfold. For this to happen, it is extremely valuable if the practitioner allows himself and his client sufficient time to approach neutral before touching and starting to listen.

In using the term 'neutral', a distinction is made between *practitioner neutral* and *client neutral*. To approach neutral means, for example, that you free yourself from expectations, desires, plans, thoughts and (e)valuations, and outwardly as well as inwardly come to rest. In many cultures, the pace of life is too fast and many things are very rationally oriented. It may therefore happen that relative beginners think they are already in neutral if, as a result of their own slowing down, there are fewer or no distractions present, or because overall there is a greater awareness. Initial relaxation and moments devoid of flowing thoughts (on the part of practitioner or client) still do not mean that neutral has been reached for the first time: however, they are welcome signposts on the road to that destination. Examples of such indicators are greater equilibrium, increased balance or elimination/reduction of conflicts.

The road to neutral requires its own time. Neutral cannot be forced. In neutral, we perceive ourselves directly as a conscious, sensitive, warm, and joyous whole. Neutral is a state of consciousness that is natural but is not routinely experienced by many people; you will perhaps be familiar with it from childhood or meditation. Even neutral can deepen in stages. The practitioner remains present, waits, stops, and allows space. He acts as a fulcrum so that the '*inherent treatment plan*' and – linked with this – the client's self-regulatory mechanisms can reveal themselves and 'take over' the session proper.

En route to neutral, or in order to deepen it, it is helpful if you *keep a constant watch for stillness*. This does not mean that the practitioner or client switch off, meditate in a rapt state or withdraw completely. Once you have connected with stillness, it is easier (in fact, only then does it become possible at all) to tune in to the expression of the Breath of Life, of the primary respiratory mechanism. It is out of stillness that the therapeutic process manifests itself, as well as the Breath of Life, which encourages health, the life force and self-regulation and breathes the divine spark of life.

The transition between the functional and the biodynamic approach to treatment is a fluid one. The more the practitioner and client approach or deepen neutral, the greater the importance of spacious and sensitive listening. Then, for example, it is possible to do away with distinguishing different body structures. Instead, you can perceive the body with its energetic shell/aura as a whole, as a fluid body.

After each release, the body will find a new balance, especially in or accompanied by spontaneous still points. At this treatment level, it is also possible to perceive rhythms that are slower than the craniosacral rhythm – the mid-tide or long-tide (see p. 8).

James S. Jealous, probably the doyen among teachers of biodynamic cranial osteopathy at the present time and a pupil of Rollin E. Becker, among others, told of an impressive experience he once had with Rollin Becker. Becker cautioned Jealous that he should only start touching and treating when *both* the practitioner *and* client are ready for it.

Tuning in to neutral gives both the practitioner and the client time and opportunity to be wholly present, to free themselves from expectations. Neutral is not a place or a point, but rather a state of consciousness. In neutral, in particular, it may happen that tissues, fluids or cells start to narrate 'stories'. Once neutral and stillness have deepened, you mainly allow the Living Matrix, the fluid body and the potency in the slow ebb-and-flow motion to do the work. It may then happen that the inherent treatment plan reveals itself.

Allowing time, slowing the pace and tuning yourself in to neutral – these things already constitute a very valuable core attitude.

4.2 The three-step healing process

The three-step healing process was defined by Rollin E. Becker, DO, a pupil of William Garner Sutherland. In his published writings (see Further Reading), the process underlying the body's spontaneous self-regulation is explained briefly and succinctly by Becker as unfolding in three essential phases. The practitioner's presence provides a safe setting in which self-regulation and, consequently, healing can take place. That which is vital and healthy, the expression of the Breath of Life and the innate potency within it rhythmically organize all tissues, fluids, the nervous system and the Living Matrix. This self-regulation is oriented, for example, around the midline and around natural fulcrums. It is also oriented around our embryological development because the consciousness in our cells joyously and lovingly remembers our primordial wholeness, and is familiar with every detail in the blueprint for healthy growth and development. The Living Matrix in its current form is able to recollect the blueprint of the Original Matrix and orients itself around this during the healing process.

The principle of this three-step healing process is followed both in the structural-functional as well as in the biodynamic approach to treatment. Change manifests itself at the level of the pulmonary respiration, the musculoskeletal system (muscles, ligaments, bones, joints), body fluids – especially the CSF – and at the energetic-fluid level. Ultimately, the practitioner's perceptual field is open to that level that directly reveals itself in the client, and so he is able to discover something about the 'inherent treatment plan'. In this process, the practitioner remains present, regulates the distance, does not intervene, and allows the rhythms and fluids to 'do the work' – self-healing takes place.

As is usual in the functional and in the biodynamic concept, the focus here is not on searching for, identifying, and resolving restrictions or dysfunctions in the craniosacral system or generally in the client's body. Also, the practitioner does not perform any active motion tests. Tissues or fluids are not confronted with restriction and limits. Instead, the practitioner listens to the free motion and to the potency in the slow body rhythms.

Using the dynamic potencies of the slow body rhythms with a frequency of 2–14 cycles/min, the Living Matrix (see p. 119) and the body fluids continuously seek for and find a new balance, a new *point of balance* or a new *state of balance*. The more the practitioner and client approach neutral and the deeper this becomes, the greater the ability of the highly intelligent whole-body matrix and the fluids themselves to implement the necessary corrections. The practitioner functions as a fulcrum, providing support through his awareness and experience.

The process of self-regulation can be explained in terms of the three-step healing process, and its stages can be identified. Respect and attentive care

are fundamental requirements because this form of self-regulation *occurs spontaneously* and cannot be forced or actively induced by the practitioner, although it can be encouraged to a high degree.

To make things easier when supporting the three-step healing process, I recommend that beginners start by tuning in and listening at a free or relatively free location.

More advanced practitioners may begin at a free or restricted location, e.g. at a knee, where there is access to the slow body rhythms: pulmonary respiration also has an important relationship with the autonomic nervous system. The cranial bones and cerebral/spinal meninges form the covering for the nervous system, which shows rhythmic motion at about 6–12 cycles/min or slower.

A brief and simple explanation of the three-step healing process

First step/phase: Listen to the tissues and fluids in terms of their motion (respiratory rhythm, craniosacral rhythm, mid-tide). Keep a watch for and cooperate with stillness. It may be that you need to tune in to stillness in yourself, then to stillness in the client, and then to stillness in the room (see p. 102). Next, observe how a new *point of balance* is being sought.

Second step/phase: Once a new point of balance has been reached, there is a change within the whole field of tissues and fluids, accompanied by stillness, a functional still point. This stillness is fundamental to the therapeutic process in which something essential happens.

Third step/phase: The tissues and fluids move more freely and re-organize themselves around natural fulcrums. The rhythmic motion is more balanced. The Living Matrix, and with it the body as a whole, seeks and finds a new *state of balance*. Make a note of any changes compared with findings beforehand.

In Phase 3, for example, the tissues feel softer, widened and warmer, and the body rhythms are perhaps stronger or slower because they are relaxed and more balanced. As you continue to listen you may find that the 'new state' (Phase 3) is beginning to stabilize and deepen, or that the first phase of a new three-step healing process is already under way.

In cases where the client's spontaneous self-regulation does not have the resources to unfold sufficiently as you go with it, a range of release techniques can be used. Once restricted structures are released as a result and a rhythm becomes manifest, you can then go with the three-step healing process before ending the session.

This three-step healing process can be used:

- for assessment, to determine the strength of the body's own capacity for self-regulation
- at the beginning of a (functional/biodynamic) treatment session
- as a treatment in itself
- to deepen the treatment
- for integration, to round off a treatment session.

4.3 The fulcrum

The human body possesses many natural fulcrums, i.e. places around which primary respiration is expressed as optimum health. A joint (such as the elbow or knee) is a helpful example to illustrate *how a natural (free) fulcrum functions*: it is the still point where different forces meet and around which movement takes place. The hub of a wheel and the eye of a hurricane are further examples of fulcrums, around which movement and force are manifested. Other fulcrums include the respiratory diaphragm, the sphenobasilar synchondrosis (SBS) and the atlanto-occipital joint.

If a body structure undergoes adhesion or hardening (regardless of whether this occurs at the level of the skin, connective tissues, muscles, bones or membranes), or if the fluid medium becomes characterized by inertia – all of which may occur as a result of traumatic factors – then an *inertial fulcrum* develops. This phenomenon can be illustrated by taking a surgical scar as our example: in this instance, natural free flow is interrupted on a physical and energetic level and the irritation is stored in the tissues as a restriction/trauma. What Dr John E. Upledger called an 'energy cyst' is referred to in the functional or biodynamic craniosacral concept as an inertial fulcrum: a densified center of inert structures that reduces freedom of motion, vital energy and the expression of the Breath of Life.

A traumatic event of a physical or psychological nature may also act as (or bring about) an inertial fulcrum for the nervous system and for the person as a whole on a physical, emotional and mental level: vital energy, awareness, and free expression of joyous living are diminished and these elements are overlaid, retained, bound, and entrapped by the trauma (to prevent further spread). Inertial fulcrums may form and resolve again particularly at the level of the connective tissues and fluids: this level constitutes a highly intelligent whole-body matrix, which senses any change and is able to react to it immediately.

As a craniosacral practitioner, you should also pay attention to your own fulcrums during treatment. These provide you with a flexible, stable, labor-saving and neutral base for your treatment. Having a grounded and centered core attitude, regulating your distance on a physical, emotional and intellectual level, checking your body posture at the treatment table and whether and how your arms/elbows are supported/placed on the table – all these are factors with which you as practitioner can create free fulcrums for yourself.

The practitioner provides the client with a safe, protected space for relaxation and self-healing. The client thus has an independent reference point – i.e. the practitioner becomes a free and yet stable fulcrum and is spaciously present.

Sensations and emotions during the session

4.4

Once your client is correctly positioned on the treatment table in a peaceful setting and has established trust in you as practitioner, she can usually remain passive during the craniosacral therapy session and enjoy not having to do anything.

Relaxation is generally deepened within 15–20 min under the influence of the parasympathetic nervous system. In most cases, the brain's frequencies slow to a rate similar to that measured during meditation, prayer, contemplation, or the relaxed waking state just before the onset of sleep. In this relaxed state, it is possible for the client to have a clearer and heightened awareness of physical, emotional, energetic, and spiritual sensations. It is equally all right if your client cannot work out or follow what is going on because the ability to do so might also be indicative of a degree of control that potentially reduces or prevents deeper self-regulation. It is commonly reported that clients are deeply relaxed and yet wide-awake and aware at the same time. Among other things, this relaxed resting at the center allows the client to focus her attention on the messages coming from her body and spirit and to sense what is happening at that moment.

The *physical sensations* may cover an extremely broad and varied range: warmth or coldness, lightness or heaviness, relaxation or tension, widening or constriction, alertness or tiredness, impulsiveness or lethargy, wholeness or disconnectedness, intensity or dullness, symptom intensification or symptom reduction, pleasure or pain, letting go and widening or pressure and compression, physical strength or weakness, and so on.

The *emotional sensations* may be just as wide-ranging, potentially including anything we are likely encounter during our lifetime: joy or sorrow, happiness or despair, contentment or frustration, confidence or doubt, a sense of security or isolation, love or hate, presence or absence, faith or resignation, emotional strength or weakness, and so on.

The *energetic sensations* may manifest themselves in very different ways, e.g. as flowing, streaming, undulation, prickling, vibration, twitching, discharging, pulsation, awareness of chakras, and so on.

Spiritual perception may furnish a rich source of important insights. This may also be stimulated against the background of physical, emotional, and energetic sensations. Occasionally, spiritual perception is revealed through a variety of sensory impressions or in deep relaxation and it can be an inspiring and telling factor in the individual's spiritual journey.

When these different levels of perception are sensed and felt collectively rather than separately, we experience the natural and spontaneous wholeness of our humanity. This may generate or deepen experiences of a spiritual, religious or existential nature. When our body is relaxed, we enjoy pleasant access to emotional, energetic, spiritual, sensory, and even transcendental perceptions and levels. By connecting with our inner wisdom and in harmony with natural laws, we discover what is useful and vital for us.

Occasionally, memories of long-forgotten situations or emotions will surface during a craniosacral therapy session. These may relate to happy events or to unresolved, suppressed issues or situations. Depending on inner preparedness, a burdensome situation from the distant past that still has repercussions for the present can be reviewed, set in perspective and receive closure in the relaxation of the here and now.

Sometimes, *sensory stimuli* can be felt more acutely. For example, a flavor or odor may resonate with accompanying memories or images. Sensations from the past may be re-lived in heightened form. In this context, all types of sensory perception are possible, e.g. a melody, the smell of anything from anesthetics (recalling a stay in hospital) through to grandma's freshly baked cakes, or mulled wine and cinnamon from those peaceful winters of childhood memory.

The *perception of time may change* during craniosacral therapy. This often happens in parallel with a broadening of perceptual awareness. The chronological time scale is abandoned because the sense of time on an emotional level, for example, is different. People entering a state of pure consciousness often report sensations of timelessness.

The peace and relaxation experienced during a treatment session often have the effect of a long, refreshing sleep. The organism as a whole, in particular the different brain regions, is in the process of re-balancing itself. Perception of different levels expands awareness and paves the way for complex experiences for body, mind and spirit. People have likened this to bathing in their own inner spring.

Using attentive therapeutic dialog, the practitioner can facilitate access to these levels. This should be done with respect and care. Therapeutic rapport is decisive if process support is to be helpful. In situations where things have become 'stuck', one solution-oriented option is to suggest making contact with the inner healer. And it is also all right to say hardly anything at all during the entire session and just occasionally to ask how the client is feeling.

There are people who are able to relax completely in their bodies and who, like shamans, can wander in the waking state between everyday reality, trance-like states and transpersonal levels. Some can identify behavioral patterns, gain access to symbols, to the collective unconscious or superconscious, and discover pathways to change/transformation. Others embark on a kind of inner visionary quest that helps them to shape the future in a positive way or to identify the background to illnesses – rather like retrieving 'lost areas of the soul' – in order for these to be fully re-lived and re-experienced in the here and now. At the same time, they are always responsive, present, and observant.

4.5 How the client can support the session:
Dedication to her own inner process

The client will decide whether she wants to consciously follow and inwardly support the session. She is also entitled to fall asleep or to stay alert and rest passively at the center.

For example, the client can inwardly support the craniosacral therapy session by:

- focusing attention on the site where the practitioner's hands are currently placed
- focusing attention on the site where noticeable sensations are occurring in her body
- attentively sensing those body areas that are soft, widened or warm
- breathing gently with an inward focus into the site that feels most pleasant
- letting her overall breathing flow, perhaps by breathing slightly more deeply, thus energizing her body and increasing her awareness of self
- consciously attempting to let go of any symptoms or pain, for example, by imagining that she is 'breathing them out' simultaneously through her slightly opened mouth and both feet.

With every touch by the practitioner on her body, the client can feel and assess the ongoing effects: How does the site in question feel? Has anything changed?

The bullet points listed above promote (body) awareness. In many cases, it is useful and immensely enriching if the client is attentive and learns to become even better acquainted with her body as the 'Temple of the Soul', to value it and to love it. In this setting too, the client's trusting dedication to her own inner process is a learning objective.

However, there are some particularly active individuals who, even during craniosacral therapy, are continuously busy externally (verbally, physically) or internally (constantly observing, incessantly thinking or visualizing). This may be a subconscious defense mechanism to help them maintain control. An obsessive need to be in control, ceaseless activity, dissociation or falling asleep may all be indicative of a lack of trust in the client's own inner process or in the practitioner. All of these strategies can also be used by people as (self-) protection after trauma. This is also permissible but it needs to be recognized by the practitioner. By issuing occasional verbal invitations, the experienced practitioner can encourage the client to try something new in this craniosacral therapy session and thus to make novel discoveries and experiences.

It can be helpful for the client not to actively monitor the entire session, to talk less and instead to feel and enjoy more, and to be relaxed in her own center.

4.6 Cell memory, therapeutic pulse and entrapped energy

Cell memory

One of the underlying premises in craniosacral therapy is that all cells possess a type of memory. Via the whole-body matrix of connective tissues and the fluids contained in them, the cells are connected with each other and in constant communication. The most recent research findings confirm this explanatory model for craniosacral therapy (see p. 119). The body as a whole reacts to physical and psychological situations that are out of the ordinary. Individual cells and cell groups can be adversely affected by *external physical factors* such as injuries, bruising, falls, lacerations, surgery, strains, and musculoskeletal lesions, and by *emotional factors* such as long-term repression of feelings or a sense of being overwhelmed. Psychological events, e.g. a fright or shock, may also leave traces behind in the body, in muscles, connective tissues, the respiratory diaphragm, breathing pattern and eyes, provoking an immediate reaction and a change in hormone secretion. It is believed that extreme or permanent psychological stress also has repercussions that extend to the bodily and cellular level.

If the natural life of the cell is adversely affected, the cell will try to protect itself by isolating itself. For example, if a part of my body receives a massively painful blow, the cells of the tissues affected will react by drawing in and isolating themselves. This self-protective mechanism helps the cell to be armed and ready for a renewed similar attack. The cells therefore store the information about the pain as a restriction. At a subconscious level, this defensive and protective patterning reaction can become the norm. It has been demonstrated that the cells – both individually and collectively – subsequently react with reduced metabolic activity.

Therapeutic pulse, therapeutic process

During a craniosacral therapy session, if your hands are placed over an area of the client's body where severely resistant, irritated or traumatized tissues are starting to release themselves from this pattern, you will often notice the onset of a rapid pounding – known as the *therapeutic pulse*. Do not confuse this with the pulse of the heartbeat or with the craniosacral rhythm. The therapeutic pulse often manifests itself as a reaction in the course of a therapeutic process whenever points of increased attention or inertial fulcrums are activated and start to change, or whenever tissues/structures are released.

At such locations, the therapeutic process may express itself under your hands in a wide variety of different ways, including:

- the therapeutic pulse
- tingling
- fine pricking
- pronounced release of warmth
- extreme feeling of coldness
- freezing, lifelessness
- sensation of being pulled down into the client's body
- sensation of being pushed away by the client's body
- a hole or irritation in the aura
- a dull feeling
- rapid breathing, marked change in the client's breathing pattern
- sweating.

If you notice any of these phenomena, leave your hands where they are. Ask the client what she senses at this site and whether you should continue your touch contact there. Before, during, and after release or a therapeutic pulse, note the qualities of the craniosacral rhythm in this area. Is a still point establishing itself?

Provided you have checked this verbally with your client, do not take your hands away until the therapeutic pulse has subsided and you have continued listening for a few moments to the tissues and to the change they have undergone. Now assess the tissue qualities – its density, warmth, and tone.

Point of increased attention

A site or region with minimal restrictions may be perceived by the practitioner and assessed as a 'point of increased attention'. The body often also responds to an energy imbalance by undergoing change at a physical level, e.g. expressed as connective tissue adhesion or pronounced connective tissue restriction. Points of increased attention are not severely traumatized and often resolve after just 1–2 min touch contact and release at the location in question.

Points of increased attention are secondary inertial fulcrums. These develop as a compensatory phenomenon as the body seeks to adapt to primary inertial fulcrums caused by energy entrapped at related body locations.

Inertial fulcrum and entrapped energy

Severely irritated and traumatized cells may manifest themselves in cell groups as 'entrapped energy' or as 'energy cysts'. Energy entrapment zones may develop, for example, following surgery or accidents. Badly traumatized body locations hold on to the pain caused at the time and act rather like a 'jamming device' in the tissues. They form a primary inertial fulcrum, which subsequently also affects adjacent or more remote zones where, after a time, they may result in a point of increased attention or secondary inertial fulcrum.

Energy cysts should not be confused with conventional cysts (walled-off fluid-filled swellings). And not every inertial fulcrum is necessarily an 'energy cyst' or has been caused by trauma. Inertial fulcrums may displace the midline and other natural fulcrums and thus reduce energy flow and self-regulation (see also p. 248).

When treating inertial fulcrums, you as the practitioner can decide (or perhaps ask the client) whether you should palpate and release the neighboring freer tissues *indirectly* or treat the inertial fulcrums *directly*. This may be done, for example, using techniques such as:

- connective tissue release
- fascial glide
- direction of energy using your hands and fingers
- process work with resource-oriented therapeutic dialog
- listening to and supporting unwinding
- still point induction
- peripheral release, e.g. at free locations on the extremities.

Unwinding 4.7

There are differing views on the subject of *unwinding*, depending on the treatment approach adopted. As used below, the term unwinding should under no circumstances be interpreted as meaning unwinding processes induced or provoked by the practitioner or client. This would not be consistent with the resource-oriented release approach being taught in the majority of craniosacral colleges in recent years. Unwinding occurs involuntarily and from the inside outward.

The unwinding described here occurs without active physical assistance from the practitioner, and should be understood, for example, as:

- an expression of letting go in the here and now
- an expression of 'un-folding', release on a physical, emotional, intellectual and spiritual level
- an expression and an attempt here and now to perceive restrictions or traumatic and unresolved events in a different (i.e. resource-oriented) way, and to provide more harmonious closure for them
- an expression of the restoration of previously absent protective and defensive mechanisms
- an experience of new qualities and sensations instead of arrested dynamics.

In chronic health problems and trauma, in particular, it is important to take things through to a resolution: whereas this may not have been sufficiently possible at the time when the event first occurred, change can now be facilitated in a setting of safety and trust. The helplessness and trauma of the past are today replaced by the potential for setting limits, feeling protected and resting in the moment, and the client is no longer overwhelmed and vulnerable to the same extent as in the past.

The role of the craniosacral practitioner is to perceive and support the client's spontaneous unwinding processes. This unwinding acts on the musculoskeletal system (and on the client as a unity) like an un-wrapping, an un-folding, a slow conscious untangling out of captivity or tension and encourages the letting-go of stored traumatic memories from the past. In this context one option is to support the extremities. Examples include: wrist or ankle, fingers or toes, elbow or knee, shoulder or hip. Alternatively the torso – in particular, the dural tube, spinal column and the entire midline – may start to release itself spontaneously from restrictions through this unwinding process.

As a visual aid to illustrate unwinding, take a 1 meter length of cling film, and fold it three times so that the different layers adhere to each other.

This is a good example showing the function of tissues such as muscles, fasciae, and ligaments, which are all interconnected. Now simulate a musculoskeletal sprain by twisting the folded cling film several turns in opposite directions and then stop without letting the film untwist. If you then twist the film even further, you will simultaneously notice the increased tension in this structure. When you let go of one end of the tightly twisted film under tension, you will clearly see what happens during tissue unwinding: the contracted, compressed or sprained area affected by adhesion, restriction or trauma frees itself *spontaneously from the inside outward*.

When a person's body is crushed by an accident or, as in the case of one client, is hurled through the air following a motorcycle accident, the musculoskeletal system and dural tube are twisted and compressed. Once the acute pain has subsided and having consulted with a physician, you may perform peripheral release with the client and attentively go with her spontaneous unwinding process. Support this process as soon as the tissues are released and this release of tension reveals itself in slow unwinding movements *from the inside outward*. You should respect every 'stop' indicated by the tissues. Is the client's breathing pattern changing? Is there any change in this specific local zone? Is the client's whole body responding to this release? If so, how? Remain alert to detect whether, when and in which direction a further wave of release reveals a new unwinding process and then go with this.

When treating symptoms of any kind whatsoever or inertial fulcrums, following injury or accidents or surgery, or in cases of severe dysfunction, feel for unwinding in the client as an expression of release and gently support this.

It is already helpful to *encourage release peripherally* and to treat transverse connective tissue layers extensively (see Figs 4.7.1 and 4.7.2). This will also influence the symptom site and its origin, which can be treated later by supporting spontaneous unwinding. Make sure that you do not work 'just' at the symptom site; wherever possible, involve neighboring zones too because in all probability these will also be vulnerable to any knock-on effects. They provide clues to further points of restriction and continuity in the body and should also be included in any comprehensive treatment.

For example, carefully and lightly lift your client's leg or arm, take its weight and so support and release the strain on the entire zone (Fig. 4.7.1A–D). Then listen but do not perform any manipulation in the process. In this position, the client does not need to contribute any effort at all; she may remain passive and relinquish the weight of her leg or arm. She may support the treatment, for example, with conscious breathing and increased sensory awareness but may otherwise remain totally passive. Sense your way into the tissues and slowly go with the leg or arm in the direction of ease. If you sense densification of the tissues or of the direction of ease, halt just before or at this point, at the barrier where the tissues tell you to stop, and wait and see what happens. It may be that the tissue memory wants to discharge itself of the trauma or

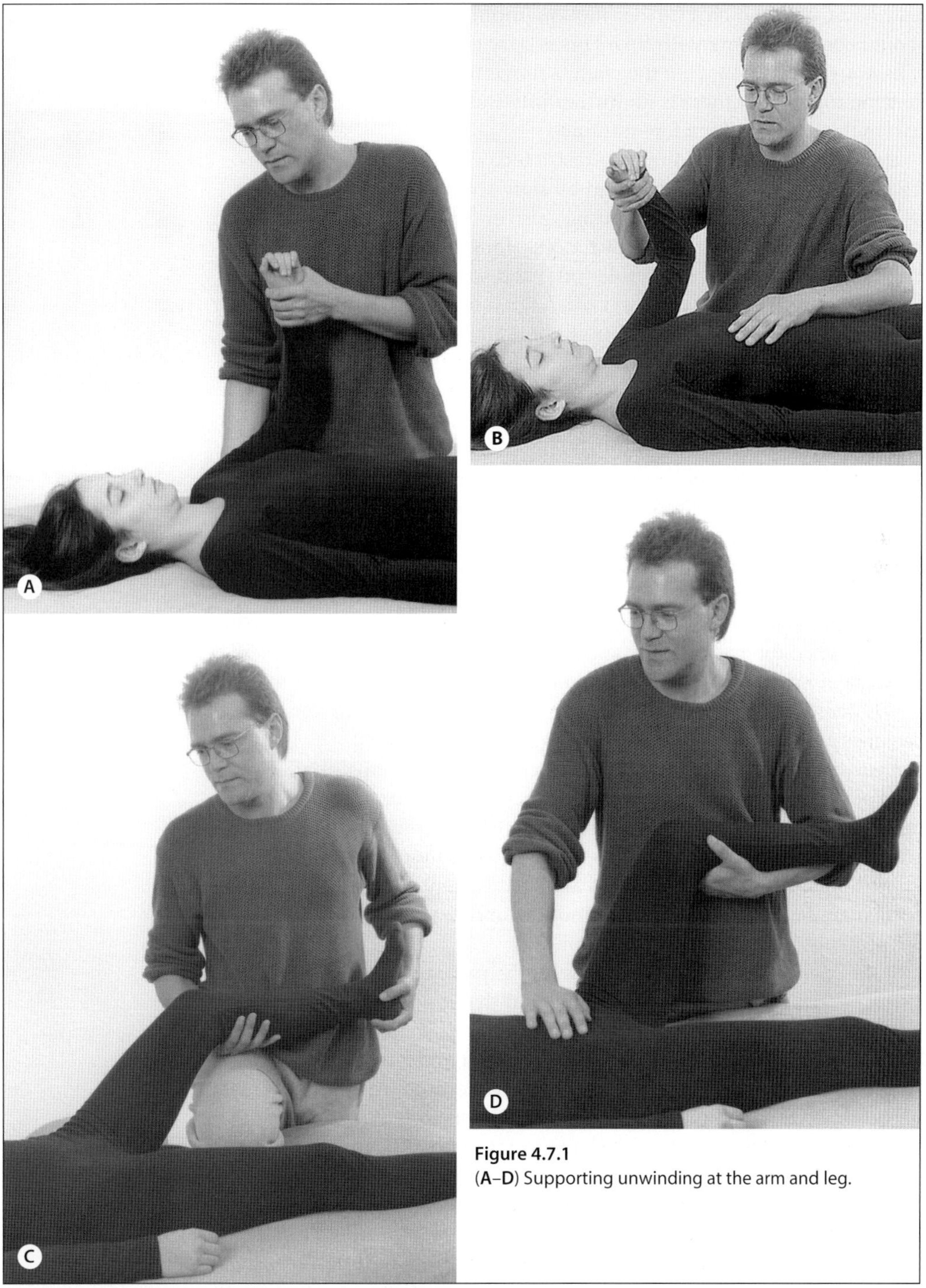

Figure 4.7.1
(**A–D**) Supporting unwinding at the arm and leg.

restriction, after which a further motion impulse may commence and you should continue going with this. This is a *simultaneous and constant process of listening to and going with* the client's movements, and this can feel like dancing together. If there is no further unwinding, keep the affected body part in this position for a few minutes.

Unwinding – the unfolding of a restricted or traumatized region – is frequently seen to be characterized by slow spiraling movements. As a fascinating analogy, this spiral form is also encountered in the microcosm and macrocosm: during the birth process, for example, a baby passes through the birth canal using rotational and spiraling movements. New leaves or blossoms in nature very often open in a spiral pattern. And our Milky Way is a cosmic spiral whirl. Energy in most forms moves in a gyratory-spiraling fashion.

During unwinding, if the client's body seems to get stuck in a longish period of continually repeating a pattern of movement or to speed up in an unruly manner, we suggest that you slow the movement down or clearly arrest it briefly, the response often being that the tissues go in a new direction of release. This is the only situation where the practitioner does not go with the movement in a wholly supportive way, but uses a deliberate therapeutic intervention to create space for the underlying impulse.

Craniosacral practitioners have achieved good treatment results – particularly in tension of the shoulder and neck muscles – by supporting passive unwinding at the neck and head (for experienced practitioners only). As it is being supported, this region (which often holds a great deal of tension) does not have to do or keep hold of anything for a few minutes, and can let go completely (Fig. 4.7.2A–G).

Every physical release and every processing of trauma also affects the level of the emotions. It often happens that the situation that originally resulted in trauma is re-lived in a similar way on a physical, emotional, and intellectual level, but this time the process is more conscious and less (or no longer) overwhelming. This allows the client to observe forgotten particulars or details, as if in slow motion, and to reconstruct and process the past injury now from a safe distance.

If the client identifies too closely with the pain, point out that she has already come through her past trauma and that it does not now have to be repeated in similarly dramatic fashion; instead it can now be resolved in a setting of perceived safety, protection, trust and letting-go.

Use of *resource-oriented therapeutic dialog* will ensure that the client does not become too 'caught up' in past events. The treatment is solution-oriented and the client remains present as far as possible in the here and now.

Following spontaneous unwinding, the client's body often automatically enters a still point, in order to produce a new *state of balance* both locally as well as overall. You may also invite a still point from outside. After the therapeutic pulse, *unwinding* and subsequent release, listen to determine the current feel of the tissues and the craniosacral rhythm. Has something also changed overall – in the client, in you the practitioner, or in the atmosphere in the room?

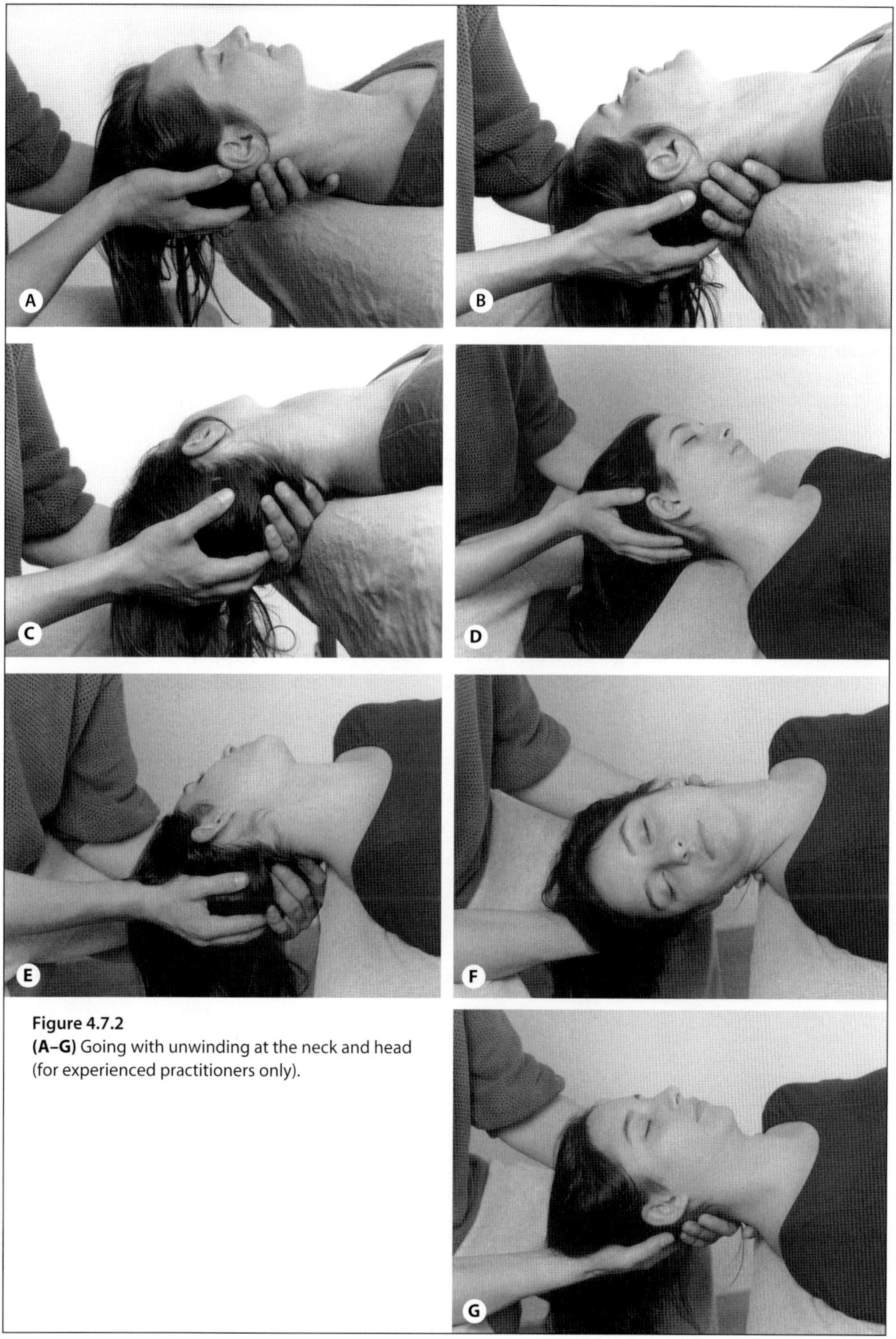

Figure 4.7.2
(A–G) Going with unwinding at the neck and head (for experienced practitioners only).

4.8 Treatment involving several practitioners (multiple hands-on)

Multiple hands-on sessions are treatments involving two or more practitioners (Fig. 4.8.1A–C). This intensifies the treatment. One practitioner assumes the role of team leader and, after a whole-body assessment, suggests a treatment position to the other co-practitioners. For example, the team leader may sit near the client's head, while the second practitioner establishes touch contact with the client's sacrum or feet, and a third practitioner with any part of the client's body that attracted particular attention during the whole-body assessment. The team leader takes responsibility for the therapeutic dialog, decides on how to support the client's process, and finishes off the session in good time to allow for integration.

When more than two hands are placed on the client's body, it is perhaps less possible for the client's hypercritical mind to keep a check on the treating hands of all practitioners. Harmonious multiple hands-on touch encourages a deeper letting-go in which the client allows things to happen and is carried along in her personal therapeutic process. Practitioners should

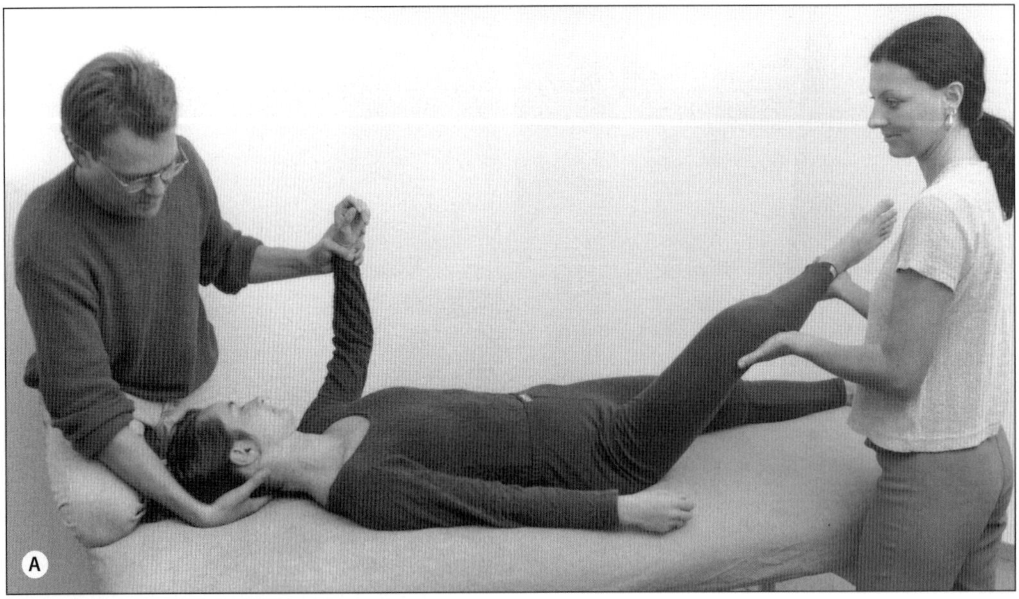

Figure 4.8.1
(**A–C**) Treatment involving two practitioners (*Continued on next page*).

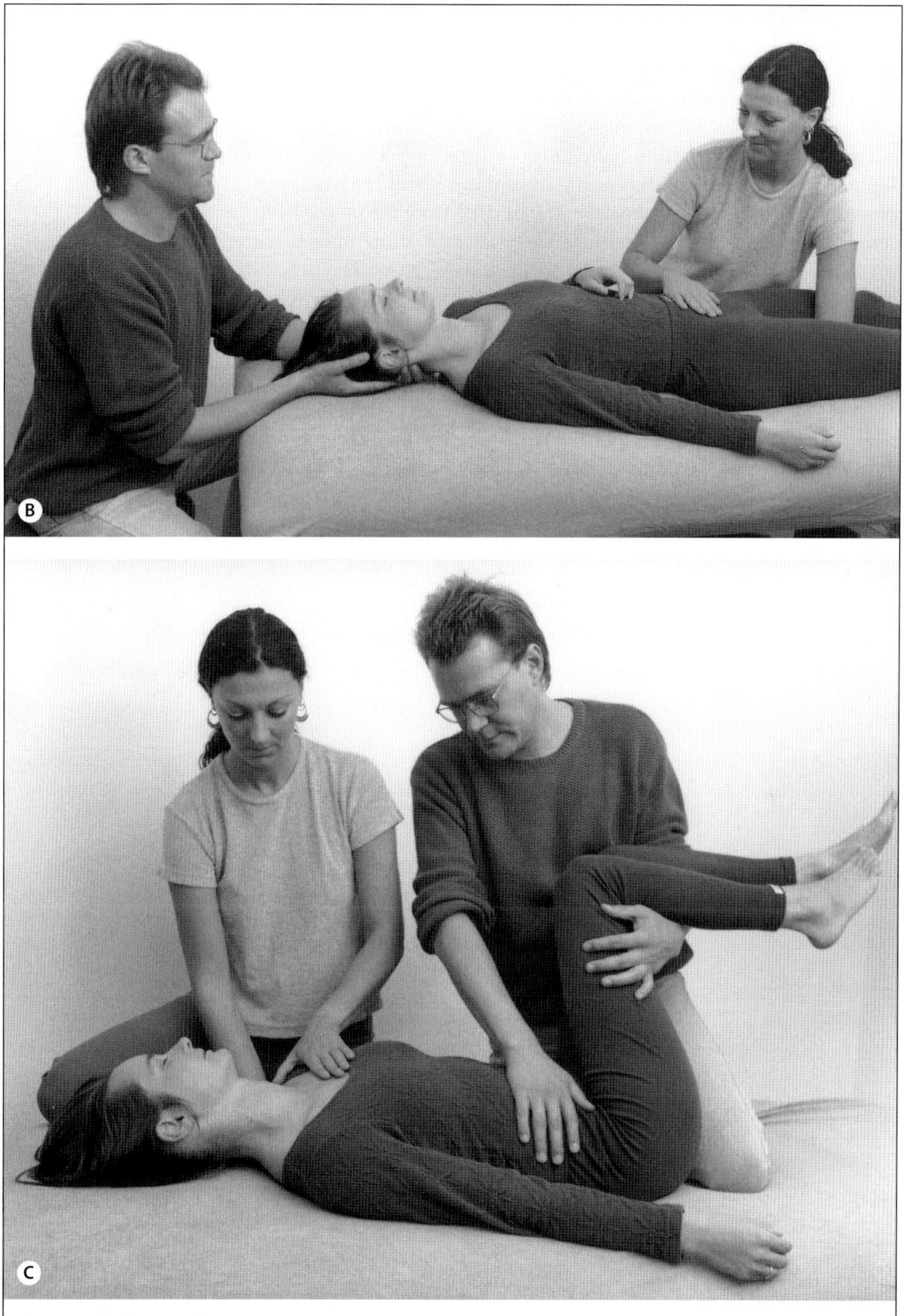

Figure 4.8.1 (*Continued*)

tune in to the tissues and the motion of the craniosacral rhythm. If they sense the spontaneous impulse as the client's body unwinds, they should support this non-intrusively. This unwinding can be extremely valuable for resolving deep-seated restrictions and trauma.

When several practitioners are supporting this spontaneous, careful unwinding, the client's body has an even greater opportunity to perform all physiologically possible movements without having to hold back one or more body parts, and can thus free itself from traumatic body memories right down to the cellular level. This can sometimes be very violent, depending on the charge of the nervous system. The practitioners should proceed with extreme caution, and force nothing: their role is to support the body movements at the legs, arms, head and neck, and throughout the torso. While this is happening they are in contact with each other and, as they listen sensitively, they go with the client's spontaneous *unwinding*. The team leader will also maintain clear verbal contact with the client, who does not backtrack but is consciously aware of the *unwinding* process most of the time.

At the end of the multiple hands-on session, the client's body will often enter a spontaneous still point or else a still point may be induced/invited from outside.

Intention and thought power 4.9

Intention

The word 'intention' has two different meanings: in common usage, it means 'the intense or concentrated direction of the powers of the intellect and psyche toward a particular aim or objective'. However, as a medical term, 'intention' also has a specific meaning in the context of wound healing and this brings us to craniosacral therapy, because craniosacral therapy supports and improves wound healing. And in the figurative sense too, this gentle body therapy heals many physical–psychological wounds.

The craniosacral method differs from other forms of manual therapy in terms of fundamental intention: the practitioner does not necessarily have to be active and do something. In craniosacral therapy, we proceed on the assumption that the client's body already possesses the answers to resolve dysfunctions, restrictions and trauma; consequently, the practitioner does not need to 'treat' the client and certainly does not need to perform excessive manipulation. By palpating the craniosacral rhythm, the practitioner tunes in to an expression of the primary respiration. Through whole-body assessment, gentle palpation of free tissues and release of restrictions, the practitioner and client arrive at a deep understanding. The experienced practitioner consequently allows himself to be led increasingly by signals and by the wisdom of the body.

The human body possesses the intelligence and the potency to heal itself. This wisdom is known as the 'inner healer' or 'inner physician': its inner endeavors are directed toward wholeness, harmony, growth, joy, and vital flow.

With this intention, the craniosacral practitioner sensitively takes up contact with the slow rhythms that are the expression of health, self-regulation and self-healing, and is equally open to all signals communicated by the inner healer. Regulating the distance, therapeutic dialog, interactive support of the client's process, and a fundamental trust that the intelligence of the whole-body matrix and the potency in the fluids will themselves perform the work – all these things are helpful here. It is not the practitioner who heals; the client heals herself as her self-healing forces are activated.

Craniosacral therapy is a living discipline. It emerged from osteopathy and its development is ongoing. With a relative emphasis on either technical or energetic aspects, both forms of treatment can be used with benefit for the client.

Additional levels can be reached, particularly if the practitioner is present and attentive and is also familiar with techniques of therapeutic dialog and interactive process support: the healing of physical symptoms is especially encouraged if the *sensations* associated with the symptoms *are experienced and processed*. This happens in craniosacral therapy particularly as a result of inner perception and letting go on a physical, mental, and spiritual level.

The more open and expansive the craniosacral practitioner's own horizons, the more able he will be to perceive the essence of these most varied verbal and non-verbal messages. In this process, he supports those impulses that are constructive and promote the client's growth. This also involves 'more negative' aspects, which may be perceived during the session. These are not reinforced but the client is allowed sufficient space and time to find positive approaches to resolution that are consistent with her inner truth. Everything is possible and everything is permissible – provided that no force is used and ethical principles (or previously negotiated agreements concerning therapy) are adhered to.

If the practitioner's philosophy and belief system are more narrowly defined, he will chiefly be able to detect, experience and go with events and situations that emanate from this familiar territory. He will be less able – or perhaps even unable – to perceive the unfamiliar, and will reject it or possibly project it on to the client.

If the practitioner has already worked extensively on his own development and has broadened his own horizons, the deep insights gained will enable him to provide even more comprehensive support to clients on their journey. The experienced practitioner will be guided intuitively to important places in the body if he has an open, clear intention, sees with the 'eyes of his heart', and treats with humility – all combined with relaxed and spacious attentiveness.

In addition, he can train himself in a kind of '3-dimensional body awareness' in which the body locations beneath or between his hands are perceived *spatially*. There are people who can sense this space. It is sometimes reported that they are able to 'see' this space or that they experience a combination of 'feeling and seeing' at the same time. This type of awareness varies greatly from one practitioner to the next and also depends on the individual's own personal level of experience and development.

Thought power

During treatment sessions, a constant stream of personal thoughts will dramatically reduce the practitioner's attentiveness for what is really happening. During the session, both practitioner *and* client should make a conscious effort to set thoughts aside. By doing so, the practitioner will be able to tune in attentively to the here and now with the client, and the client in turn may gain a deeper understanding and valuable information about herself. It is primarily a matter of *sensing and bodily sensations*, not of thinking, reason or control.

Clear thought power, and intention can be used by the practitioner as one of many elements in craniosacral therapy. As a prelude to gentle, manual release, some practitioners first 'treat' using thought/intention and listening to the structure to see if anything is changing.

Thoughts are also energy. Brain frequencies can be measured. If the practitioner is resting in himself, and is in a meditative and attentive state, there is a fall in his brain frequencies, heart rate and respiratory rhythm. The parasympathetic system switches the nerves and muscles over to relaxation.

When thought, power, and intuition are combined, they are very effective: clear thoughts and intentions can help to release restrictions. When you focus on a particular location or situation, this has the effect of energetic intensification. This is not desirable in every situation or in every client: too much focus may even prevent/obstruct or interrupt a natural release process and be experienced by the client as pressure or as 'too much'.

If your mind is swimming with thoughts instead of sensing, perceiving, and recognizing, collect your thoughts again and re-focus them in a way that is relevant to the treatment. This has an entirely different effect from not being present and thinking about your next trip to the cinema or about bad news. Re-focusing helps you not to be mentally over-taxed but to remain listening and present and in appropriate physical and verbal contact with the client. The more the client's body and the client as a whole person relaxes, the less useful intention and thought power become: even a well-meant intention or a mentally transmitted thought can be invasive and reduce or interfere with the natural process of inherent self-regulation.

The less busy or absorbed you are on an exclusively technical level or in some other way, and the more you invite release and balance, the more the treatment session will be helped by intention and by your broad, spacious perceptual field.

4.10 Intuition

The more familiar you become with the basic treatment and with the further treatment options, the less you will have to think about what the next step should be. Building on a foundation of anatomical and structural competence, coupled with experience gained from further craniosacral training and supervision, you will develop the necessary confidence to broaden your perception even more. Narrowing your perceptual field is not beneficial either for you or for your client.

- If during treatment – in addition to placing your hand on the transverse connective tissue layers as you have been taught – you feel inspired, for example, to position your hand a little more in one particular direction, do so. Without intuition, which is a premonition or the spontaneous ability to grasp a situation, the treatment would turn into purely technical repair work. Trust your intuition!

Visual findings, palpatory findings, and internal 'conversation' with the client's body (see p. 267), taken in conjunction with practitioner intuition, will often enable you to treat at sites where the client wishes or that she feels are important (without her having communicated this verbally).

At the same time, it is important in the process that you do not become detached but remain present, listening to everything that the tissues and your collective senses want to tell you. Make certain, if necessary by checking with the client, that an intuitive hand position actually also feels pleasant. In craniosacral therapy, intuition and intention usually go hand-in-hand.

The therapeutic dialog II: Dialog, imagination and mental pictures

4.11

Transference/projection

Before you ask the client a question, ask yourself first what this question has to do with you. In particular, ask yourself whether and why it is useful to the client.

Solution- and resource-oriented activity

The therapeutic dialog should be a solution- and resource-oriented activity and should not be driven by your private personal agenda. Be imaginative and above all listen very closely so that, together with the client, you can discover what is important for her.

Using the subjunctive

In any kind of impasse or if your client has reached a point in her process where there is no obvious way forward, questions using the subjunctive can be helpful, such as: 'What would happen if …?' or 'How would it be if …?'.

Repeat the client's answers and ask further probing questions

You may take the client's answers and repeat them as a statement. You can then add a further question (e.g. 'How's that for you?').

Contacting the inner healer

At the right time it may be useful to suggest that a client makes contact with the inner healer, inner physician, wise woman or shaman, e.g. 'If there was a power within you that knew precisely what is good for you, what would you be most likely to call it?', 'How would it be if you were to try and make contact with your inner healer?', 'Let's suppose that your inner healer has a name or a particular appearance: would you like to describe this?', 'What would he say to you if he were to speak to you?' or 'What would he write down for you if he were to write?'. After contact has been established, the inner healer may, for example, listen to the state of body areas and organs and perhaps give important clues pointing to release.

Internal 'conversation' with the client's body

Some practitioners enter into an internal 'conversation' with the client's body and receive non-verbal answers, e.g. 'Would the system like to go into a spontaneous still point?'; 'Should I continue at this site or …?'

Perceiving and anchoring insights and bodily changes

Insights and changes arising during treatment can be reinforced by asking the client and thus become securely anchored. Support the client in finding useful and appropriate implementation strategies for everyday living. Perhaps you might suggest trying this out before her 'inner eye' as a test to discover how this might feel. New stimuli and sensations create new conduction pathways in our nervous system: when you imagine a delicious dinner, the mental picture alone can stimulate your appetite and increase the production of saliva and gastric juices. If in your mind's eye you smell a rose from the garden, this can alter your mood.

4.12 Treatment continues to take effect after the session

Reactions following a craniosacral therapy session are extremely varied and highly individual: some clients feel ready for action and wide awake, while others feel pleasantly sleepy. Some are extremely vigorous and euphoric, others pleasantly relaxed and centered, with nothing being able to dislodge them from this sense of peace. Each craniosacral therapy session is again uniquely different and the after-effects will vary. If the subconscious level has been addressed, this can also manifest itself in everyday life through sudden memories or dreams. Sometimes the after-effects can be unanticipated and occur on other levels which are hardly perceived at all by the client.

It is important that clients take care of themselves after the session. Sometimes after a session, people are very open and vulnerable emotionally. In such cases, it is important that they find themselves a suitable haven to retreat to for a while. After the session, the client should check that she has returned to reality before venturing out on to the roads. Clients should always drink plenty of fresh water after a session.

Craniosacral therapy delivers important input to central body systems in terms of the restoration of balance, and this continues to take effect after the session proper has ended. Depending on the client and her momentary frame of mind or current life situation, this may last for a few hours, several days or as long as 2–3 weeks.

As a rule, the treatment and its after-effects are perceived in positive terms. For example, clients report improved sleep, pleasant body awareness and greater calm and they derive greater pleasure from life. After several sessions, others are again better able to sense what is good or less good for their own body and their inner growth. As a result, substitute strategies may be recognized or are spontaneously no longer needed. In many cases, obstinate physical problems are only resolved when habits are also altered or discarded in the everyday routine of life.

4.13 Intensification of symptoms due to re-organization

An experienced craniosacral practitioner knows that he must not provoke or force anything with his treatment. The client's body will indicate those areas that are free or at all restricted. The practitioner's touch does not forcefully break through restrictions but gently encourages them to melt away. Provided that the experienced practitioner uses his background knowledge during treatment to regulate physical and emotional distance, does not treat too long or too intensively, and occasionally asks for feedback, any initial deterioration due to faulty treatment can be virtually ruled out.

However, it is possible that pleasant as well as unpleasant sensations may make themselves felt. Any obstacle to the natural streaming flow of energy or anything that stands in the way of the sensation of wholeness and joy, may present itself as a challenging opportunity for growth on all levels. The client should be warned about this during the initial interview so as not to be totally surprised if this happens. Just like symptom reduction, the intensification of symptoms during or after treatment should in most cases be understood as reflecting *re-organization* due to improved self-regulation. Initial worsening is rarely an expression of faulty treatment, but is more likely to be indicative of change, of a healing crisis.

The connective tissues and nervous system (including the amygdaloid nucleus, a part of the limbic system) have stored up countless experiences, which the rational mind has often repressed and forgotten; during craniosacral therapy, these may free themselves from the subconscious and from the cell memory. The content does not always have to be worked through in verbal psychotherapy: the resource- and solution-oriented approach enables the individual to experience this differently and more holistically in a protected therapeutic setting in the here and now. The client can become consciously aware of this process through interactive therapeutic dialog.

It seems paradoxical that while the client wishes to experience an improvement through craniosacral therapy, the treatment may first usher in a degree of uncertainty and discomfort. The client has to assume responsibility for these individual and unique processes. For example, during the self-correction process (e.g. after an examination), the body often first exhibits tension and nervousness, only later to be followed by a relaxing balance. Some people are hardly aware of their body at all and perceive it as heavy or even 'leaden' after a treatment session because they have only just become aware of their years of tension and restriction.

The intensification and reduction of symptoms due to re-organization may last for seconds, hours or in rare cases several days. If the sense of being unwell persists for longer, a consultation with the attending craniosacral practitioner or a shorter follow-up course of integrative treatment should be considered.

Perhaps it is helpful to understand that changes to old patterns and structures may be accompanied by a crisis. At the same time, a brief period of uncertainty, accompanied by physical discomfort and emotional highs and lows, may signal the beginning of a vital re-orientation and transformation.

For example, if a body that has been permanently tense for decades is released in one craniosacral therapy session, this can produce feelings rather similar to muscle cramp. If the individual concerned is more clearly aware of musculoskeletal tension after the session, this may understandably also feel uncomfortable and constricting. Long-forgotten events from the distant past and the body areas affected may be spontaneously recalled to the conscious mind.

The tension was not triggered or provoked by the craniosacral therapy session but was already there and became accessible to experience as a result of the treatment. A habitually unhealthy lifestyle first needs to be deliberately shaken, sometimes to its very foundations, in order for release and necessary change to become possible. It takes an individually variable length of time before a person re-adjusts to a healthier and more agreeable lifestyle. Involvement of the emotional level and an understanding of this aspect can be helpful here. Sometimes the emotional component also wants to be processed and a more appropriate setting created so that the person as a whole is ready and able also to resolve the physical symptoms. This may have a transforming feel, almost like a butterfly emerging from its chrysalis.

4.14 Guided meditation to increase CSF flow in the body

Consciousness-related processes cause physiological-neurological activation of brain regions including the thalamus, hypothalamus, hippocampus, and brainstem. Complex neurological circuits are known to interconnect all areas of the brain. These brain regions are constantly bathed in a nourishing liquid known as the cerebrospinal fluid (CSF). CSF is produced in the walls of the four cerebral ventricles from where it is transported by rhythmic pulsation: in the occipital region, close to the cerebellum and parts of the brainstem, the clear CSF emerges through three apertures and then flows around the brain and spinal cord.

The cerebral membranes (or meninges) are located on the inner surface of the cranial bones. The outermost membrane, the dura mater, protects the brain. The CSF flows in the subarachnoid space between the middle and innermost membrane layers, the arachnoid and the pia mater. CSF protects and nourishes the brain, which is covered by the pia mater. On the dura mater, especially in the central region of the cranial vault, there are tiny granulations through which the CSF is reabsorbed into venous sinuses.

Our spinal column and connective tissues carry and support us. Nourishing CSF flows along the spinal cord, and even at its center, in the central canal. Away from the central canal, the CSF bathes all the nerve roots that emerge from the spinal cord and then travel onward into tissues, muscles and organs.

(Before embarking on the guided tour of the body you may find it helpful to study the section on The anatomy – an illustrated account, on p. 15.)

Guided tour of the body

Sit or lie down comfortably in a quiet area where you will not be disturbed and close your eyes if you wish. If you still feel a little tense, briefly increase the tension in your whole body – powerfully tense your extremities and entire torso, hold for about 3 seconds and then let go completely. Take a few deep breaths. Again make sure that you are optimally positioned so that you can spend the next 15 min undisturbed. In the course of this journey into your brain and along your spinal cord, you are invited to listen attentively to your body. Even if you cannot sense the suggested sites or movements at the first attempt, body touring and quiet listening will train your body awareness. Perhaps the guided meditation will help you to compose yourself better and to relax.

1. Allow the movement of your breathing to flow like a wave through your body. Breathe in and out slightly more deeply, from your abdomen up to

your thorax. It is all right to exhale with your mouth slightly open. In addition, your lower jaw may slowly drop a little. Now for a while there is no longer anything active for you to do.

Focus your attention entirely inward, to the center of your torso: sense your pelvis, your spine, your occiput, the whole midline from your coccyx up to your head as far as the front end of the falx cerebri, i.e. the ethmoid between your eyes and immediately above the area of the 'Third Eye': How do you perceive these body regions? Where does it feel pleasant? Remain there and listen.

2. Now focus your attention to the center of your head where the third ventricle is located, a kind of treasure chamber of the consciousness. From there travel up a little and now sense the two hemispheres of your brain on the right and left sides. Each of these hemispheres houses a chamber known as the lateral ventricle. Try to locate your two lateral ventricles. Stay a while with your left and right lateral ventricles. Can you perceive a slight flowing sensation or anything else?

   Again follow the two channels connecting the lateral ventricles with the center of the brain, the third ventricle. Stay a while with your third ventricle. What can you sense there? From there now follow the channel leading slightly obliquely downward, toward the back of your head, to the fourth ventricle. Stay a while with your fourth ventricle. What can you sense there?

   Perhaps you are able to perceive your head as a whole: as a next step, focus your attention on *all four cerebral ventricles*, which are interconnected and in the walls of which fresh CSF is continuously being produced by fine venous networks known as plexuses.
3. Now try to sense your *cranial bones* from outside, then from inside. What can you perceive? Now connect with the *meninges*, immediately beneath the bones of your cranial vault, where the *CSF*, the brain fluid, moves with a gentle rhythm. Its specific gravity allows your brain to float almost weightlessly. Your CSF and brain move in rhythmic synchronicity.
4. Now direct your attention to all the structures mentioned together: your interconnected cerebral ventricles, the meninges attached to the inner surface of the cranium, filled with CSF, and then your entire brain with all its structures. All these locations are continuously bathed by fresh CSF. Its slow rhythm transmits its slow-motion ebb-and-flow movements to the entire head and body.
5. Now direct your attention to your spine, then to the spinal meninges inside it that encase the spinal cord (a continuation of the cerebral meninges) from top to bottom, from your occiput down to the tip of your sacrum in the lower pelvic region. Throughout this whole area the protective, nutritive and cleansing CSF is constantly circulating.

   Next, turn your attention to the center of your spinal cord. Here too, in the central canal of your spinal cord, some CSF is continually flowing. What can you sense in this area?

Can you perceive how *all the areas mentioned are continuously bathed by fresh CSF and are also moving gently in time with the craniosacral rhythm?*

6. Now perceive your entire craniosacral system, from cranium to sacrum. Can you sense how the CSF is gently circulating everywhere, so setting the entire craniosacral system into slow, delicate motion, and how this gentle motion is subtly transferred to the entire body, down to the level of each individual cell?
7. If you sense that certain body areas are restricted, direct your attention there and ask the respiratory and craniosacral rhythms to use their movements to soften and release the restriction. Take the feeling of tension or restriction and consciously breathe it out through your mouth and via your legs and feet.
8. Where now in your body is the most pleasant feeling? How can you sense this? Are there any other body areas/regions that feel similarly pleasant? Can you sense the craniosacral rhythm? If so: where and how?

Now consider your entire body – as a whole entity.

At the end of this body tour, has something changed compared with how things were at the beginning?

And even when you open your eyes again after a while, stretch a little, perhaps yawn and then slowly start to move about again, you know that the CSF is continuously being produced and is flowing rhythmically throughout your entire craniosacral system.

Self-treatment techniques for the torso

4.15

Loosening the tissues around the sacrum and sacroiliac joint (side-lying)

Lie down comfortably on one side. Rest your head on a pillow or on your arm. Position your free hand above your gluteal fold and feel for your sacrum. Gently massage the skin and connective tissues around your sacrum. Also feel the tissues in this area using slow circular movements and appropriate pressure. In the area at the sides of your sacrum allow your broad fingertip contact to go more deeply. If you sense resistance in the structure, gently vibrate your hand (by moving from your shoulder) to work on this zone.

If this position becomes uncomfortable, change to lying on your other side and continue massaging your sacrum using your other hand.

This loosening technique can also be performed as you lie supine in the bath.

Relaxing the pelvic region

You can also practice sacroiliac joint relaxation on yourself. To do this, lie comfortably in a good position on your back, with your arms beside your body. Feel for your iliac crests on your right and left side.

Place your left hand on your left iliac crest, and your right hand on your right iliac crest. Allow yourself sufficient time so that via the skin and connective tissues you are able to establish deeper definite contact with the *bony sides of your pelvis* and to blend with these. Relax and listen for a while. Now, use both hands to deliver even compression that is *simultaneously directed inward and upward*. Hold this position for about 1 min, keeping your arms and shoulders relaxed. This then gently stretches the sacroiliac joints (see also p. 149).

This self-treatment technique can also be performed in the bath.

Relaxing connective tissues (supine, seated)

At any time, you can use one or both hands to feel your way into your own connective tissues. As you lie on your back, this is best done at the front of your body wherever you can comfortably reach with your hands without straining.

Sense the padded surface underneath your body. Allow your weight to sink downward. Now use your hands to feel your way into your connective tissues (as you did when releasing connective tissue restrictions in your client, see p. 120). A gentle fascial glide (p. 116) and deliberate breathing into the affected area will also help to release tensions in the tissues. You can also sense deeply with your hands, listen and train yourself in 3-dimensional body awareness.

By leaving your hands in position on your body and turning over on to your front, your own body weight will provide assistance in this self-treatment. It may also be comfortable to use a pillow to raise your thoracic region and relieve any strain on your cervical spine.

Full details of craniosacral self-treatment techniques are described in my book *Harmonizing your Craniosacral System: An Easy and Effective Self-Treatment* (see Further Reading). The craniosacral self-treatments are also available on CD (see p. 345).

Section 5

Advanced treatment

5.1 Basic treatment for advanced practitioners

Before you start

As a prelude to the structural basic techniques for advanced practitioners outlined here, you should first check whether your qualifications entitle you to treat people with health problems and whether a physician's referral is necessary.

Before you move on to the following treatment options and more sophisticated techniques, you will have mastered the release of restrictions in transverse connective tissue layers and learned to palpate the craniosacral rhythm at the head for several cycles.

You will also have attended a number of craniosacral courses involving supervised tuition and will be skilled in allowing the craniosacral rhythm and the body's inherent self-corrective processes to do the work. It will already be clear to you that while the craniosacral system can be treated specifically, it cannot be fixed or provoked merely with technical proficiency. In fact, the opposite is true: your part is to rest quietly in stillness and to listen sensitively. When you think back to the most recent treatments you have given, how has the feedback been from your practice partners or clients?

The following treatment options and techniques are designed to supplement the structural basic treatment (see pp. 106–201). However, they are only advisable and – as far as your client is concerned – helpful if you have largely mastered everything that has gone before.

Three treatment options

1. *Functional:* For several minutes, *exclusively* listen to and go with the *free motion* of the craniosacral rhythm *without using any corrections and techniques*. Your intention for the rhythm to become stronger, freer, broader, and more balanced will often be sufficient for minor compensatory restrictions to start to release. As you do this, you will be automatically encouraging the release of the craniosacral system. The qualities of the rhythm will become more balanced (see also p. 51).
2. *Functional-structural:* Listen to the craniosacral rhythm for several cycles and go with it. Is the palpated motion similar or the same over several cycles? Support it as you continue to go with the craniosacral rhythm, and occasionally deliver just a hint of amplification to exaggerate its

motion gently. As you do this, always go with the current motion of the craniosacral system, which you subtly amplify for a few moments. Make sure that this *gentle amplification* of craniosacral motion always occurs in time *with the craniosacral rhythm*. Afterwards, continue to listen to the rhythm for a few more cycles and palpate to determine whether and how this is more balanced.

3. *Structural:* Listen to the craniosacral rhythm for several cycles and go with it. If the palpated motion of the structure is clear and recurring, gently deliver just a suggestion of compression–decompression or use the indirect–direct technique to invite the structure to free itself from restrictions. To do this, go with the motion pattern, exaggerate it slightly, and then slightly amplify the opposite motion. Details on this are outlined below.

- Start with the first treatment option listed and also use the second option occasionally if you are practicing at an advanced level.

The third option is still gentle for the craniosacral system but it is the most invasive of the three. Because you are *merely inviting* the structure or, *at the head, treating with a pressure of 3g at most*, the second and third options are still very delicate in comparison with other treatment options/release techniques, for example, which operate with the direct method and use treatment pressures in excess of 5g.

Because the first two treatment options are relatively straightforward, it is mainly the third option that is described in detail in the following pages.

For the structural basic treatment (for advanced practitioners) described here, it is assumed *that you are able to palpate the craniosacral rhythm reliably at the sphenoid, the occiput and the paired temporal and parietal bones over several cycles*. You should be able to feel the 'neutral position' in the motion physiology, i.e. the approximate mid-point of the motion into flexion/external rotation (ER) and extension/internal rotation (IR). As an experience base, it is recommended that you will have already attended specialist courses, delivered about 50 treatments using the options listed above, and received about 20 treatment sessions yourself at the hands of other craniosacral practitioners.

As already mentioned, touch contact at the sphenoid is extremely subtle and yet clear at the same time. The sphenoid occupies the most central position of all the cranial bones. It runs transversely through the cranium and can be palpated laterally at its two greater wings in the temporal region. Its motion in time with the craniosacral rhythm decisively influences the movements of all the other cranial bones.

Do not start with the *basic treatment for advanced practitioners* until you have accumulated sufficient experience with the earlier basic treatment for beginners in healthy subjects and have received positive feedback (duty of care).

Supplementary techniques

Sphenoid: Compression–decompression

- Practitioner's finger position: sphenoid and occiput (see p. 181).

Neutral position: Using both thumbs (or index fingers) go with the tilting motion of the sphenoid and, with your two little fingers, simultaneously palpate the motion of the craniosacral rhythm at the occiput. Where is the neutral position, i.e. the midpoint of flexion and extension?

Compression: Hold the sphenoid in the neutral position, and for a few seconds deliver a gentle hint of compression (≈1 g) down toward the treatment table, i.e. posteriorly in relation to the client's head. Use your two little fingers to stabilize the occiput in this process. This delicate compression on the sphenoid acts on the sphenobasilar synchondrosis (SBS), which forms the articulation between the sphenoid and the occiput. Briefly and lightly amplify the identified restriction pattern.

Decompression: Immediately follow this brief compression with more prolonged decompression in the opposite direction, toward the ceiling, i.e. anteriorly in relation to the client's head. Using traction of 1 g, perform this decompression very gently and continuously for between 30 seconds and 1 min maximum. During the process, continue to listen and accept any 'stop' indicated by the tissues. Perform brief manual compression–decompression without simultaneously listening to the structure. As you deliver just a suggestion of decompression, can you sense whether one side of the sphenoid is freer or more restricted than the other?

Go with the craniosacral rhythm: After decompression, go again with flexion and extension and listen: Has this changed? If so, in what way? Is the craniosacral rhythm now more balanced? Is the travel into flexion and extension approximately the same?

Remove your thumbs/index fingers and little fingers, ideally in the neutral position.

To follow, we recommend the cradle hold and/or the cranial vault hold. Make a before-and-after comparison of motility and mobility.

Temporal bones: Amplifying physiological motion using the finger-in-ear position

- Practitioner's finger position: finger-in-ear position at the temporal bone (see p. 184).

After some practice, you will be able to support the tilting motion of the craniosacral rhythm at the paired temporal bones by gently amplifying the movements at their extreme rotation points, i.e. in full ER and in full IR. For this, use your index and ring fingers on each hand *to slightly prolong and exaggerate* the direction of motion *at the end of rotation*. This supports the flexibility and mobility of the temporal bones: the ER/IR movements often become larger and more balanced.

Alternatively, you may also increase the craniosacral motion of the temporal bones. *Starting from the neutral position* (i.e. from the approximate midpoint of ER and IR), go with this motion into the respective rotations and gently amplify these for a few moments. With this alternative option, you will not obstruct the craniosacral rhythm, something that tends to happen with the amplification/exaggeration of rotation at the end of full ER or IR, as described above.

Mastoid processes: Amplifying physiological motion

- Practitioner's finger position: thenar eminences on mastoid processes of the temporal bones (see p. 185).

As for the gentle compression technique you learned originally, place your thenar eminences immediately behind your client's ears and palpate the craniosacral rhythm at the two mastoid processes.

To illustrate this more clearly: During ER of the squamous part of the temporal bones, the mastoid processes move into IR medially, while IR of the temporal bones moves the mastoid processes into ER laterally. Go with these ER/IR movements *of the mastoid processes* laterally and medially for several cycles. After performing even medial compression (during IR of the mastoid processes, toward the middle of the client's head, *always with* the craniosacral rhythm, see p. 188), palpate the motion of the two mastoid processes again – are internal and external rotation now symmetrical on the left and right side?

During the next rotation of the mastoid processes toward the middle of the head medially, amplify this motion slightly, alternating between the right and left sides. First, using your thenar eminence during IR of the mastoid processes, deliver gentle compression *on one side* so as to amplify the motion on this side. (With your other hand, go with IR without pressure and listen.) At the innermost point of IR, additionally deliver brief compression medially, toward the middle, and then allow the mastoid process to rotate again into ER. Afterwards, perform unilateral mastoid process compression *on the other side* in the same way. You may perform one or two repetitions of this unilateral exaggeration technique using medial mastoid process compression during IR. Among other things, it amplifies lateral fluctuation and increases the flexibility of the tentorium cerebelli.

After you have treated both sides individually, listen again to the craniosacral rhythm for several cycles – it may no longer in fact be necessary to repeat this alternating compression.

Finally, as in the starting position at the mastoid processes, use both thenar eminences *simultaneously* to deliver *gentle* compression toward the middle of the client's head: while both mastoid processes are at the deepest point of IR, briefly deliver even medial compression with both thenar eminences.

Now remove all compression and listen to the craniosacral rhythm at both mastoid processes for several cycles: How is their radius of motion now? Has ER/IR changed? If so, how? Are the left and right sides now more balanced?

This amplification technique may be combined with the finger-in-ear technique and the gentle ear pull.

Structural treatment sequence for experienced practitioners

- Do not move on to the structural basic treatment shown in Table 5.1.1 until you have frequently used the simpler basic treatment for beginners (see p. 218) in different clients and have received positive feedback about this.

All release techniques are very gentle (weight of touch: 1–3 g). Terms such as 'lift' or 'compression' should be understood more as a hint, a subtle invitation to release, and not as manipulative maneuvers in a physiotherapy sense, for example. Start with the cradle hold or invite a still point.

After your treatment, listen to the craniosacral rhythm at several palpation stations. Has it changed? If so, how and in which body areas is this particularly pronounced? Are there any other differences compared with the situation before?

If the client wishes, she may finish off the session by lying on her side and taking time to enjoy the ongoing effects of treatment.

Table 5.1.1 ● Structural treatment sequence for experienced practitioners

Whole-body assessment

Listen to the craniosacral rhythm connective tissue layer release at:

Torso, hyoid bone, atlanto-occipital joint, lumbosacral region, sacrum, sacroiliac joints

Treating the head

Support craniosacral rhythm at the:	***Technique***
Frontal bone	Gentle lift
Parietal bones	Gentle compression in IR, gentle lift in cranial direction
Sphenoid	Go with tilting motion: Where is the neutral position? Which is greater – flexion or extension? Gentle compression in neutral position (brief, down toward treatment table, posteriorly) Gentle decompression in neutral position (more prolonged, up toward ceiling, anteriorly) Palpate flexion/extension: before-and-after comparison Listen to other movements and motion patterns
Temporal bones	Finger-in-ear position, listen to craniosacral rhythm: Where is the neutral position? Which is greater – IR or ER? Exaggerate/amplify ER/IR Go with mastoid process motion: support IR of mastoid processes by gentle medial compression, in IR slight medial amplification (perhaps alternating between right and left sides) Gentle posterolateral ear pull
Masticatory muscles	Massage and stroking: upward at side of auditory canal, downward below TMJ
Lower jaw (mandible)	Gentle hint of compression (brief, toward ear/TMJ) Gentle decompression (more prolonged, at 45°, diagonally toward ceiling/client's feet)

Conclude treatment of the head with the gentle ear pull and the cranial vault hold or cradle hold. Invite a still point.

Integration of head and torso

Comparison: before and after

5.2 Taking treatment further

Motion patterns of the sphenoid and occiput and how to balance them

The sphenoid and the occiput together form the 'key bones' of the cranial base. They articulate via the *sphenobasilar synchondrosis* (sphenobasilar joint) (Fig. 5.2.1). As the central bone in the cranium, the sphenoid is able to – and indeed often has to – compensate for positional anomalies and dysfunctions of other cranial components. The potential positional anomalies of the sphenoid itself are in most cases minimal but they may be sufficient to reduce well-being enormously and to cause headaches and disturbances of vision and learning.

These positional anomalies are only treated after other sites in the craniosacral system (e.g. the sacrum and occiput) have been treated. Using the broad-based contact of your index fingers or thumbs, you must be able to clearly palpate the craniosacral rhythm at the sphenoid for several cycles. The craniosacral motion of the occiput is palpated with your two little fingers.

First, listen to the free directions of motion. By doing this, you will learn also to recognize any motion restrictions. With this intention, however,

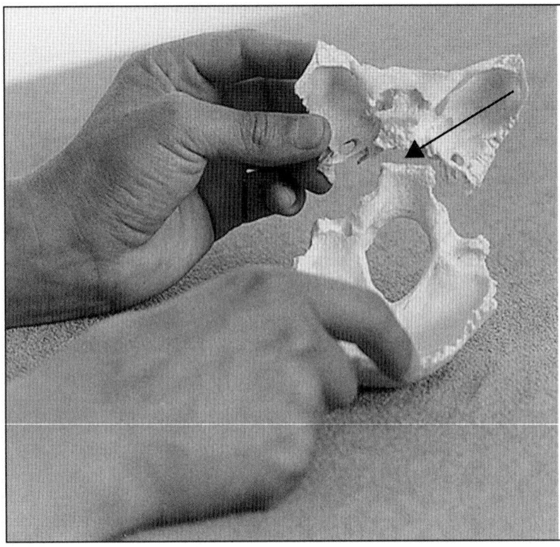

Figure 5.2.1
The sphenobasilar synchondrosis.

listen primarily to the movements that reveal themselves; these express functional potential and hence aspects of what is healthy. Consequently, you are not exclusively on the look-out for dysfunction but are primarily appreciating and looking for function and health.

Dysfunctions of the sphenobasilar synchondrosis (SBS) can be corrected in different ways

Version 1: For several minutes *do nothing except listen to and go with the free motion* of the craniosacral rhythm (*employ no techniques and have no intention of performing a correction*). As you do this, note whether and how the 3-step healing process (see p. 246) is encouraging self-regulation.

Version 2: Listen to and go with the craniosacral rhythm and gently exaggerate its motion, almost merely as a suggestion. This *gentle amplification* of craniosacral motion *always* takes place *with* the craniosacral rhythm. Then make a before-and-after comparison and perhaps repeat the process of going with and gently amplifying the rhythm.

Version 3: Once the palpated motion potential is known, use a gentle suggestion of compression–decompression or the indirect–direct technique to invite release from restrictions.

Version 4: Over a period of about 5 min, listen to and go with the craniosacral rhythm with two fingers placed on each side at the greater sphenoid wings and the occiput, issuing an invitation with the intention that *these four points become balanced* in their motion.

Versions 2–4 are very delicate and are, as it were, *suggested* to the structure, not performed with any pressure. Stabilize the occiput using your two little fingers: this is of course the cranial bone with which the sphenoid forms the sphenobasilar synchondrosis. It is often the case that all the motion restrictions and positional anomalies of the sphenoid and occiput cannot be released in a single session. After each release as described in Versions 2 or 3, listen to sphenoid and occipital motion in flexion and extension for 2–3 cycles before moving on to treat the next pattern. To conclude, go with the craniosacral motion of the sphenoid and occiput and check whether the motion is clear and as balanced as possible. Use of the gentle ear pull, cradle hold and still point induction may encourage the new balance of the structures.

- Motion patterns and dysfunctions involving the SBS are often caused by compensatory adaptation. They result either from restrictions elsewhere in the body or from external physical cranial trauma, for example, caused by a fall or collision

In craniosacral therapy, a lesion or dysfunction is defined as a recurring, exaggerated motion pattern. In the following sections, the motion patterns are explained deliberately in very simple terms and only in relation to the sphenoid. A single or multiple motion pattern will invariably also affect the occiput and other cranial bones because these together form the cranium as a unit. For simplicity, in this introductory practical manual, we will not be discussing the simultaneous compensatory pattern of the occiput. Any explanation of rotational axes has been intentionally avoided here. These aspects are covered in detail in more advanced craniosacral textbooks (see Further Reading). The explanations are intended to give an insight into possible positional anomalies and dysfunctions.

In practice, we always encounter *combinations of motion patterns*. These are unique to each individual and it is important to evaluate and treat them without being fixated on the patterns and their resolution.

The neutral position is the approximate midpoint of flexion and extension. In neutral, there tends to be minimal tension on all the structures involved. After the SBS has been released, the temporal bones, the head as a whole, and the torso and sacrum should also be included for purposes of integration.

Motion patterns/dysfunctions of the SBS include

- flexion/extension
- compression of compensatory origin
- torsion
- sidebending.

These four motion patterns are of compensatory origin. Consequently, the atlanto-occipital joint and the torso should also be included in the treatment, as appropriate.

- lateral strain
- vertical strain
- compression due to external physical trauma.

These dysfunctions are due to external physical trauma, e.g. a blow, fall, collision, or accident involving severe compression.

Correction of motion patterns as described in Versions 1, 2 and 4 is recommended more at the beginning because they are less invasive than Version 3, the indirect–direct technique. In each case, this will be explained after the individual exaggerated motion patterns have been described.

Flexion or extension patterns

We speak of a *flexion dysfunction* in cases where the sphenoid moves predominantly into flexion (i.e. caudally, toward the client's feet), but hardly at all into extension (i.e. cranially, toward the top of the client's head).

In an *extension dysfunction*, the sphenoid moves predominantly into extension, but hardly at all into flexion.

Flexion or extension dysfunctions are mostly of compensatory origin. You will automatically palpate the dysfunctions/motion patterns if you go with and listen to the motion of the sphenoid and occiput. Listen to the motion at the occiput using your two little fingers, which merely stabilize the occiput briefly during sphenoid release, as described in Versions 2 and 3.

For release, as described in Version 3, first go with the flexion–extension motion for several cycles. At the limit of the direction of motion, gently amplify the exaggerated pattern for a moment. Then go with the sphenoid back to the neutral position, to the midpoint, and then again into the direction previously found to be restricted on palpation. Hold the sphenoid at the point of restriction – the 'tissue stop' – for a brief moment and then invite it to move slightly further in the restricted direction. To do this, *exaggerate* this directional movement merely *as a gentle suggestion*.

Afterwards, go with flexion–extension again: now test whether these have already become more balanced.

Alternatively, the craniosacral motion of the sphenoid can also become stronger and freer *if you gently amplify its motion starting from the neutral position into the direction of restriction* (according to Version 2). In this way, you will not impede the craniosacral rhythm, which can happen during amplification of the direction of motion in full flexion or extension. After you have gently amplified flexion and extension, starting from the neutral position and going with the craniosacral rhythm, test whether flexion and extension have already become more balanced. Then, as in Version 1, listen to the self-corrective process for a few cycles. If the dysfunction is still present, you may repeat the described correction a further two or three times.

Torsion

We speak of torsion in situations where the two greater wings of the sphenoid are no longer horizontal. In such circumstances, the sphenoid undergoes torsion in a clockwise or counterclockwise direction. In the client's face (viewed from the front), one side wing of the sphenoid is slightly higher, and the other is slightly lower: one sphenoid wing has moved more cranially (i.e. higher, up toward the top of the head), and the other has moved more caudally (i.e. lower, down toward the maxillae/feet). The torsion is named after whichever sphenoid wing is *higher*; this dysfunction is almost invariably of compensatory origin.

Test for torsion as follows: in the neutral position, use the surfaces of your thumbs or index fingers briefly to exert a gentle hint of traction caudally on one side and cranially on the other, and then change immediately and go in the opposite direction. As you do this, take note of any free slippage or resistance in the structure. In the process, stabilize the occiput with your two little fingers.

For release using the indirect–direct technique, begin ideally in the neutral position. Start by imperceptibly and briefly amplifying the exaggerated pattern. With your thumb/index finger, guide this sphenoid wing slightly downward (caudally) and the other sphenoid wing simultaneously upward (cranially). Immediately afterwards, gently and more protractedly propose the opposite directional motion. Then palpate to check whether the torsion has already become balanced and listen to the craniosacral rhythm for a few cycles, as in Version 1.

Sidebending

We speak of sidebending when the sphenoid undergoes lateral torsion. In sidebending, one sphenoid wing has moved more toward the orbit, and the other more toward the temporal and parietal bones, or occiput. A convexity develops on the left or right side, i.e. the sphenoid and occiput are bowed outward slightly on one side. This dysfunction is almost invariably of compensatory origin and may lead, for example, to cross-bite. Test for sidebending in the neutral position.

To perform the indirect–direct technique, start by imperceptibly and briefly amplifying the exaggerated motion pattern: with your thumb/index finger invite one sphenoid wing to glide more toward the orbit (anteriorly) and the other sphenoid wing more toward the temporal/parietal bone (posteriorly). Immediately afterwards propose the opposite directional motion. Hold this for slightly longer and gently exaggerate. Then test to establish whether the sidebending lesion has already become balanced and listen to the craniosacral rhythm for a few cycles, as in Version 1.

Lateral strain

Lateral strain tends to cause the entire sphenoid to be displaced to one side; this exerts tension on the SBS. Left or right lateral strain is caused by trauma, e.g. a blow, fall, or collision impact on one side of the head. In most cases, this also results in slight sidebending. Left or right lateral strain is named after the direction of lateral displacement of the sphenoid.

Test for lateral strain as follows: in the neutral position, use your thumbs/index fingers to perform a clear, brief suggestion of lateral glide on one side, and immediately afterward on the other side. Can you detect a tendency to displacement toward either side? This is indicative of a lateral strain in that direction.

To correct this, begin with the indirect–direct technique. Stabilize the occiput with your two little fingers. Start by imperceptibly and briefly amplifying the lateral strain, i.e. the direction of traction on the sphenoid: using your thumbs/index fingers go with one sphenoid wing to the side (laterally) and with the other toward the center of the head (medially). Immediately afterwards, propose the opposite directional traction. Hold this for slightly longer and gently exaggerate. Then test to establish whether the lateral strain has already become balanced and listen to the craniosacral rhythm for a few cycles, as in Version 1.

Vertical strain

Vertical strain displaces the sphenoid upward (superiorly) or downward (inferiorly) in relation to the occiput at the SBS. Vertical strain is caused by cranial trauma, e.g. during the birth process or due to a violent blow, fall or collision impact on the head. The client's forehead may show a greater tendency to be prominent (where there is upward traction on the sphenoid) or to be lower and displaced slightly backward (where there is downward traction on the sphenoid). In vertical strain, the falx cerebri and the tentorium cerebelli are under pronounced tension.

Palpate the flexion and extension motion. In cases of vertical strain, these will feel very sluggish or heavy by comparison with normal flexion/extension. If the sphenoid wings descend toward the orbits and at the same time markedly downward (caudally) in flexion but hardly at all in extension, a superior (upward) vertical strain of the sphenoid body is present. If the sphenoid wings move markedly in a cranial–posterior direction toward the treatment table in extension, but hardly at all in flexion, an inferior (downward) vertical strain of the sphenoid body is present.

If you use the indirect–direct technique, stabilize the occiput using your two little fingers. Go with the greater sphenoid wings into the dysfunction/vertical strain and briefly suggest a slight exaggeration of this motion. Afterwards, encourage the sphenoid wings in the opposite direction and gently exaggerate this direction. After a short time, again go with the sphenoid in its flexion–extension for several cycles and listen to check whether flexion and extension of the sphenoid and occiput are already revealing themselves to be more balanced.

If the corrections using the indirect–direct treatment method are not efficient, gentle direct corrections may be used. Before performing direct release techniques, however, it is advisable to listen at all the key bones in the craniosacral system (sacrum, occiput, sphenoid) and to comprehensively treat the connective tissues in the upper torso as well as the entire cranium, including the horizontal and vertical membranes. In lateral and vertical strain, both the intracranial membranes and the elasticity of the cranial sutures should be tested because in most cases the dysfunction is caused by external physical factors.

Releasing the facial bones

The bones of the face articulate with each other in a complex manner. They form our face and also serve as a buffer zone for the sphenoid and brain, e.g. in the event of frontal impact. They are not directly continuous with the cranial meninges, but they move principally due to the rhythmic craniosacral motion of the sphenoid and ethmoid. Problems involving the area of the facial bones are sometimes caused by trauma or inflammation; compression of the facial bones may therefore hamper the free motion of the cranial bones behind them.

The following techniques may release restrictions and help to relieve visual disturbances, pressure around the eyes, or headaches in the frontal lobe region. Each of these release techniques can be applied for 1–2 min. This gentle stretching and widening extends into the deep parts of the orbit, which is formed by seven bones altogether. During the following release techniques, ask the client how she feels and encourage her to provide feedback if anything changes, or if something feels pleasant or unpleasant. In the facial region in particular, attentive touch that is pleasant for the client is extremely important.

Before establishing touch contact, check your own position at the treatment table and regulate your distance vis-à-vis the client.

Releasing the zygomatic bone

The zygomatic (cheek) bone articulates with the temporal bone via the zygomatic arch. It also has articulations with the maxilla, where it helps to form the lower part of the orbit, and above with the frontal bone. Together with the frontal bone, the zygomatic bone forms the lateral rims of the orbits. The zygomatic bone also articulates with the sphenoid. Before performing release on the zygomatic bone, you should already have treated the frontal bone, parietal bones, and sphenoid, as well as the masseter muscles, as described previously.

In preparation, you might try using your fingers to palpate your own paired zygomatic bones in the upper cheek region and allow your lower jaw to drop as you do this. The motion of the craniosacral rhythm at the zygomatic bone is determined and decisively influenced by the various cranial bones mentioned.

As you sit at your client's head, perform a brief visual inspection. Then palpate with your fingers the client's paired zygomatic bones. Are her left and right zygomatic bones symmetrical, are they located on the same level or on different levels (high/low)? If so, how do they feel?

Take up a position at the top end of the treatment table. To eliminate any tremor, rest both your elbows on the treatment table. If an arm extension comes as an accessory with your treatment table, this would be useful now. If not, the client can perhaps shift down the table slightly so that you can comfortably position one elbow close to the client's head. Check your seat height and distance *before* you take up contact. Now first treat the zygomatic bone around the eye on one side, followed by the other.

At a sufficient distance from the head end, position one arm close to your client's frontal bone but without touching her head. Then touch her eyebrow with the terminal phalanges of your index and middle fingers, turning them gently and carefully toward her eye so that you can feel the bony edge of the frontal bone. Starting from this point, now position your fingertips to establish broad contact at the upper *inner edge of the orbit*.

Position your other arm, supported at the elbow, to one side of your client's head at eye level, in such a way that your thumb can comfortably touch the lower *lateral* edge of the orbit (of the same eye). With your thumb, gently locate the bony margin of the zygomatic bone, well to the side close to the bottom of the orbit. The tip of your thumb should be pointing toward the client's nose and be positioned 1–2 cm lateral to the middle of the bottom edge of the orbit. Your thumb should provide broad-based contact. So as to locate your thumb in the best possible way at the inner edge of the zygomatic bone, rotate your thumb surface slightly toward the eye. In this way you will hook on to the edge of the zygomatic bone, your contact will have a better purchase and you will avoid compression or slipping off. The client's eyeball itself is not touched either by your index and middle fingers at the upper edge of the orbit or by your thumb at the edge of the zygomatic bone.

While your thumb at the edge of the zygomatic bone stabilizes this, use your index and middle fingers of the other hand to deliver a gentle stretch at the edge of the frontal bone, simultaneously toward *the top of the client's head and the ceiling*, i.e. diagonally upward (at about 45° in an anterior–cranial direction) (Fig. 5.2.2A, B overleaf).

Then with your index and middle fingers stabilizing the edge of the frontal bone, *use your thumb in broad contact at the edge of the zygomatic bone to deliver a gentle stretch in a diagonal direction*. Afterwards, deliver gentle, even releasing traction *diagonally in both directions, i.e. on the frontal and zygomatic bones simultaneously, drawing them apart*.

Then change sides to treat the other zygomatic bone.

Releasing the nasal bones

In preparation, you might first try using your thumb and index finger to palpate your own nasal bones for a few moments. Make sure you establish clear contact at the bone level. The two nasal bones articulate primarily with the maxillae, and their upper part also articulates with the frontal bone. The following technique releases the sutures between the nasal bones, frontal bone, maxillae, and lacrimal bones and also gives the ethmoid bone more space and freedom to move. In addition, it relieves tension on the falx cerebri.

Take up a position level with the client's head, to one side or at the head of the treatment table. To eliminate any tremor, place both your elbows on the treatment table, as above.

From the head of the table, bring one arm over your client's frontal bone without touching her head. With the tips of the index and middle fingers of this hand, establish contact with the frontal bone at the upper inner edge of the left and right orbits. Using the thumb and index finger of your other hand, placed at the side of the client's head, now gently and clearly feel for the two nasal bones (Fig. 5.2.3A–C overleaf). By exerting light, even traction with both hands away from each other, release the frontonasal suture from adhesions and compression. The optimal direction of traction for your two hands is at an angle of about 45°: your index and middle finger on the frontal bone stretch diagonally upward, i.e. simultaneously up toward the ceiling and toward the top of

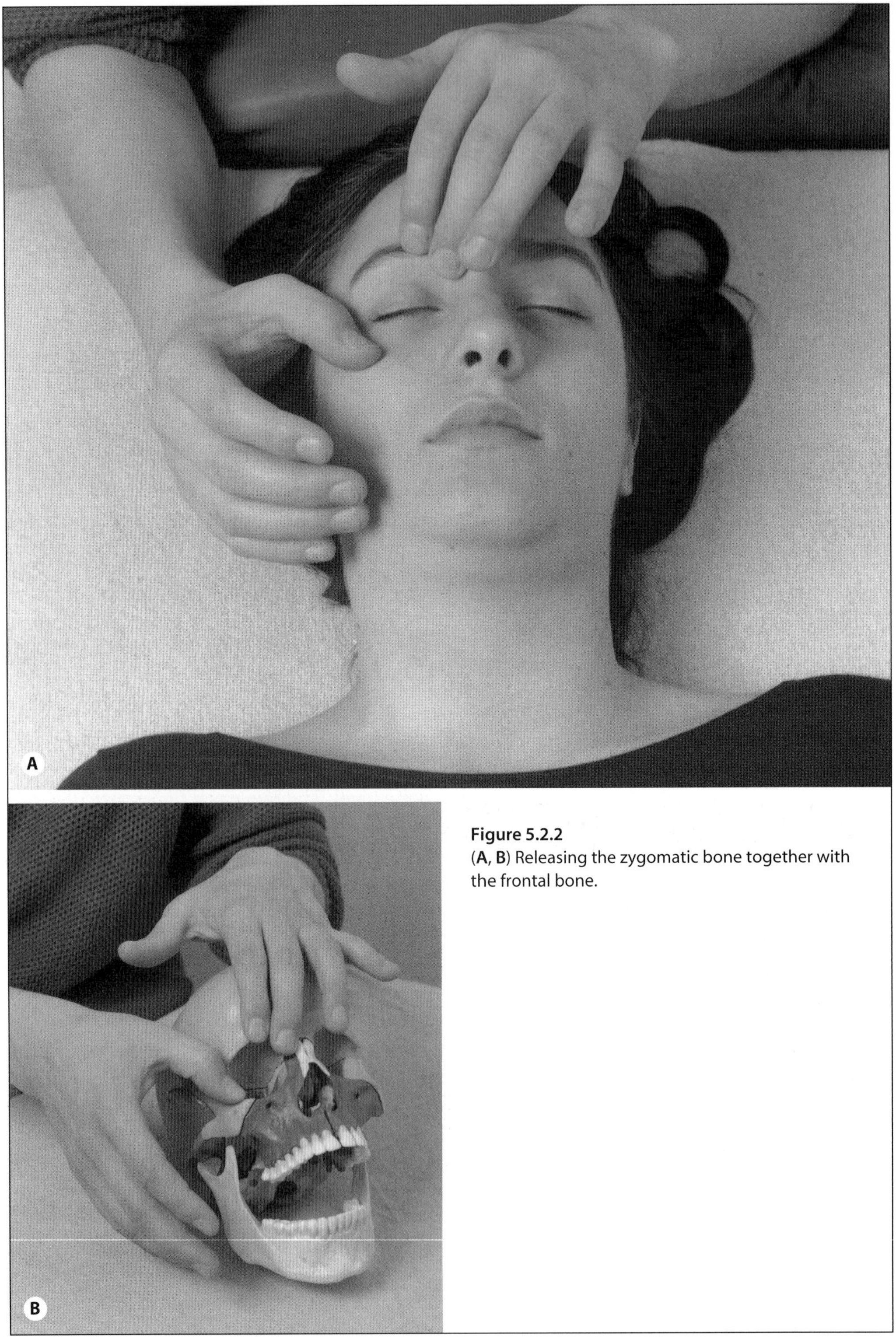

Figure 5.2.2
(**A**, **B**) Releasing the zygomatic bone together with the frontal bone.

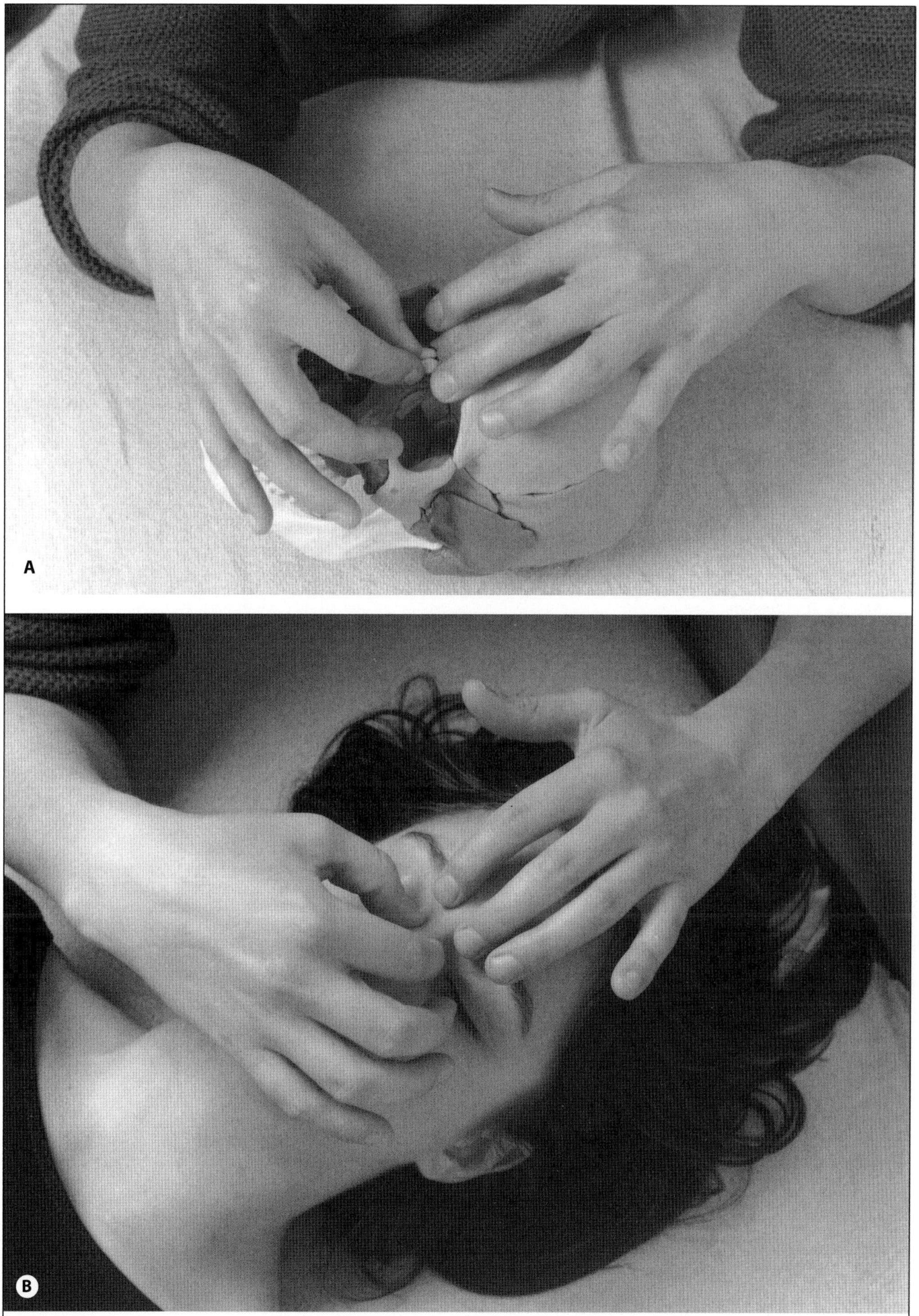

Figure 5.2.3
(**A–C**) Releasing the nasal bones, frontal bone, and maxillae (*Continued overleaf*).

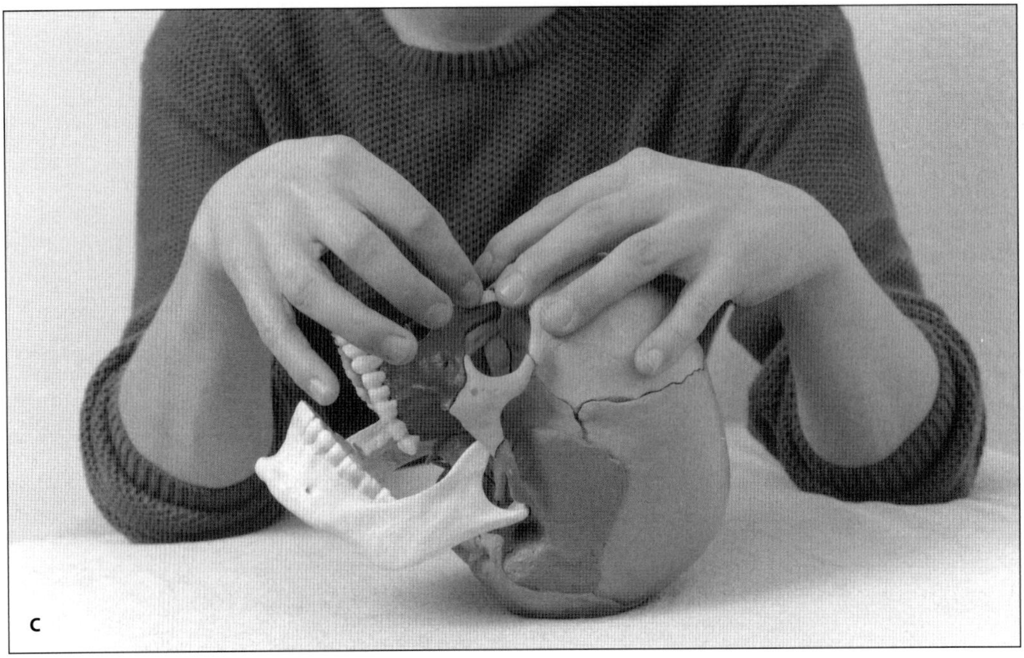

Figure 5.2.3 (*Continued*)

the client's head (anteriorly and cranially), while the thumb and index finger of your other hand simultaneously lift the nasal bones diagonally upward (anteriorly and caudally), i.e. toward the ceiling and toward the torso of the supine client.

For spectacle wearers, this release technique for the frontal and nasal bones is a helpful self-treatment method.

Intraoral treatment

Before performing intraoral treatment, first palpate the cranial bones as a whole. Also listen to the motion of the sphenoid because it is primarily the craniosacral rhythm of the sphenoid and temporal bones that is transmitted to the maxillae. It is also beneficial to massage the masticatory muscles beforehand and to perform temporomandibular joint (TMJ) release via the lower jaw.

The mouth is a very intimate and sensitive area. Where intraoral craniosacral therapy is recommended, in response to the wishes of or the particular problem communicated by the client, the practitioner should be able to provide this option. Intraoral work presupposes the client's trust and consent. Treatment is always performed using single-finger or full-hand examination gloves.

Ask the client whether she wears dentures. Remove these before treatment and return them to the client when the session is over.

It is useful to agree with your client a sign (e.g. raising a hand) to indicate that intraoral treatment should be interrupted. The client should be able to continue breathing in the same rhythm. If her breathing becomes very hesitant or if she holds her breath, then take a short rest. Ask what she felt and how she feels now. Allow both the client and yourself as practitioner plenty of time. Respect the client's tempo as well as your own. Only make a start once you yourself are grounded, centered, relaxed and in a calm, unhurried frame of mind. Your own contact with stillness here is often helpful.

It is important for you to attend craniosacral courses offering opportunities for intraoral treatment practice (under specialist supervision); this affords a new experience of touch and tension release not only to dentists, dental assistants and other specialist personnel but also to their patients.

Take up a position at one side of the head of the treatment table. Ensure that your seat is sufficiently high so that you do not have to tense your shoulders. If the client lies *diagonally* on the table, you do not have to lean over the table to perform intraoral treatment, and this increases treatment comfort both for you and the client. A roll of padding behind the client's knees takes the strain off her torso, and this effect extends indirectly up to the cranial base and mouth.

The vomer

The *vomer* – which takes its name from the Latin word for a 'plowshare' – is a thin, flat bone situated beneath the ethmoid and in front of and below the sphenoid. Its lower edge articulates with the median palatine suture. In particular, the motion of the sphenoid is transmitted to the vomer because the vomer is attached to the rostrum of the sphenoid. This motion transmission occurs in a vertical direction; as a result, the paired maxillae in flexion are moved outward slightly. The flexion motion of the sphenoid moves the vomer slightly upward in the anterior palatine region and slightly downward in the posterior palatine region.

When treating the vomer, support the client by placing your 'more cranial' hand transversely under her neck muscles or flat across her frontal bone. Advanced practitioners will be able to locate their thumb and middle finger pads precisely and gently over the greater wings of the client's sphenoid. The client should voluntarily consent to intraoral treatment. She has a say in whether this should take place and how long it should last. To signal when treatment should start, ask the client to open her mouth when she is ready.

Establish broad contact with the pad of your index finger and locate the vomer via the median suture of the anterior palate. Again, allow yourself sufficient time to be able to feel the structure clearly and definitely. Then listen to determine whether you can sense the craniosacral motion. Does this go further into flexion or extension? Is the vomer displaced slightly sideways? If so, is it displaced along its entire lower surface (sideward/transverse displacement) or more in the anterior part of the palate (torsion)? These positional anomalies can be treated using the indirect–direct method by briefly issuing a hint of amplification to the positional anomaly of the vomer and then immediately inviting correction in the other direction.

Decompression of the vomer releases its position and simultaneously reduces positional anomalies overall

With your 'more cranial' hand, transversely support the client's neck muscles from underneath, span her frontal bone or touch the sphenoid wings with your thumb and middle finger. When the client is ready, she will open her mouth. With the terminal phalanx of the index finger of your other hand, establish broad contact with the anterior part of the midline of the maxillae (*median palatine suture*). The surface of your index finger thus makes intraoral contact with the vomer. Place the thumb of this hand immediately under the client's nose. Via the tissues of the upper orbicular muscle of the mouth, this thumb should be in contact with the *bony maxillae* (not with the teeth) (Fig. 5.2.4).

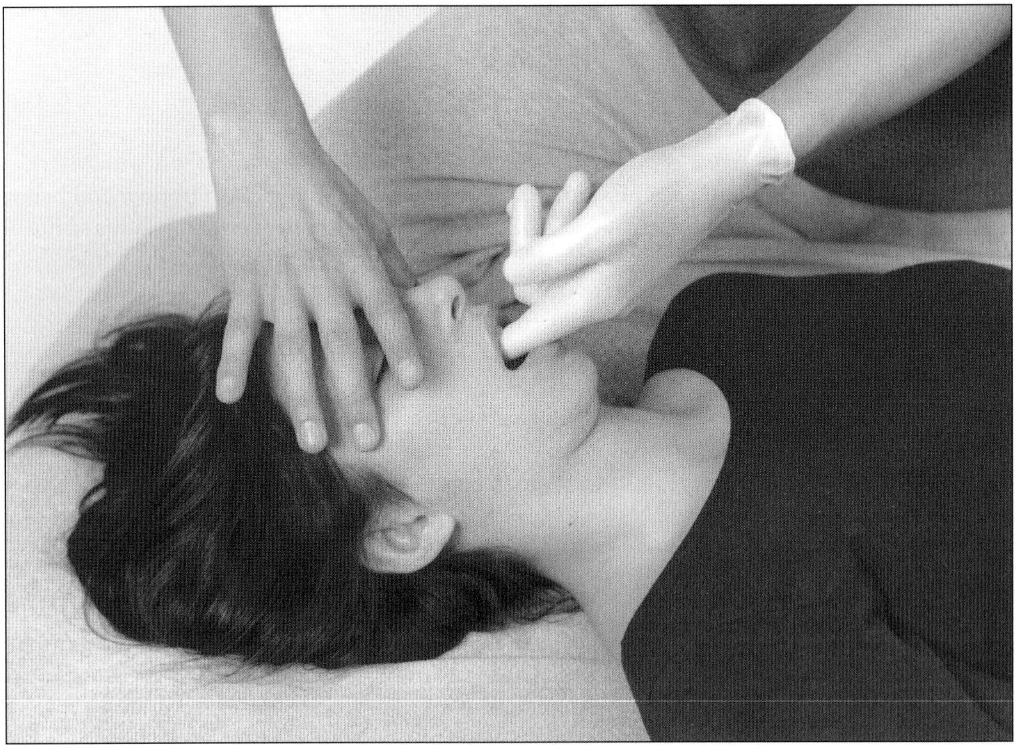

Figure 5.2.4
Palpating the sphenoid and vomer.

Ensure that your own body posture is relaxed. Allow yourself sufficient time so that your touching points (index finger and thumb) have very clear contact with the client's palate/vomer and maxillae. Also, the touch of your other hand at the neck, frontal bone or sphenoid should remain clear and yet spaciously gentle at the same time.

Using your index finger and thumb, slowly start to perform gentle decompression on the maxillae (with simultaneous support on the vomer), if possible without slipping off. *Perform decompression at an angle of 45°*, i.e. diagonally away from the torso, toward the client's feet, and simultaneously up toward the ceiling (anteriorly and caudally). This is approximately the same as the angle of inclination of your index finger. This gentle decompression may last for about 1–2 min and is then slowly released again.

After intraoral treatment, listen to the motion of the sphenoid and occiput and again invite correction and balance. It is also recommended that you invite a still point, use the cranial vault hold or cradle hold, and perform head-torso integration (including the sacrum).

Masticatory muscles

The large, powerful masseter muscles and the medial and lateral pterygoid muscles located at either the side of the oral cavity are among the strongest masticatory muscles. They are often under severe tension. Some of the masticatory muscles are attached to the pterygoid process of the sphenoid. If the masticatory muscles are severely restricted, they will limit the craniosacral motion of numerous cranial bones, particularly the sphenoid.

Before you start the treatment, first locate your own masticatory muscles on the outside of your cheeks and then with your little finger or index finger inside your mouth, at the sides outside your molars. If you briefly bite and release several times, you will clearly feel the masseter, for example.

First, treat one side, and then the other. The client will open her mouth when she is ready. Slowly slide your index finger or little finger gently back along the bottom or top row of teeth, then out to the side to carefully locate the masseter muscle outside her molars (Fig. 5.2.5). With a light touch, broadly place the pad of your index finger against her masticatory muscles, but without pressing her teeth or tissues in the process. If the client does not feel that your other hand under her neck is supportive, you can place the fingers of your free hand outside on her cheek over her masticatory muscles. With two fingers in a V-spread outside on her cheek, directing energy with the tip of your index finger intraorally can encourage further release (Fig. 5.2.6). You may touch the masticatory muscles intraorally for 1–2 min on each side. The client's lower jaw can relax in the process because your index finger is located *outside* her molars. Occasionally the client may slowly open and close her mouth slightly.

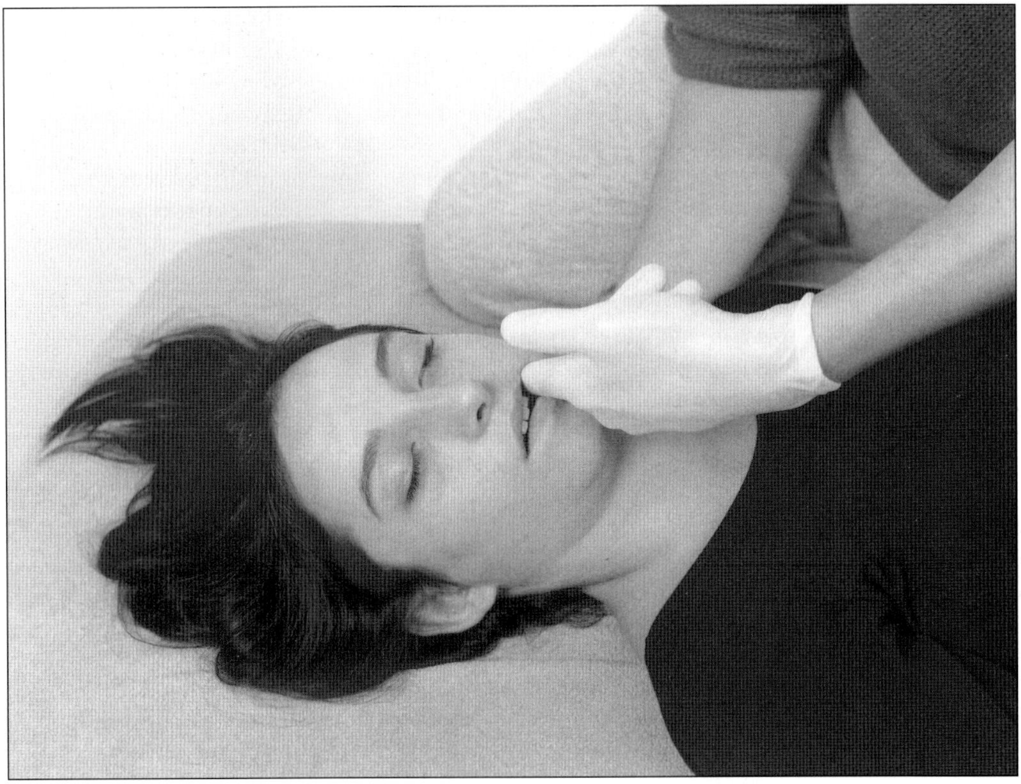

Figure 5.2.5
Touching the masticatory muscles intraorally.

Afterward allow your client sufficient time to enjoy the ongoing effects throughout her body and to perceive the release. Listen using the cranial vault hold. Grounding and balancing touch contact at the torso and legs (e.g. at both sides of the pelvis, thighs or knees) is usually very pleasant for the client.

Intraoral support for lower-jaw unwinding

Unwinding of the lower jaw should only be used after multiple treatments of the head and lower jaw, as already outlined. The technique presupposes an understanding of going with the body's spontaneous unwinding at the extremities and an in-depth personal experience of craniosacral therapy. On a practical level, disposable gloves are also required. Before and during treatment of the lower jaw, make sure that your own TMJs are relaxed and allow your own lower jaw to drop slightly. An unhurried and open-minded approach is especially valuable in this setting.

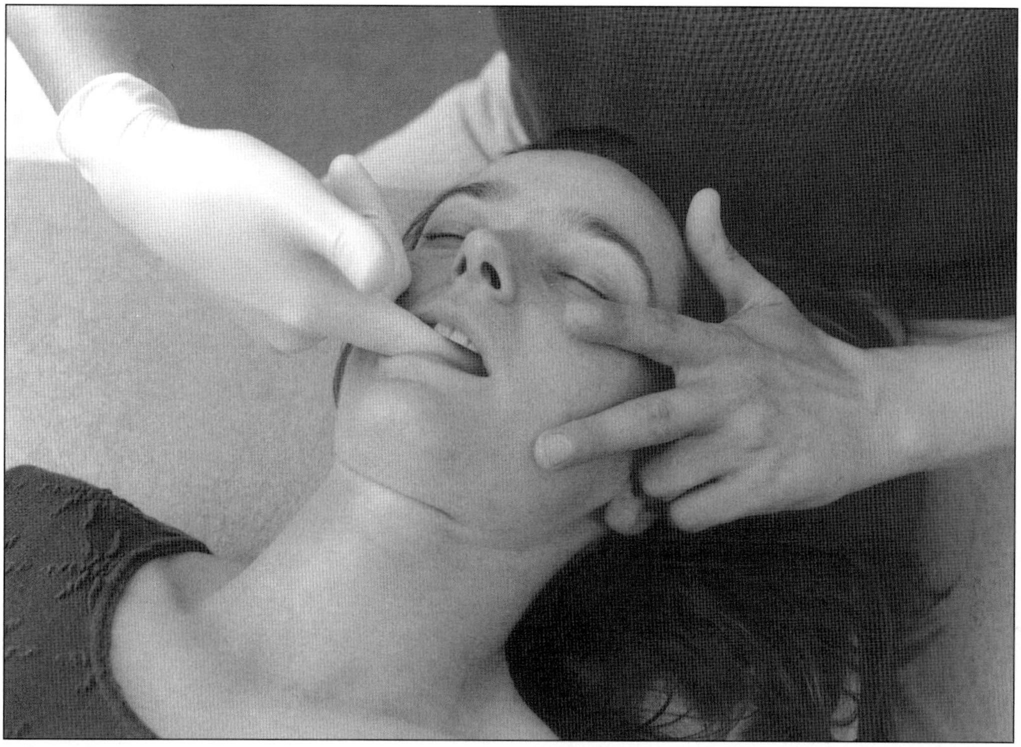

Figure 5.2.6
Touching the masticatory muscles combined with direction of energy.

Take up a position beside the treatment table, level with the client's shoulders. The client should be lying diagonally on the table, with her upper body/head close to you. After the client has opened her mouth, place one of your thumbs on her bottom row of teeth on one side, and your other thumb on the other side (Fig. 5.2.7). Your thumb contact should be broad-based and without pressure. Your two index fingers should take up broad contact with the outside surface of the lower jaw. This gives the client and you a clear, compact quality of touch at the lower jaw without compressing it. Ask the client to raise her hand, for example, to indicate if your touch feels too intensive or a rest is required.

Again, allow sufficient time for your palpatory awareness to blend with the contact points and then really *listen* so that you *never* treat using pressure or deliberate movement.

In this position, you may perform the previously described compression–decompression in an unhurried manner, while listening simultaneously, or you may directly invite the lower jaw to widen, i.e. in the direction of decompression, before you listen to the body's spontaneous unwinding.

If you already have experience of unwinding at the extremities, you will know how gentle this feels. At the lower jaw, you should be particularly attentive and spacious as you listen to and go with this

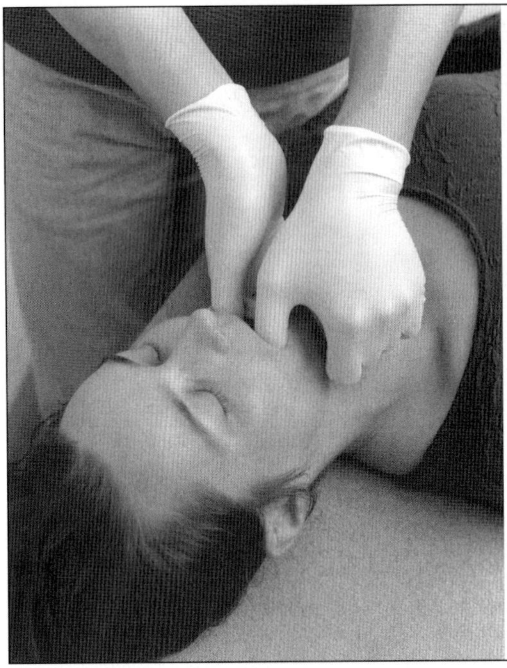

Figure 5.2.7
Going with unwinding at the lower jaw.

unwinding. Go with the spontaneous motion of the lower jaw for a period of about 2–5 min. As you do this, respect every 'stop' indicated by the tissues, pause and only support new movements if these occur spontaneously, i.e. if they come from the client.

Afterwards, it is recommended that you listen to the motion of the two temporal bones (are they rotating synchronously in ER/IR?) and that you harmonize this, where necessary. You may use the gentle ear pull and the cranial vault hold or cradle hold and invite a still point.

Advanced self-treatment techniques

5.3

Self-treatment for the masticatory muscles

Locating the masticatory muscles from outside

With the palms and fingers of both hands, take up broad contact with your right and left cheeks and lower jaw. Perform several chewing movements. As you do this, trace the entire course of these masticatory muscles (the masseter muscles) and note their position.

Stroking and massaging the masticatory muscles (seated)

Place your hands on the sides of your face so that your fingertips are about 2 cm to the side of your auditory canal and temporomandibular joint (TMJ). Now let your arms become heavy. As you do this, notice how your elbows are slowly drawn toward the floor by the 'dead weight' of your arms; while this is happening, use as broad a finger contact as possible to exert perceptible downward traction along the course of the masticatory muscles. To conclude, use your fingers to slightly stretch your lower jaw downward.

Repeat this stroking several times. Take care to ensure a pleasant weight of pressure and vary your speed. Slower stroking is mostly felt to be more intensive. Deliberate exhaling of perceived tension through your slightly open mouth will enhance the relaxing effect.

Intraoral technique for locating and relaxing the masticatory muscles

You can also use the intraoral method for the masticatory muscles as a self-treatment technique (see p. 297). A supine position is helpful here, for example, after you have used the various self-treatment techniques described previously.

Wash your hands first or use single-finger examination gloves (as protection against transmissible diseases). With your mouth relaxed and slightly open, use your index finger to locate the firm muscles outside the row of teeth. Slightly opening and closing the mouth slowly will help you locate the powerful masticatory muscles precisely. As well as the powerful masseter muscles inside your left and right cheeks, you will also feel the other masticatory muscles (e.g. those located more toward the TMJs). If the space is too confined, use your little finger instead of your index finger. Using clear and gentle touch, invite space and widening and allow yourself and the structure sufficient time for the natural balancing of tone. Then move your contact slightly by a few millimeters and continue with this form of tension release. Use this intraoral technique to explore your masticatory muscles and release any tension there.

From time to time, deliberately make sure that your perceptual field also includes your flow of breathing and the sensations in your body as a whole.

Intraoral technique for locating your masticatory muscles and directing energy

With the tip of your index finger in broad contact, gently touch the masticatory muscles without exerting pressure. Exhale any perceived tension through your open mouth. The more relaxed your index finger, wrist, arm, and shoulder, the clearer the invitation to the muscle being touched to also become relaxed. Out of this relaxed state, start to direct releasing energy with your index finger. You may position your other hand outside on your cheek. Place it gently and with as broad a contact as possible immediately over the area being treated intraorally, or alternatively form a V-spread with two fingers (see p. 213).

Self-treatment for tension relief in headache (for advanced practitioners)

For mild tension in the shoulder–neck region or for mild sensations of pressure in the head, it is possible to combine various craniosacral techniques and self-treatments described in this book. A supine position is helpful, especially for still point induction using juggling balls or tennis balls. The choice and sequence of self-treatments for headache is up to you: you yourself decide how long to perform a particular technique and with what intensity of touch. Among other things, it is important for your breathing to be calm and fluid and for you to exhale with your mouth slightly open. Picture to yourself that you are dissipating the mild tension through your body to the padded surface of the treatment table and to your pelvis, and from there to your legs and feet. It is also recommended that you perform touch contact and release on your own pelvic region/torso so that any excessive build-up of energy in the head can be diverted away to your torso and then to your pelvis.

Allopathic medical clarification should be sought if poor health or headache persists.

Suggested self-treatment sequence for tension relief in headache

Release transverse connective tissue layers in your torso, massage and stroke your masticatory muscles, massage muscle attachments at the occipital ridge (including the occipital region), induce a still point, occasionally listen to the stillness, perform arm bridge at pelvis, massage sacral border while side-lying, breathe down into your feet, yawn, deliberately exhale, gently lift frontal bone, gently lift parietal bones, lift the nasal bone and frontal bone together and away from each other, perform gentle ear pull, touch your costal arch (diaphragm region, possibly also solar plexus/stomach zone), perhaps induce a still point, palpate both sides of your pelvis: sense your sacrum, legs and feet, take time to enjoy the ongoing effects while side-lying, with one hand positioned below your navel. Make a before-and-after comparison of your body awareness: What has changed? How do you sense this? Where do things feel most pleasant? How do you perceive your body as a whole?

Section 6

Further applications

6.1 Pregnancy and childbirth

Midwives and body therapists in increasing numbers have come to recognize the many versatile applications of craniosacral therapy and are employing it before, during and after the birth process.

For couples seeking to become pregnant, craniosacral therapy improves potency in men and helps women become more likely to conceive by reducing stress levels. This goal is promoted in particular by the resolution of restrictions in the pelvic region, for example, through the release of transverse connective tissue layers and fascial glides at varying depth levels, combined with visceral therapy and therapeutic dialog to support the process.

During pregnancy, craniosacral therapy eases the strain on the entire musculoskeletal apparatus and on the pulmonary breathing of the mother-to-be. In particular, the zones of the cranial base, shoulder–neck, respiratory diaphragm, lumbosacral region, and the entire pelvis – including the sacroiliac joints and pubic symphysis – are suitable for treatment and release. This serves to optimize pelvic function and to balance the collective mechanical forces acting on the body and can help to alleviate back pain.

Purely as a precautionary measure, it is advisable not to induce any still points before the end of month 3 or after month 7 of pregnancy (see 'Contraindications', p. 66.

Craniosacral therapy may be used alone or in combination with other preparatory techniques to make childbirth easier. In this context, the client's position merits special attention: in the advanced stages of pregnancy, the mother-to-be should not remain supine for longer than 10–15 min. Treatment with the client side-lying (see p. 202) is felt to be very pleasant. A 30-min treatment session is often sufficient, depending on the week of pregnancy and the pregnant woman's disposition. Sitting up slowly from the side-lying position, taking in her surroundings in a stress-free manner, and then slowly walking a few paces while noting the positive changes, is just as valuable as the treatment itself. The mother-to-be often feels that her body is lighter and is once again more 'whole'. As a result of release, she experiences noticeably greater degrees of relief, calm, trust, and confidence during the many different internal and external changes that occur in pregnancy.

Particularly during or after difficult phases of a pregnancy, craniosacral therapy helps to transform agitation into centered relaxation. This emotional and organic support is also beneficial for the unborn child; although it exists within a certain protected environment, it is nevertheless aware of its mother's moods and external factors.

On grounds of safety, treatment in a high-risk pregnancy should only be given if expressly recommended by the midwife or gynecologist. (For example, from month 7 of pregnancy onward, I personally only give treatment if the cervix is closed – something that can be ascertained with the pregnant woman by the aforementioned specialists at each consultation.)

Midwives with further training in craniosacral therapy have reported several cases to me where a cesarean section had already been scheduled because of the baby's presentation. However, in response to non-invasive craniosacral therapy and the verbal invitation of the practitioner, some of the babies re-positioned themselves and were able to be born naturally and without any complications through the mother's flexible pelvis.

After week 40 of pregnancy, a midwife with extensive craniosacral experience can attempt by multiple still point induction to invite and encourage the birth process from outside. In this way, it may be possible to avoid use of labor-hastening medication or cesarean section.

During the birth process, obstetricians with craniosacral experience can induce still points at the sacrum or head from outside. Still points may encourage uterine contractions and so intensify labor, thus facilitating natural delivery for mother and baby. In the event of exhaustion during delivery, still point induction and other craniosacral techniques may release fresh reserves of strength and energy.

Postnatal care of mother and baby incorporating craniosacral therapy is highly recommended, particularly following problem births (cesarean section, forceps delivery, ventouse delivery). In such circumstances, a valuable stimulus toward healing can often be given by gentle therapeutic support, which should also be based on experience in pediatric craniosacral therapy gained through training courses and practical implementation.

After delivery, craniosacral therapy encourages regeneration in general and provides valuable support for the mother during the immediate postnatal period. Craniosacral therapy combined with visceral therapy is extremely effective for balancing the collective mechanical forces of the maternal pelvis and other organs, especially during the weeks and months after delivery. Structural regeneration mediated by craniosacral therapy and the simultaneous resource-oriented, emotional processing of childbirth are also valuable to the mother in preventing later problems involving the musculoskeletal system, organs, and nervous system in general. For example, this can foster the resumption of pain-free and fulfilled sexual activity after pregnancy.

Many mothers and families would benefit if greater account were taken of these regenerative and preventive aspects. The repercussions of birth trauma can be minimized or resolved at an early stage, with hugely positive spin-offs for the future of both mother and baby. Seen in the long term, implementation of craniosacral therapy in this setting would also ease the load on ensuing generations, both in terms of individual development and social interaction. In addition, by unburdening the nervous system and by processing/resolving trauma, it might also prevent a post-traumatic stress syndrome. This would decisively reduce the associated consequences and costs – which are generally underestimated; and the healthcare service would also benefit as a result.

It is not unusual for complications to arise during pregnancy and at the time of delivery; however, the baby's cranial vessels and nerves may also be compressed during normal births. The still very mobile cranial bones may overlap during the birth process – in the case of the parietal bones by as much as 1.5 cm. Cranial asymmetries can often be reduced after a few treatment sessions. The occiput with its four component parts is also exposed to major stresses during birth and may become compressed and displaced as a result. If the area around the foramen magnum is compromised, thus hindering communication between the brain and the rest of the body, the CSF is less able to flow freely into the dural tube. For example, compression of the vagus nerve may increase the incidence of colic or allergies.

Where the baby has difficulty negotiating the birth canal, excessive torsion and simultaneous compression of the head and cervical spine can be harmful. This may subsequently reduce the supply of blood to the brain or lead to torticollis (wryneck) in which the suboccipital region, among others, is affected.

Anesthesia, amniocentesis, premature birth, cesarean section, ventouse delivery, forceps delivery, an excessively rapid or slow birth process, and immunizations that are too numerous or too early can lead to: allergies, asthma, respiratory distress, autism, cerebral developmental disorders with motor deficit, disturbed CNS regulation, cough, infections, sleep disorders, growth disorders, and bonding problems.

Treating children 6.2

Soon after birth or during the first 12 months of life, every infant should experience a few craniosacral therapy sessions. This would be an important and ideal gift to ensure as carefree a start in life as possible. During the various phases of development, too, craniosacral therapy is a great help to growing children. In the long term, this comprehensive form of prevention would certainly save billions in terms of sickness and invalidity – thus benefiting the health of the nation and the economy – and would also be to the profit and advantage of every individual.

The founder and pioneer of craniosacral osteopathy, William Garner Sutherland, treated many children. He it was who originated the statement: 'As a twig is bent, so the tree inclines'. In a study conducted in children with behavioral problems, Viola Frymann, a pupil of W.G. Sutherland and a pioneer of pediatric cranial osteopathy, noted that among other ailments, the vast majority of her patients had a dysfunction of the sphenobasilar synchondrosis (SBS), the articulation between the sphenoid and the occiput.

Time and again in babies and toddlers, in particular, it is impressive to see how much can change for the better. The initial changes often occur after just a short time. Depending on the course of pregnancy and childbirth, relatively few treatment sessions are required to encourage the infant's inherent homeostasis and bonding.

The practitioner should always allow sufficient time for the parents and child, although craniosacral therapy in infants is generally significantly shorter than in adolescents and adults. Here too, harmonious treatment is more important than a plethora of techniques or a major time investment. It requires patience and trust from all parties involved, empathy for the child, and attentive tuning in to the child's tempo.

Crying babies are often also affected by suckling problems, abdominal colic, and fragmented sleep patterns. Their crying reflects their need to draw attention to something important. After a full medical examination, muscle tone problems (increased, reduced) and asymmetries (of the head, spine, shoulders, pelvis) should also be treated at the earliest possible stage. The growth centers of the cranial bones and their capacity for free expansion enable the brain to grow unhindered. In children with a squint (strabismus), ophthalmological treatment can be supported by craniosacral therapy. Children suffering from psychological or apparently irrational fears can experience a climate of trust in the context of craniosacral therapy and be encouraged to let go and relax in a safe, protected setting.

Craniosacral therapy is also finding increasing use in the areas of special education and speech therapy.

Up until the early 1990s, children who had experienced a problem birth, for example, because their umbilical cord was tangled around their neck, were often termed POS (psycho-organic syndrome) or MCD (minimal cerebral dysfunction) children. In recent years, the terms ADD (attention deficit disorder) and ADHD (attention deficit hyperactivity disorder) have come to the fore. The growing incidence of children and adults with concentration disorders and specific learning difficulties is particularly striking.

In actual fact, the true cause is almost always rooted in pre- and perinatal complications. Another contributing factor in this context is the virtually incessant 'tidal wave' of stimuli so characteristic of modern life – the infant's or child's nervous system is all too often under strain and overstretched. The general atmosphere in the home also plays a role: how balanced or unbalanced are the parents and siblings, are they themselves constantly in action or do they allow themselves sufficient time to rest quietly sometimes – these aspects will impinge on the child in question. Alongside the capacity for relaxation, if there is some guarantee that the child can actively embody joy and strength in an appropriate and creative way, then its nervous system will be familiar with both activity and perceptive passivity and will be better equipped to achieve spontaneous balance.

My own observations over the past decade have often revealed that on top of the child's hectic and over-stressed home environment, there is additionally a pressure to perform, for example, in terms of school, sports, hobbies – causing many children to be overstretched over a fairly long period, a natural reaction and yet one with adverse implications. In recent years, the widespread prescription of medicines to schoolchildren has become a hotly debated issue; manufacturers produce several tons of these medicines each year. In some schools in the USA, it is already routine for children to require daily medication to stay 'healthy' or to calm them down. It is estimated that some 10 million children worldwide are taking medication on a daily basis to help them cope with the pressure to perform or to combat hyperactivity. Even if some parents have reported improved concentration in their children, long-term solutions are needed which not only combat symptoms but also seek to alleviate or resolve the underlying causes.

My experience with ADD/ADHD children is that they are frequently very gifted and creative – sometimes even above average for their age. As a descriptor in this connection, the term 'indigo children' is gaining some popularity. This label is truly applicable to only a few of the young children in my practice identified as suffering from ADD. What they really lack is sufficient opportunity to experience and express their energy and creativity free from pressure and duress.

Many anomalies, deficits, health problems, and symptoms are an expression of a post-traumatic stress disorder. People generally manage to repress a post-traumatic stress syndrome (PTSS) so that they can function properly and hold their own in everyday life. If the PTSS and its causes are dismantled or resolved, there is generally also a subsequent improvement in those everyday areas that are (subconsciously) associated with it.

- Treatment of babies, preschool and school-age children should be performed by trained specialists. Practitioners intending to treat children must have many years of experience in craniosacral therapy with adults and adolescents.

Depending on the treatment approach adopted, slowly go with and listen to the spontaneous motion at the head and the body's spontaneous *unwinding*. In cases where asymmetries, postural anomalies and motion patterns are to be corrected in babies and preschool children, this should be done *directly* into the direction for release *without previous compression* and without using the 'indirect–direct technique' (Fig. 6.2.1A–E).

Treatment duration in terms of pure hands-on time is definitely shorter than with adolescents or adults. In babies, invite still points at the occiput using your index and middle fingers.

Support the child's spontaneous unwinding, for example, by placing one hand in the sacrum–pelvis region and one hand in the neck-occiput region. The dural tube, which is often twisted and compressed due to the birth process, can unfold and rock itself free by spontaneous unwinding (Fig. 6.2.2A–F).

Treatment involving the head is performed largely via the bone level *at meningeal and fluid level*. In most cases, it is not just the purely mechanical–structural levels that have to be taken into account in the resolution of birth trauma, but also the high and sometimes life-threatening intensity

Figure 6.2.1
(**A–E**) Palpating the craniosacral rhythm
(*Continued overleaf*).

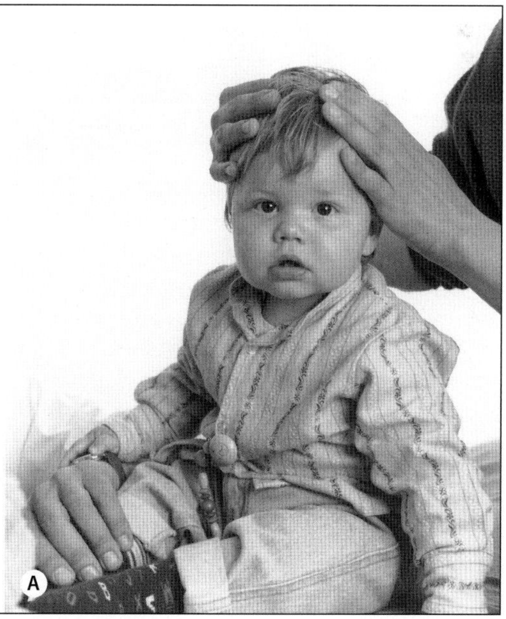

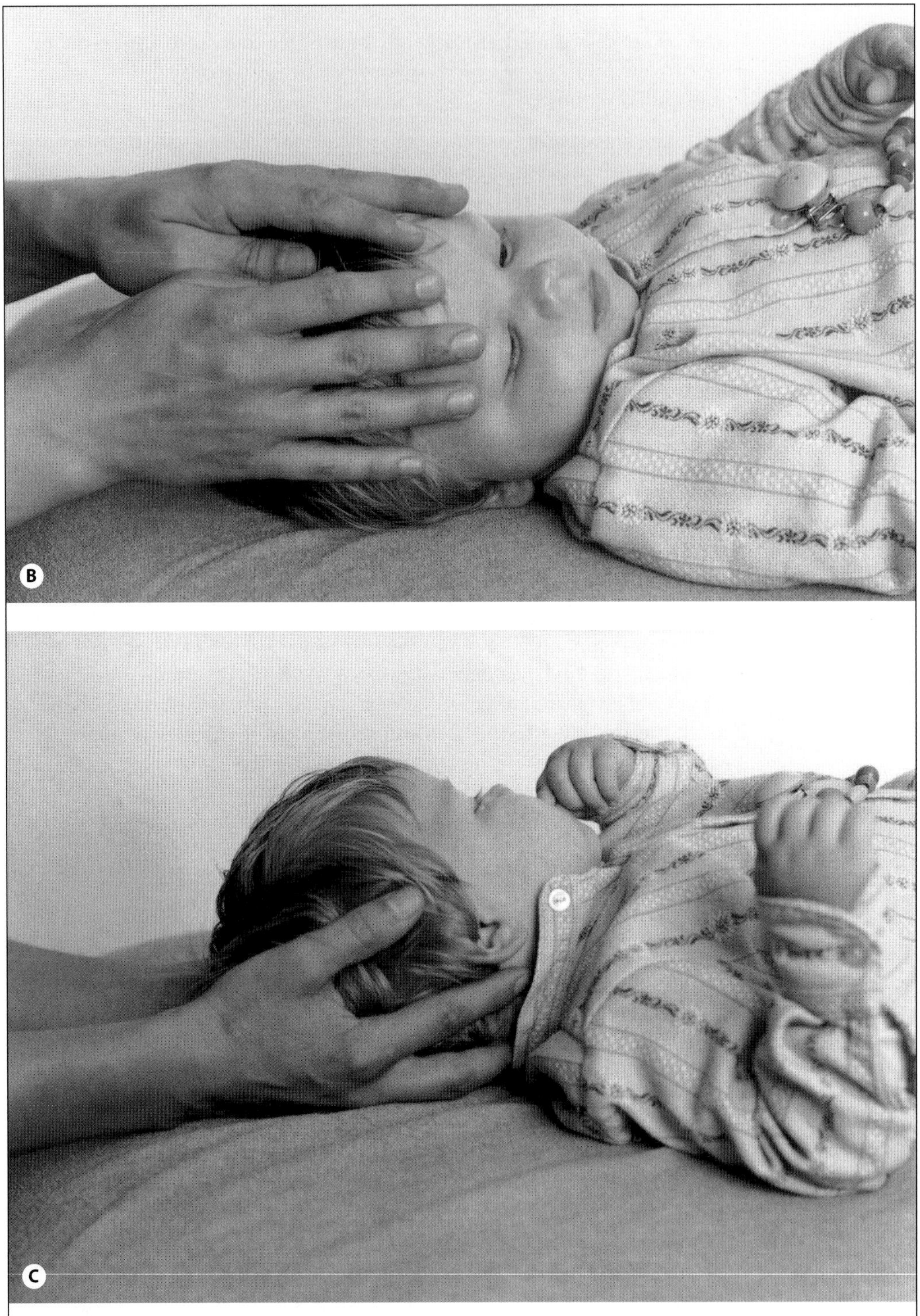

Figure 6.2.1 (*Continued*)

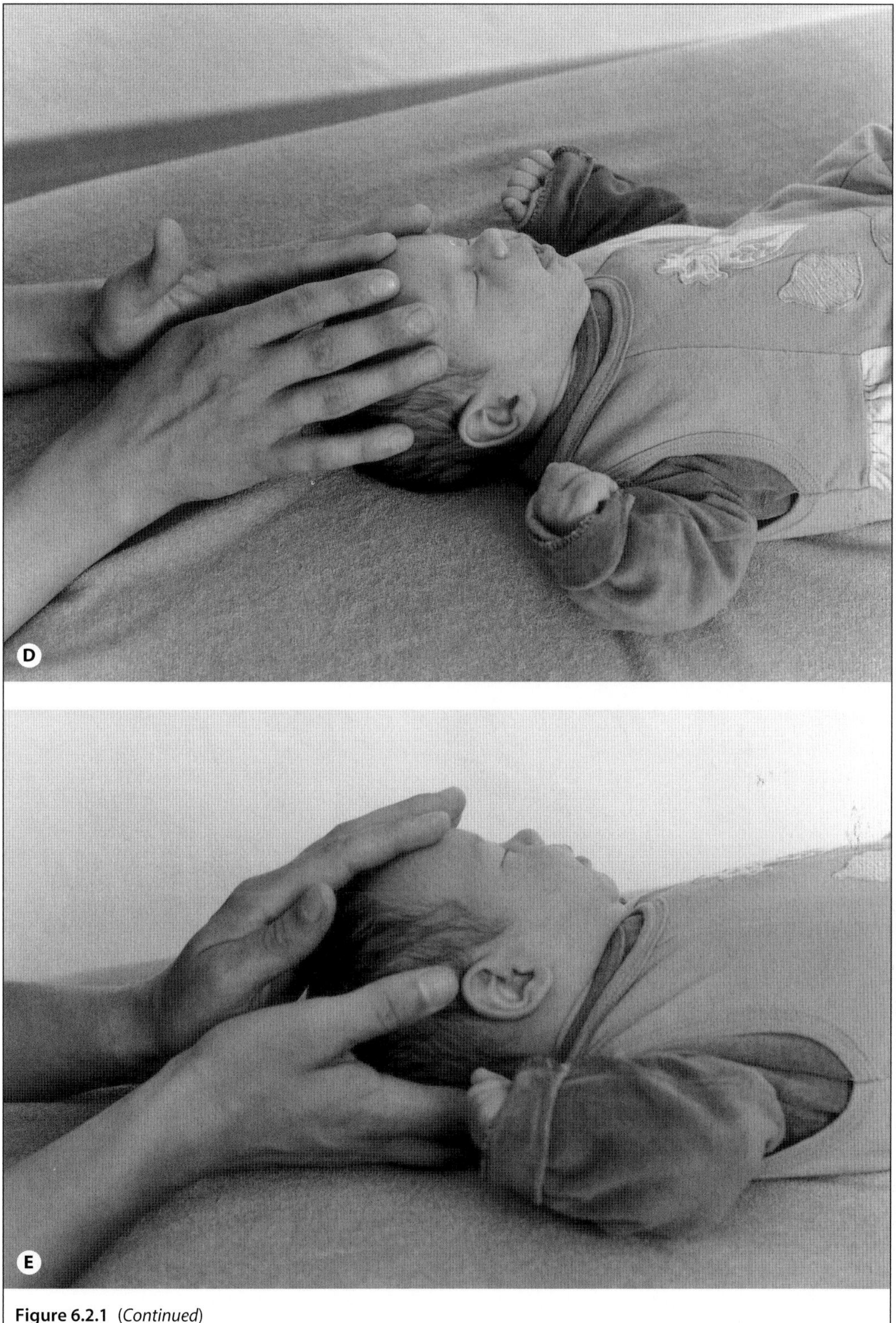

Figure 6.2.1 (*Continued*)

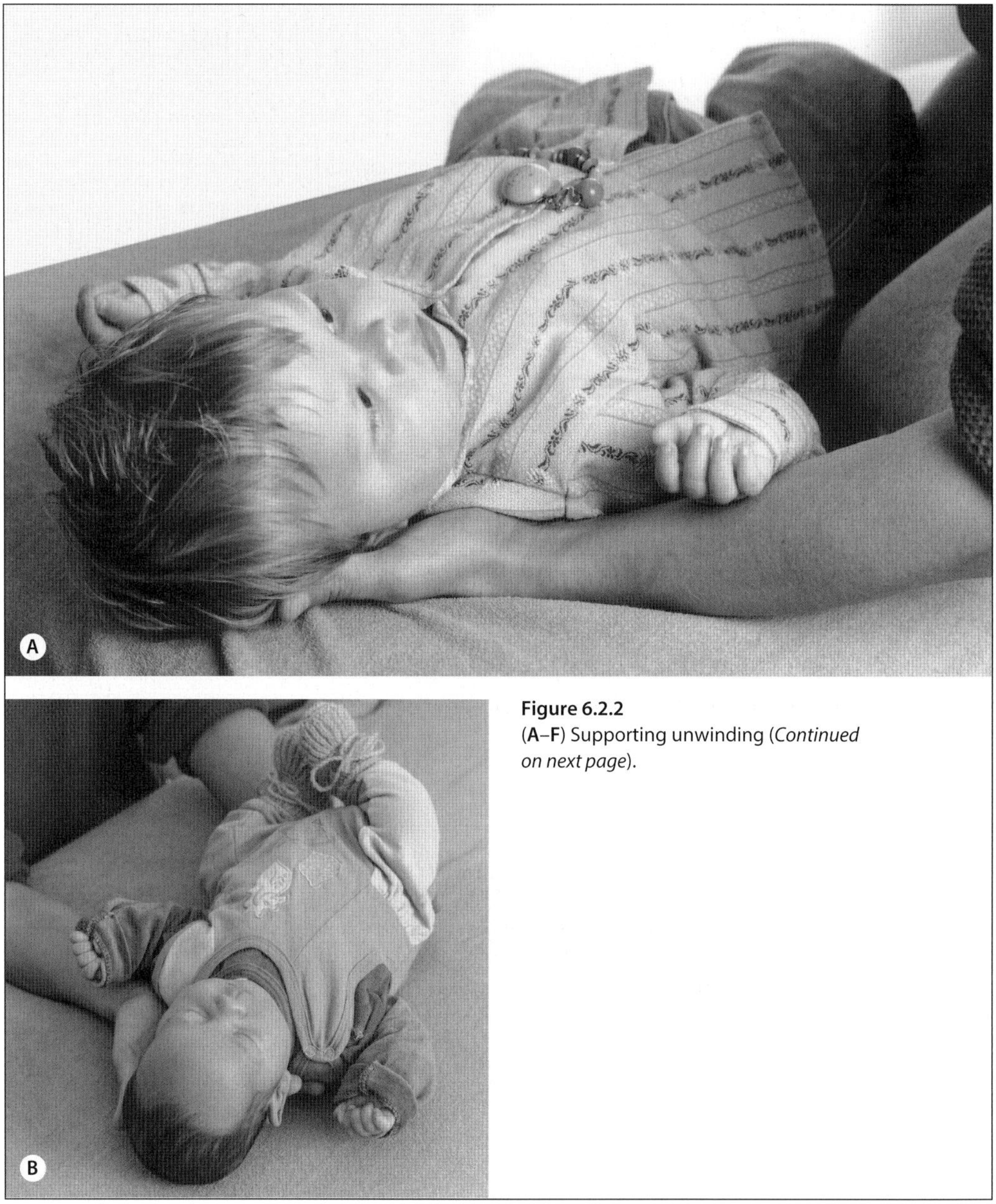

Figure 6.2.2
(**A–F**) Supporting unwinding (*Continued on next page*).

of the trauma at the time, which is stored *in the nervous system and in the tissues* down to the cellular level. Crying or shouting may be an expression of this stored memory. Eye contact, verbal contact, and harmonious touch have a connecting and trauma-healing effect. They enable the child, in the secure presence of its mother and the practitioner, to experience and relax in the here and now.

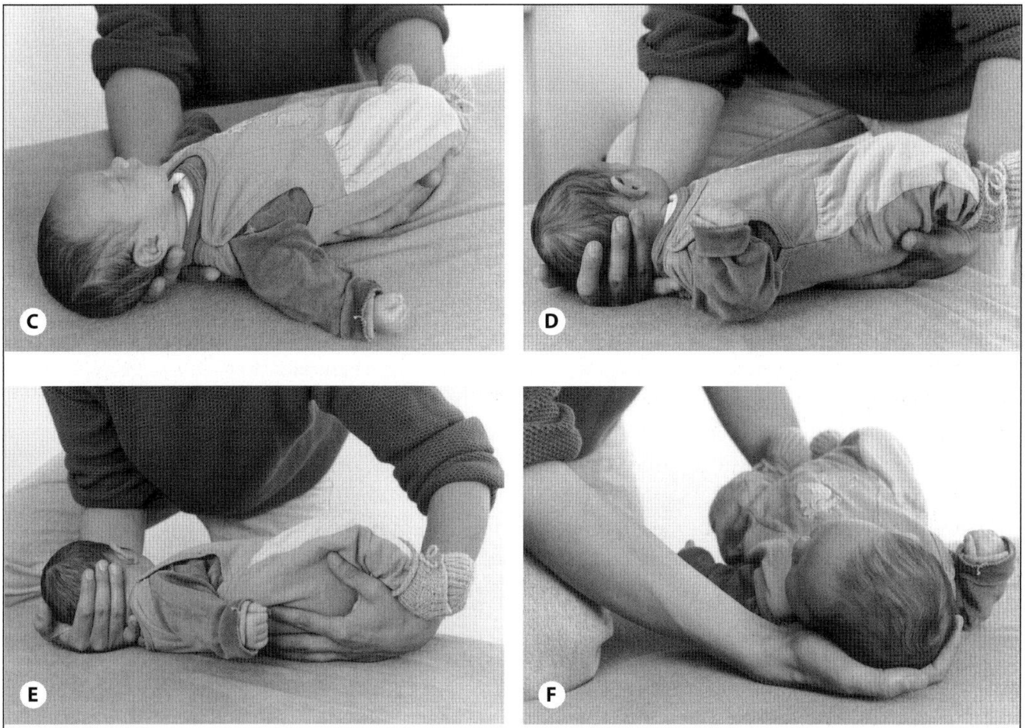

Figure 6.2.2 (*Continued*)

In addition, according to the findings and opinions of many practitioners experienced in pediatric craniosacral therapy, *the parents too* should be supported and *included in the treatment*, because parents and children together form an intimate family system. In a stressful situation, particularly where there are complications, the parents may feel more deeply affected, overtaxed, annoyed, powerless, helpless or else they repress these feelings instead of utilizing them as a springboard for personal and shared growth. Once the parents relax, the child notices this change very quickly, and vice versa.

This is a key reason why it is better for parents to bring their child to a craniosacral practitioner for treatment – so that they too can find some benefit – than to treat their child themselves.

Naturally, it makes sound sense for children to be touched by immediate family members who have attended craniosacral therapy courses – provided that they are content for this to happen. In this context, it is often found to be supportive if, in peaceful surroundings, the parents listen to the child's craniosacral rhythm and invite a still point. Children also often like to lie on their side for treatment (see p. 202).

Craniosacral therapy encourages children in all growth and transformation processes. Particularly after falls, accidents, shocks, as well as before or after surgery, craniosacral therapy is recommended to avoid compensatory dysfunctions and later illnesses and to promote good health overall. Compression and positional anomalies of the cranial bones have been detected in many children with concentration and learning difficulties.

Before craniosacral therapy or a series of sessions, the desires and expectations of parents *and* children should be addressed. I personally set great store by voluntary compliance. It is usually counter-productive to force a child into something, possibly because the parents wish it. I touch and treat children only if they wish me to and for as long as they permit.

The transformation through to greater calm and relaxation can often be perceived even while the treatment is in progress. Sometimes it may take several sessions before the child gets used to it and the craniosacral system accepts the invitation to release offered by the practitioner. Changes are indicated by a freer, more balanced craniosacral rhythm, altered pulmonary respiration, altered musculoskeletal tone, or falling asleep. Treatment may also simultaneously affect the emotional level in that children become happier, easier, more vibrant, develop new aspects to their personality, become more creative or sociable, or define themselves increasingly in a healthy manner and communicate their needs.

Provided that the framework conditions are defined and the practitioner supports the baby, child or adolescent respectfully in spontaneous relaxation, trust is strengthened (and attention is perhaps no longer fixed on peripheral phenomena) and the way is opened up again to a natural inner reconnection with the essential core. If the child's contact with reference persons and its immediate environment (and the expression of this) is encouraged, and if its capacity for inward flow and connectedness is strengthened, then the body as a whole is better able to regulate itself, to heal itself and to remain healthy.

Because body, mind, and spirit form a unit, harmonization on one level also always has a supportive and healing effect on other levels.

Recent years have witnessed the publication of several books on craniosacral therapy for babies and children. The subject of pre- and perinatal psychology and trauma healing has also produced its own extensive literature (see Further Reading).

Tooth and jaw problems 6.3

There can be hardly anyone who does not have unpleasant memories of going to the dentist. For some people, because of past experiences, just thinking about it is enough: their nervous system undergoes marked instinctive activation, their pulse rate quickens and endogenous stress hormones are circulated throughout their body in their bloodstream and cerebrospinal fluid (CSF). Against this background, it probably comes as a surprise and an incredible relief to many clients when they experience entirely new types of touch and sensation in and around their mouth during craniosacral therapy.

In clients with tooth and jaw problems, treatment should always include the pelvis/sacrum, torso and in particular the region from about vertebra Th5 up to the cranial base, together with the hyoid bone and atlanto-occipital joint release.

Preferential chewing on one side may cause major tension in the muscles on that side. The particular cranial and facial bones to which tense muscles are attached may therefore be impeded in their natural craniosacral motion. A temporomandibular joint (TMJ) dysfunction is very unpleasant and TMJ restrictions can be extremely painful.

Following a blow to the head, for example, the cranial bones will seek to achieve the best possible compensatory configuration. In a worst-case scenario, the position of the temporal bones may be altered: as a result, the TMJs will have a different angle of inclination and this will have implications for the lower jaw and lead to problems affecting the concerted action of the upper and lower jaw. Releasing restrictions in the lower and upper jaw may have repercussions on the craniosacral motion of the temporal bones, and vice versa. In some cases, orthodontic work to correct tooth and jaw problems may result in feelings of compression, headache, learning difficulties or a reduced blood supply to the brain and, where restrictions persist for many years, in organic disease (among other things, due to an underactive or overactive pituitary).

Many children and adolescents have orthodontic work done. This may be advisable on prosthetic grounds but may restrict the natural free motion of the craniosacral rhythm. The reduction in craniosacral motion at the maxillae also has repercussions on the sphenoid and this in turn has implications for the entire cranial base and indirectly for the sacrum. In children and adolescents, the bones are still relatively flexible and therefore can be molded. Necessary corrections have been achieved in many cases through regular craniosacral therapy sessions, including intraoral work and harmonization of the entire craniosacral system. This is not always possible but it is often worth attempting a course of 4–9 sessions. If craniosacral therapy fails to achieve the desired optimal correction, experience indicates that subsequent orthodontic correction is at least better tolerated and compensated. In any event, the sessions will have an ongoing effect in many parts of the body and the entire craniosacral system and the individual as a whole will become more balanced.

Of course, teeth must sit firmly and yet be flexible at the same time to absorb any impact that may occur. Therefore unwinding can be supported at each individual tooth.

In light of this, it is desirable for dentists, dental assistants, and orthodontists to acquire some knowledge of craniosacral therapy or to collaborate increasingly with experienced craniosacral practitioners so as to broaden the range of treatment options for the benefit of children and adults.

Accidents and illnesses 6.4

Illnesses can often be an expression of loss of polarity and wholeness at one and the same time, or of a prolonged imbalance between 'inside' and 'outside', activity and passivity. Symptoms or illnesses may also be seen as an attempt by our nervous system/body to prevent further fragmentation.

Precise allopathic medical diagnosis and a physician's referral are required following accidents or in the event of illness. The craniosacral practitioner treats each person as an individual. This involves resource-oriented, interactive therapeutic dialog and support for the client's process, perhaps incorporating specific advanced techniques. In many cases, to facilitate optimum recovery, an understanding of trauma healing is very important for treatment following an *accident* or *surgery* or in chronic health problems. There is no standard treatment for each individual indication because it is the person and his or her craniosacral system that is being treated. Each person responds differently to craniosacral therapy.

It is the whole treatment, which acts on the different body systems and so is helpful in a wide range of health problems.

The extensive variety of advanced techniques offers additional highly effective options to successfully alleviate illnesses and the consequences of accidents and to bolster self-healing. Even partial success can often be very valuable. *For patients in a persistent vegetative state*, it is helpful if spasms can be reduced and minimized. For patients, *the alleviation of pain* (and with it the possible reduction or discontinuation of medication) is a major plus factor.

In the treatment of *whiplash injury*, for example inviting still points at the feet or gentle treatment of the connective tissues with the client side-lying can have a calming effect. However, there are cases in which the body has first to recover from the shock and cannot tolerate any touch on the torso or head. In such circumstances, peripheral craniosacral touch with resource-oriented therapeutic dialog is helpful. As far as I am concerned, regions that feel unpleasant should not be treated until the client's resources have been sufficiently strengthened and touch is desired, even if this does not happen until 2–6 weeks after the event. In any case, it is better to start at the periphery (e.g. feet, legs, pelvis, sacrum, possibly also respiratory diaphragm, thorax, arms. *Note*: make sure your client's head is supported) and not to treat for too long to begin with (this will be different for each individual, e.g. 20–40 min). In this way, you can first assess the reaction of the affected region to release before establishing with the client whether and how her shoulder, neck and head can be gently touched. This type of indication requires extensive experience and an unhurried, patient approach on the part of the craniosacral practitioner.

Before or after *surgery*, craniosacral therapy helps the client to cope. Before surgery, perform connective tissue release so that less tissue becomes tense and affected. After surgery, craniosacral therapy promotes wound healing, and the cells are able to discharge the trauma.

In the fields of rehabilitation, in nursing care and pain clinics (in Switzerland and in a few European countries), amazing treatment successes are increasingly being reported following craniosacral therapy.

6.5 Shock, trauma, and post-traumatic stress syndrome

In many cases, a shock or trauma experienced in the past can be the underlying, hidden cause of symptoms, illnesses, and seemingly tragic accidents. In such circumstances, we tend to speak about a post-traumatic stress syndrome (PTSS). If a symptom in an allopathic medical diagnosis is considered and treated merely in a fragmented, isolated way instead of holistically, there is little prospect of success in the long term and any success that is achieved will be short-lived. There are still allopathic medical treatment modalities that merely combat symptoms; if the underlying cause is not identified and dealt with, these symptoms will re-surface later in a new form or as syndromes. Sadly, although it is often not recognized as such, the true cause of constantly recurring health problems, illnesses, and accidents may be a hidden PTSS, and in extreme cases, this can lead to absence from work and invalidity.

Fear is a normal emotion that is part and parcel of life. It is important for survival and forms an 'alarm system' that protects us from danger. Nature has given us the ability to sense fear and pain. However, the rapidity, frequency, and intensity with which these emotions flare up – and whether in the circumstances they are justified or without foundation – will vary from person to person and depend on past experiences and how these have been handled. If permanent or fairly prolonged, fears and anxieties will produce feelings of tension, sweating, dizziness, headache or stomach ache, digestive problems, heart ailments, panic attacks, and sleep disturbances. The loss of any sense of security after a severe shock may lead to an anxiety disorder: excessive anxious tension remains in the body and expresses itself in the form of symptoms – the body itself becomes a source of danger. Such patients tend to do the rounds from physician to physician or give up completely. A resource- and solution-oriented treatment approach helps these people to regain their self-confidence, to assume personal responsibility and to draw on fresh reserves of trust.

Instead of bottling up and suppressing anxiety and having to mount a permanent and excessive defense strategy, it is more helpful to expose the nervous system to new, positive experiences. Patients who have undergone severe trauma or PTSS have often lost a healthy relationship with fear; they feel overwhelmed and helpless and compensate by adopting the other extreme. Their mind is powerless against imagined dangers – and with time, their anxiety becomes transferred to other areas of their life. In many cases, such people feel that their ability to handle stress has diminished and that they can no longer cope with the demands of their private or professional lives. They feel overstretched by the pace of the age in which we live, and this may generate fears about losing their job or their social status, for example, which in turn produces new anxieties or deepens pre-existing ones. Illnesses may also intensify anxiety or a sense of being threatened.

Trauma constitutes a violation of our borders. It is also a sign of 'too fast and too much': our conscious mind becomes too rapidly overwhelmed by intense impressions and it rigidifies or collapses. Shock is also a protective mechanism against too much pain or being inundated with even more stimuli. In the wake of shock and trauma, it is often the case that defense and avoidance strategies (to fend off fears) assume a central role. It would be useful here to work with an experienced practitioner to develop the individual's resources. In such therapy, the emotions that provoke fear can be felt briefly, and then the individual's resources can be deliberately tapped again and their surroundings perceived. This has the effect of scaling down the fear and in due course enables the trauma to be transformed.

As a practitioner, it is important to remain present, to maintain a safe space and to go with the client's timing – in particular, this should be unhurried to allow the client to perceive the positives – instead of you wanting to achieve something or allowing yourself to be carried away by the rapidity of the trauma.

For the client (and for the practitioner), a deepened physical awareness of personal resources in the safety of the here and now also forms an antithesis to the traumatic memory and provides the basis for lasting trauma healing.

Recent insights into the healing of shock and trauma have also enriched the resource- and solution-oriented body therapies that work with momentary bodily sensations – especially with the activation and deactivation of the nervous system – rather than with overly intellectualized, rational analysis. A great many body therapists and psychotherapists have acquired knowledge and experience in trauma healing.

Personal shock and trauma

Recent research has shown that even before birth, the unborn child is able to pick up on its mother's surroundings and emotional state via her hormones and using its own senses. The child's nervous system is already starting to develop and take shape before birth. Pre- and perinatal complications (see p. 307) will have a varyingly traumatizing effect on the fetus or newborn child, with highly individual implications for body, mind and spirit.

During the various phases of the child's physical, mental, and spiritual development, sudden unforeseen events may occur that cause the child to be overwhelmed, shocked, paralyzed, frozen with fear, or traumatized – this may be a physical injury due to external force or a deep emotional shock. The child's life force is often so strong that in the best-case scenario it can express its feelings and then forget the incident and grow out of it.

Fortunately, we humans have at our disposal various conscious and subconscious options for handling shock and trauma. We are able to accept that there has been a serious infringement and violation of our borders and, with professional help, we deliberately face up to the past event – or we efficiently repress it for as long as we can, make compensatory adjustments and at some point even appear to 'forget' it. However, our body remembers shocking, traumatic events from the past: our body incorporates them into its structure, right down to the level of cell memory. As a result, for example, the free flow of vital energy and of all body fluids may be impaired. Miraculously, however, numerous self-regulatory mechanisms efficiently help to compensate for trauma at a bodily level.

Falls while learning to walk and ride a bicycle, accidents sustained in the course of leisure activities, sport, hobbies and work, as well as deep-rooted psychological shocks and trauma – all of these add up to reducing the life force and its strength of expression. The implications of this, i.e. the body's efficiency at making compensatory adjustments, are reflected among other things also in the strength of expression of the craniosacral rhythm and in its qualities (strength, amplitude, symmetry, cyclic form).

Similarly, *our subconscious, our instinct, and our nervous system* have never forgotten anything that is (life-)threatening. Motivated by fear and in order to protect us from further shock or trauma (or to weaken their effects in a timely manner), these faculties are on permanent 24/7 alert – often even years later, when the event itself has long been forgotten.

When difficult and stressful life phases or new traumatic situations arise over the course of time, our past experiences may be *reactivated and experienced again with similar intensity*. For example, depending on the particular situation, our nervous system may become highly agitated (fight or flight response, often associated with a marked increase in muscle tone) or paradoxically it may quickly start to shut down, in a kind of 'playing dead' reflex, characterized by rigidity or flaccidity.

Suppressing past events may give temporary protection against further trauma. The suppression or compensation of past trauma on the one hand and the ongoing desire to prevent fresh trauma on the other both absorb a huge amount of strength and attention. People who have been severely traumatized are often no longer able to cope with stress to the same degree, their immune system is more labile and their health is therefore chronically under attack. If such individuals do not seek professional help, the true cause of symptoms and illnesses is rarely resolved. In fact, the very opposite happens: the cause is suppressed – with momentous consequences – and the symptoms are addressed superficially. Because such people are less robust, the resultant associated stress tends in turn to reinforce adverse trends: e.g. the body subjectively announces stress even though there appear to be no outward signs of stress at all. Consequently, the body as a whole, including the nervous and hormonal systems, is 'whipped up' by endogenous endorphins.

There are people who are addicted to regular 'kicks' of adrenaline/ noradrenaline and endorphin. The body – which is in fact a complex miracle – cannot be perpetually used like a machine without allowing it to compensate appropriately and naturally.

Basically, this *'no longer feeling secure' reduces our capacity for deep relaxation and self-regulation*. Unresolved issues remain pent-up on a physical, energetic, and mental–spiritual level and subsequently present themselves to us personally (or to our immediate environment) in different guises – perhaps as an opportunity for growth so that we can become more aware or healthy in the sense of 'whole'.

Via the bodily level – relaxed and inviting – the craniosacral practitioner is in direct contact with the client's nervous system where the shocks and trauma of the past are stored. Old wounds sustained on a physical, mental or spiritual level can heal: instead of being viewed as fragments in isolation, the body as a whole is increasingly rediscovered as a unity or, put another way, the 'body-mind-spirit' continuum is directly *experienced as a unity*. The nervous system stores these new positive sensations.

Collective shock and trauma

Examples of collective trauma are not only familiar to us from history books or from the last century. They may involve smaller or larger groups or communities, people living in villages, towns, districts, nations, and entire continents – in fact anyone, regardless of skin color, culture, religion, and social status.

Concrete examples include: a multi-vehicle pile-up on the motorway; witnessing a hold-up with hostage-taking; a plane crash over a built-up area; a ceiling collapse at an indoor swimming pool during public opening hours; a catastrophe alarm following a chemicals accident; the abduction and murder of well-known celebrities; kidnapping of schoolchildren and teachers, theatre-goers or members of parliament.

For the civilian population affected, the repercussions of war constitute a personal and collective trauma of incalculable magnitude. People killed or wounded in war as well as their relatives, together with thousands of displaced military families, and war veterans poisoned by chemical weapons are all victims of collective trauma.

The victims of terrorist attacks, their families and numerous emergency service workers may be collectively traumatized, in most cases for life and in a radical way. Here too it is often the case that those affected no longer feel safe, are hardly able to relax any more and are unable to recharge their batteries adequately.

In recent decades, certain regions of our world have also been plagued increasingly by environmental and natural disasters: earthquakes and tsunamis, tidal waves, flood disasters, avalanches, storms, and hurricanes. Of course, such events have always happened and yet the human contribution to the growing accumulation of such catastrophes, e.g. following decades of underground bomb tests or climate change/global warming, is less and less in dispute because it has been scientifically proven and corroborated. Glaciers that have been there for millennia are melting at an alarming rate, and there is currently much evidence to suggest that these natural disasters are on the increase.

I draw attention to this collective trauma potential because as 'human animals' (a term coined by Wilhelm Reich) we are all – together with the flora and fauna – affected by this, both locally as well as globally. As individuals, we can bring only limited influence to bear on this situation and we find ourselves relatively helpless in the face of all these phenomena.

In the meantime, however, through trauma healing and resource-oriented body therapies as well as craniosacral therapy, we have at our disposal tried and tested methods with which the effects and consequences of personal and collective shock and trauma can be reduced or transformed. As well as signifying the start of a lasting change, leading to fresh hope and greater joy, to calmness and confidence in life and existence, this can also bring with it a transforming effect. The greater our personal and collective understanding of systemic and traumatological relationships and dynamics, the more effectively and naturally we will be able to help our fellow human beings to process personal and collective trauma.

6.6 Combination with methods of allopathic and energy medicine

Many body therapists and physiotherapists treat health problems using craniosacral therapy. It is an effective supplementary option, particularly in cases where classic therapies do not bring any improvement. Appropriately trained health practitioners, naturopaths and ancillary medical staff also successfully employ the gentle art of craniosacral therapy.

Therapeutic modalities such as kinesiology or polarity therapy have integrated aspects of craniosacral therapy and cranial osteopathy into their training and treatment. In numerous other forms of 'hands-on' treatment, e.g. massage, lymph drainage, Rolfing, shiatsu or Reiki, craniosacral therapy is used as an add-on feature in that practitioners also listen to the craniosacral rhythm and specifically and gently release restrictions in the craniosacral system.

Body-oriented therapies such as Feldenkrais, Alexander technique or sensory awareness operate principally using an instructional approach, perception and body awareness. They can be supplemented and amplified with craniosacral therapy. Because craniosacral therapy and its perceptual and self-help exercises promote the life force and its flow, it is also readily used by experienced practitioners of yoga, Tai Chi or Qigong.

Massaging the feet (e.g. reflexology, antenatal foot massage) can be supplemented with the craniosacral method by palpating the craniosacral rhythm and inviting a still point at the feet. Chiropractors, atlas therapists and practitioners of the Dorn-Breuss back massage method value craniosacral therapy as a combination method or as a gentle alternative.

Speech therapists, occupational therapists, and special needs teachers also attend craniosacral courses to enable them to use this gentle body therapy – possibly in combination with their traditional rehabilitative methods – in children, adolescents and adults.

In craniosacral therapy, a key emphasis is placed on harmonizing the craniosacral system and those structures associated with it. At the same time, the practitioner's hands are occasionally placed on the chakras (energy centers in the body), on acupuncture points at meridians, or on the marma points of Ayurveda massage. These 'subtle energy' body systems – known in Asia for thousands of years – are gently balanced as the motion of the craniosacral rhythm becomes freer and stronger.

Unfortunately, broad labels such as 'Craniosacral treatment', 'Craniosacral therapy' and the like may also include practices that are only remotely connected with the true principles of the method (e.g. 'structure and function affect each other mutually') or that adhere too rigidly to a dogmatic concept.

Treatments are often offered by unqualified individuals with little first-hand experience of training courses, practical implementation or personal exposure to the techniques involved.

Even though the craniosacral method can be combined with other modalities, it is important not to mix too many treatment methods with each other: our body and its subtle energy system should not be irritated or 'overdosed' with too many impulses or stimuli.

To me, it seems extremely important that craniosacral therapy with all its demands should be comprehensively learned and practiced under expert guidance before it is combined free-style and mixed (too early) with other methods. For the practitioner as well as the client, it is advisable to start by treating or being treated comprehensively with one method, so as to be able to establish whether – and how – a particular treatment method and approach is effective.

6.7 Treating animals

All mammals have a craniosacral system and hence a craniosacral rhythm. Animal healers with experience in the craniosacral method also use this in animals, especially domestic pets. In horses, craniosacral therapy is particularly suitable in combination with the Tellington (TTouch®) method. Osteopaths, as well as craniosacral therapists have reported success in treating horses that are particularly nervous or suffer from autonomic disturbances.

I personally have occasionally had opportunities to treat cats and dogs spontaneously on my garden terrace, on walks in the countryside, or when I am on vacation. Here too my activity is governed by respect for the animal, and its willing compliance. Animals will very quickly let you know whether and for how long they wish to be touched.

Once when I was on vacation, a dog suffering from chronic digestive problems and occasional loss of appetite regularly came up to me and my partner (who is also experienced in craniosacral and visceral therapy) and allowed itself to be 'treated' by us. The animal would usually lie down on its side or even on its back and often rolled its eyes blissfully while stretching and yawning. Then it became quiet and receptive to our craniosacral touch. It was noticeable how it was able to connect internally and how its pulmonary respiratory rhythm changed after a short time, on each occasion accompanied by occasional slow exhalation. Clearly audible gastrointestinal sounds developed, and the dog's mood became peaceful and quiet. Occasionally it would change position, so indicating to us those places where it also wanted to be touched. In this way, we sometimes specifically treated organs, body segments, transverse connective tissue layers, the sacral region, and masseter muscles. The sessions often concluded with the dog rolling over several times and performing some 'yoga-like' tricks, before stretching and yawning, getting up and trotting off.

On the day after the very first session, we discovered from the dog's owner that the animal had regained its appetite and wanted to eat. After 3 weeks and several touch sessions, in each case 'requested' by the dog, its eating and digestive problems had disappeared completely and permanently. Thanks to these sessions, coupled with a change of diet, treatment with expensive chemical medication became unnecessary. The dog's restless, aggressive and loud behavior faded, to be replaced by a more even underlying temperament.

Cats too enjoy this kind of touch, for example, in the region of the occiput and sacrum, and around their neck and masticatory muscles. They often clearly indicate where and for how long they wish to be touched, and they accompany this by purring, yawning and sinking into a deeply relaxed, semi-sleeping state.

In animals too, there are benefits to be derived from this unhurried, unobtrusive touch therapy based on voluntary participation. We make this touch therapy available but do not impose.

6.8 Concluding remarks

Many health problems can be avoided if we allow ourselves sufficient time to relax naturally. This has the effect of supporting our day-to-day autonomic balance, which regulates numerous body functions. Provided that our body's signals are recognized and we act accordingly, the result will be less tension and dysfunction. This is helpful for the craniosacral system, craniosacral rhythm and homeostasis. Rhythm and motion are of core significance for healing and health.

Perhaps you might like to try an experiment: Now and every hour on the hour check to see which muscles you are tensing excessively and needlessly, and let them relax. Is your lower jaw relaxed? Yawning, for example, is very healthy but is often stifled. Are your buttock muscles relaxed or clenched? Does the weight of your body draw you down? Does your sternum move slightly each time you breathe in and out?

Instead of persisting in unhealthy habits, we can do ourselves a world of good by pursuing healthy habits such as yawning, having a good stretch, self-massage, swimming, walking, and taking notice of the natural world around us. Treat yourself occasionally to a craniosacral therapy session before the processes of self-regulation and natural deep relaxation start to decline.

As a supplement to craniosacral sessions delivered by a practitioner, the self-treatment techniques described in this volume – if used regularly – will promote the craniosacral rhythm and re-balance the autonomic nervous system. Simply listening to the different slow rhythms in our body is a relaxing inner journey and has a regenerating effect. In the main, preventive healthcare starts with ourselves. It does not need to be complicated or expensive – quite the opposite, in fact: it can bring relaxation, have an element of fun to it, and help to foster an attentive approach to ourselves and others.

In this way, craniosacral therapy and craniosacral self-treatment techniques – both of which operate using the element of perception in the sense of 'awareness through touch' – become more than just a successful way of combating symptoms. They enable us to connect increasingly with our inner core, and to sense in the here and now our body-mind-spirit unity, while at the same time experiencing this unity as part of a greater whole. Out of this natural experience of non-separate-ness, of connected-ness (being whole = being healthy) and out of stillness, we develop strength, attentiveness, respect for the miracle of life, and a renewed zest for living. Mental and emotional experiences increasingly foster our personal growth, our inner understanding and spiritual experience. And like children, we will regain a sense of wonder at everything we can perceive as sentient beings.

When we listen to our breath and to the slower rhythms of our body, we are directly in contact with health, with vitality, and with an expression of the Breath of Life, which constantly animates us with the divine spark.

Appendices

Craniosacral treatment record

Client's name:		Health insurance provider:
Address:		Details of any surgery:
Post code and town:		
Private tel.:	Work tel.:	Details of any accidents:
Mobile:	E-mail:	
Date:	Session no.:	Other information:
Practitioner's name:		
Treatment requested by:		Treatment duration:

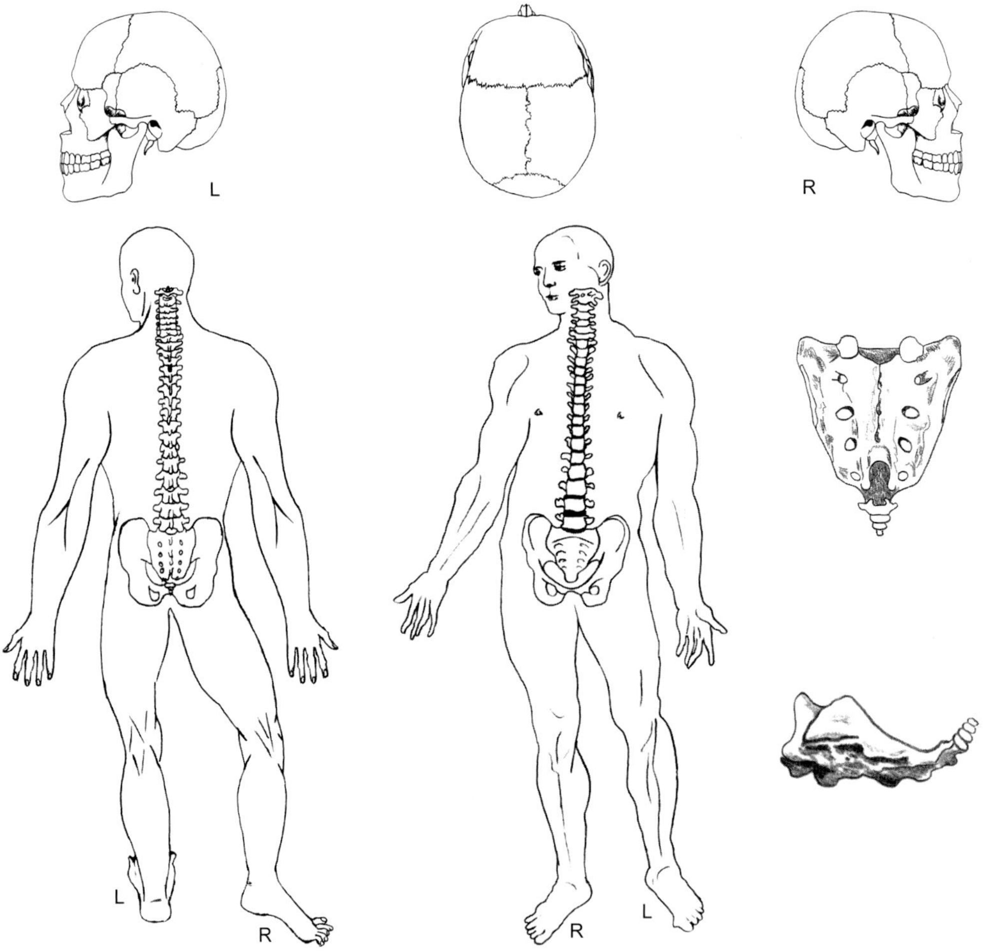

Fl.	Flexion	+	Free CS rhythm		Direction of connective tissue/ musculoskeletal traction
Ex.	Extension		CS rhythm easy to palpate		Alarm point(s), pain point(s)
ER	External rotation	−	CS rhythm restricted		Point(s) of attention
IR	Internal rotation		Amplitude of CS rhythm	IF	Inertial fulcrum (energy cyst)
			Amplitude of CS rhythm and restrictions	a/p	anterior/posterior

Application/treatment

Initial dialog + brief history (detailed initial history on separate sheet)	What the practitioner detects	What the client feels/expresses
Listening stations		
Treatment sequence (torso, neck, head, extremities)		
Other comments		
Finishing-off		
Follow-up dialog		
Notes for next session		
Inner reflection: time management, other		

© Sphinx Craniosacral Institute

A list of indications

The word 'Indications' here is used in the broader sense of 'When is craniosacral therapy appropriate?' and not just in the medical–pathological sense.

It is not possible here to go into detail about the specific treatment of individual medical conditions. This book is intended primarily as an entry-level text to the treatment of healthy individuals. For the specific treatment of medical conditions, comprehensive basic training and in-depth experience are indispensable.

Several treatment options are presented in this book. With regular treatment sessions you will support the *craniosacral system as a whole*, and over the ensuing days, weeks and months this has positive implications for all the indications listed. There is little to recommend the exclusive use of individual techniques in isolation because their possible consequences can be assessed only by practitioners. Wherever possible, the goal should be for the craniosacral rhythm to become *more balanced in the system as a whole* once you have completed one (or many) structural treatment session(s).

- Only ever treat to the level of your experience.

  Before craniosacral therapy, medical clarification is required where clients are ill or have experienced longer periods of poor health. In such circumstances any treatment should be implemented as instructed by a physician/naturopath.

  It is essential that you note the contra-indications listed in Chapter 1.8

Indications for craniosacral therapy include:

Accidents
Addiction
Allergies
Anemia
Anxiety states
Apathy
Asthma

Back pain
Back problems
Balance disorders
Birth trauma
Breathing difficulties
Bronchitis
Burn-out syndrome

Cardiovascular problems
Carpal tunnel syndrome
Chest tightness
Childbirth, preparing for and aftercare
Circulation, unstable
Coldness, sensations of
Coma
Concentration problems
Constipation

Dental alignment problems
Depression
Diabetes
Digestive problems
Dizziness
Down's syndrome
Dysfunctions, chronic

Ear problems
Emotional trauma
Eye problems, chronic
Exhaustion states

Facial palsy
Falls
Fear of flying
Fever
Frontal sinuses, blocked,
Frontal sinuses, inflamed

Gastric upset
Gastritis (not acute inflammation)

Headache
Hearing disorders
Hip problems
Hormonal disorders
Hyperactivity
Hypertension

Immune system, to boost defences
Impotence
Increased muscle tone
Inflammation, chronic

Jet lag
Joint problems and restrictions

Kyphosis

Learning difficulties
Libido, disturbed
Lumbago

Menstrual problems
Mercury poisoning, consequences of
Metabolic disorders
Migraine
Motor disturbances
Muscle tension (hypertonus)

Nervousness
Neuralgia, chronic

Organic brain syndrome
Organs, chronic complaints
Overwork

Pain, chronic
Pain symptoms without pathological findings
Palpitations
Panic attacks
Paralysis, signs of
Paranasal sinuses, blocked
Paranasal sinuses, inflamed
Pelvic tilt
Phantom limb pain
Postnatal period, immediate
Postural problems
Pregnancy (no still points, see Contraindications)
Prolapsed intervertebral disc
Psychological problems
Psychosomatic complaints
Psychovegetative disorders

Reading and writing difficulties
Recovery, aid to
Regeneration
Relaxation, promotion of

Scarring
Scheuermann's disease
Scoliosis
Self-healing forces, strengthening of
Sense of smell, impaired
Sensitivity to light
Shock sequelae
Skin problems
Sleep disturbances
Spasms
Speech disorders
Spinal problems (scoliosis, lordosis, kyphosis)
Squint
Stiff neck
Stomach complaints
Stress
Stutter
Surgery, preparation for and aftercare
Swallowing difficulties

Teeth grinding (bruxism)
Temperature sensation, disturbed
Tendon sheath inflammation
Tennis arm (tennis elbow)
Tinnitus (ringing in the ears)
Tiredness, chronic
Temporomandibular joint (TMJ) problems
Torticollis
Trigeminal neuralgia

Uneasy feelings

Vision disturbances
Vomiting

Whiplash injury

As described in Chapter 1.8, a distinction is made between absolute and relative contraindications. Please read through the comments there carefully. It will depend on a variety of client- and practitioner-related factors as to whether treatment for medical conditions such as Alzheimer's disease, Parkinson's disease, multiple sclerosis, epilepsy, Crohn's disease, and certain central nervous system (CNS) disorders is recommended or contraindicated.

At this point, it is recommended as a precautionary measure that you do *not* treat potential clients suffering from these medical conditions. As an exception to this general rule, this statement does not apply if you have many years' experience with these medical conditions and with craniosacral therapy and you are delivering the treatment on the instructions of a physician.

Observance of a duty of care is important for you, your client, the further spread of craniosacral therapy and for naturopathic medicine as a whole. As a practitioner, if there is the *merest suspicion* that something is not right with a client, you have an obligation to withhold treatment until an allopathic medical diagnosis has been made and the client has been referred by a physician.

The treatment and ongoing care of people who are the victims of tragedy, shock, and trauma demands many years of professional experience – also to ensure practitioner protection so that you do not overtax yourself and so that you yourself stay healthy. You must take full responsibility for any treatment you give.

Glossary

ADD	Attention deficit disorder
ADHD	Attention deficit hyperactivity disorder
Amplitude	Breadth of range, width
Anatomy	Science of the structure of the body and its parts
Anterior	Toward the ventral surface of the body, from the middle forward
Aqueduct, cerebral of mesencephalon of Sylvius	Narrow channel carrying CSF from the third to the fourth cerebral ventricle
Arachnoid (mater)	Delicate membrane between the dura mater and pia mater
Atlas	First cervical vertebra
Atlanto-occipital joint	Articulation between the atlas and the occiput
Autonomic	Self-controlling, functionally independent, not under voluntary control
Autonomic nervous system (ANS)	The totality of nerves and ganglial cells not subject to the control of the will and the conscious mind
Breath of Life	A term coined by Dr W.G. Sutherland to denote our essential life force
Bregma	Point on the skull surface at the junction of the coronal and sagittal sutures
C	Denoting vertebrae in the cervical spine (C1–7 = cervical vertebrae 1–7)
Calvaria	Cranial vault
Caudal	Downward, denoting the inferior end of the body (from L. cauda = tail)
Cell memory	Capacity of the body's cells to store past events
Choroid plexus	Infoldings of blood vessels of the pia mater, which produce CSF
CNS	Central nervous system
Compensatory	Restoring balance
Contraindication	Any circumstance that makes the use of a particular medicine or diagnostic/therapeutic procedure undesirable
Corpus amygdaloideum	Amygdaloid body, a part of the limbic system
Cranial	Upward, toward the (top of the) head
Cranium	Skull
CSF	Cerebrospinal fluid

Decompression	Relief of pressure
Diagonal	Having an oblique direction, slanting
Diametric	Opposite
Diaphragm	Respiratory diaphragm; or more generally, a transverse separating structure
Diencephalon	Interbrain
Dorsal	Toward the back, posterior
Dura mater encephali	Dura mater covering the brain
Dura mater spinalis	Dura mater covering the spinal cord, the dural tube
Dysfunction	A disturbance, impairment or abnormality of function
ER/IR	External rotation/internal rotation (outer–inner rotation)
Encephalon	The brain
Endocrine system	The hormonal system
Energy cyst	Entrapped trauma energy, inertial fulcrum
Epiphysis	Pineal body or gland
Extension	Stretching, drawing apart
Falx cerebelli	The small fold of dura mater in the midline of the posterior cranial fossa
Falx cerebri	The sickle-shaped fold of dura mater extending downward in the longitudinal cerebral fissure
Fascia	A sheet or band of connective tissue
Flexion	Bending
Foramen magnum	The large opening in the anterior and inferior part of the occiput
Fulcrum	A point around which motion takes place
Humoral physiology	The science of the body fluids
Hypophysis	Pituitary gland
Hypothalamus	The ventral part of the diencephalon, the center controlling and integrating the autonomic nervous system
Indication	A sign or circumstance suggesting a remedial course of action, a reason for using a particular diagnostic or therapeutic procedure
Inertial fulcrum	A place of stasis containing unresolved forces that organize patterns of restriction in the body
Intracranial membranes	In particular, the vertical and horizontal membranes that envelope the brain
Intraoral	Inside the mouth
Lateral	To the side, away from the midline of a structure
Lesion	Any pathological or traumatic disturbance or loss of function
Ligament	A band of fibrous tissues that connects bones or cartilages
Long tide	Expression of the Breath of Life that moves rhythmically at about 100 seconds/cycle

LS	Lumbar spine
L1–L5	Lumbar vertebrae 1–5
L5–S1	Lumbar vertebra 5–sacral vertebra 1, the lumbosacral junction
Medial	Toward the midline of the body
Meninges	The membranes covering the brain and spinal cord
Mid-tide	An expression of the Breath of Life, having a rhythmic motion of 2–3 cycles/min
Mobility	Movement of one structure in relation to another
Motility	Inherent motion
Motor	Producing motion
Multiple hands-on	Treatment by more than one practitioner
Muscle:	
masseter	main masticatory muscle in the cheek
pterygoid	wing-shaped masticatory muscle
rectus abdominis	large abdominal muscle
temporalis	temporalis muscle, one of the masticatory muscles
Neurocranium	Part of the cranium that encloses the brain
Occlusion	Degree of closure achieved by the contact surfaces of the teeth in the upper and lower jaws
Palpate	To examine by touch
Palpation	The act of sensing through the hands/fingers
Pathological	Indicative of or caused by disease or illness
Peristalsis	The movement by which the gastrointestinal tract propels its contents
Pia mater	The innermost of the three membranes (meninges) covering the brain and spinal cord
Pineal gland	Epiphysis cerebri
Posterior	Toward the dorsal surface of the body, from the middle backward
Potency	Strength, force or power, also the potency in the CSF or Breath of Life
PRM	Primary respiratory mechanism
Receptors	Molecular structures within the organism characterized by selective binding and a specific physiological effect; sensory nerve terminals that respond to stimuli of various kinds
Regulation	Adjustment of the organ systems of a living organism by various control mechanisms (e.g. hormones, nerves), the autonomous adaptation of a living being to changing environmental conditions while maintaining a physiological state of equilibrium in the organism

Resorb	To take up or absorb again
Resource	Source of strength or help
Rhythm	Regular movement; periodic change, regular recurrence of natural processes
Sacroiliac joint	The joint between the iliac bone of the pelvis and the sacrum
Sacrum	The triangular bone just below the lumbar vertebrae
Salutogenesis	The body's capacity to keep itself healthy
Self-palpation	The act of self-examining by touch
Sensory	Involving or referring to the senses
Sinus	Cavity, depression or hollow space; also used to denote closed channels, dilated areas of veins and lymph vessels, and air-filled spaces in bone
Solar plexus	A prevertebral plexus located on the front and sides of the aorta
Sphenobasilar joint/ sphenobasilar synchondrosis (SBS)	Important articulation between the sphenoid and occiput
Sternum	The breastbone
Still point	A temporary pause of the craniosacral rhythm
Superior sagittal sinus	Venous sinus running on the inner surface of the cranial vault along the attachment of the falx cerebri
Sutura, suture	Cranial suture, forming a joint
Symptom	Evidence of illness, a pathological change that is characteristic of a particular disease or belongs to a particular condition
Tentorium cerebelli	The process of dura mater that supports the occipital lobes and covers the cerebellum
T	Denoting vertebrae in the thoracic spine (T1–T12 = thoracic vertebrae 1–12)
Thalamus	A large ovoid mass in the posterior part of the diencephalon forming most of each lateral wall of the third ventricle
Therapeutic pulse	A physical/energetic sign indicative of tissue relaxation
Thoracic inlet	Thoracic aperture
TMJ	Temporomandibular joint
Trochanter major	Greater trochanter, a broad flat process at the upper end of the lateral surface of the femur
Unwinding	Involuntary movements of the tissue to release tensions and entanglements
Vagus nerve	The tenth cranial nerve
Ventral	From the midline toward the front of the body

Ventricle, cerebral	A cavity within the brain (filled with CSF)
Visceral	Pertaining to the viscera
Viscerocranium	The facial bones of the skull
Visualize	To picture something in the mind's eye
Vomer	The unpaired flat bone that forms the inferior and posterior part of the nasal septum
V-spread technique	An energy-directing technique to release tension, pressure, dysfunction or pain

Further reading

Agustoni D. *Harmonizing your craniosacral system: an easy and effective self-treatment*. Findhorn Press, Forres, ISBN 1844091171

Becker RE. *The stillness of life*. Stillness Press, Portland, ISBN 0-9675851-1-2

Becker RE. *Life in motion*. Stillness Press, Portland, ISBN 0-9675851-0-4

Chaitow L. *Palpation and assessment skills: assessment through touch*. Churchill Livingstone, Edinburgh, ISBN 0-443-07218-3

Cohen D. *An introduction to craniosacral therapy: anatomy, function and treatment*. North Atlantic Books, Berkeley, ISBN 1-55643-183-X

Calais-Germain B. *Anatomy of movement*. Eastland Press, Vista, ISBN 0-939616-17-3

Damasio A. *Descartes' error: emotion, reason and the human brain*. Quill/HarperCollins, New York, ISBN 0-399-13894-3

Damasio A. *The feeling of what happens: body and emotion in the making of consciousness*. Harcourt, New York, ISBN 0-15-100369-6

Gehin A. *Atlas of manipulative techniques for the cranium and face*. Eastland Press, Vista, ISBN 0-939616-02-5

Gershon M. *The second brain*. HarperPerennial, New York, ISBN 0-06-018252-0

Grey A. *Sacred mirrors: the visionary art of Alex Grey*. Inner Traditions, Rochester, ISBN 0-89281-257-5

Handoll N. *Anatomy of potency*. Osteopathic Supplies, Hereford, ISBN 0-9511-3565-1

Heller DP, Heller LS. *Crash course: a self-healing guide to auto accident trauma and recovery*. North Atlantic Books, ISBN 1-55643-372-7

Kern, M. *Wisdom in the body*. North Atlantic Books, Berkeley, ISBN 1-55643-559-2

Levine PA, Frederick A. *Waking the tiger: healing trauma*. North Atlantic Books, Berkeley, ISBN 1-55643-233-X

Levine PA, Kline M. *Trauma through a child's eyes: awakening the ordinary miracle of healing*. North Atlantic Books, Berkeley, ISBN 1-55643-630-0

Liem T. *Craniosacral osteopathy: principles and practice*. Elsevier, Edinburgh, ISBN 0-443-07499-2

Lipton B. *The biology of belief: unleashing the power of consciousness, matter and miracles*. Mountain of Love/Elite Books, Santa Rosa, ISBN 0-9759914-7-7

Magoun HI. *Osteopathy in the cranial field*. Original edition, Sutherland Cranial Teaching Foundation, Denver, ISBN 1-930298-03-X

Milne H. *The heart of listening*. North Atlantic Books, Berkeley, ISBN 1-55643-279-8

Oschman JL. *Energy medicine: the scientific basis*. Churchill Livingstone, Edinburgh, ISBN 0-443-06261-7

Oschman JL. *Energy medicine in therapeutics and human performance*. Butterworth/Heinemann, Oxford, ISBN 0-7506-5400-7

Pert CB. *Molecules of emotion: why you feel the way you feel*. Scribner, New York, ISBN 0-684-83187-2

Sills F. *Craniosacral biodynamics: the breath of life, biodynamics and fundamental skills*. North Atlantic Books, Berkeley, ISBN 1-55643-354-9

Sills F. *Craniosacral biodynamics, Vol. 2*. North Atlantic Books, Berkeley, ISBN 1-55643-390-5

Sutherland WG. *Contributions of thought: the collected writings of WG Sutherland*. Sutherland Cranial Teaching Foundation, Rudra Press, Portland, ISBN 0-915801-74-4

Sutherland WG. *Teachings in the science of osteopathy*. Sutherland Cranial Teaching Foundation, CSTA, ISBN 0-930298-00-5

Sutherland WG. *The cranial bowl*. Free Press Company, Mankato reprint, 1939

Sutherland WG. *With thinking fingers*. The Cranial Academy, Indianapolis reprint, 1962

Upledger JE, Vredevoogd JD. *Craniosacral therapy*. Eastland Press, Vista, ISBN 0-939616-01-7

Upledger JE. *Craniosacral therapy II: Beyond the dura*. Eastland Press, Vista, ISBN 0-939616-05-X

Upledger JE. *SomatoEmotional release: deciphering the language of life*. North Atlantic Books, Berkeley, ISBN 1-55643-412-X

Upledger JE. *Cell talk: talking to your cell(f)*. North Atlantic Books, Berkeley, ISBN 1-55643-461-8

Upledger JE. *A brain is born: exploring the birth and development of the central nervous system*. North Atlantic Books, Berkeley, ISBN 1-55643-236-4

Music (a selection):

Agustoni Daniel. *Harmonizing Your Craniosacral System; 17 Exercises for Relaxation & Self-Treatment.* Findhorn Press, ISBN 978-1-84409-126-3

Deuter Chaitanya H. *REIKI – Hands of light.* New Earth Records, NE 9806-2

Deuter Chaitanya H. *Wind & Mountain, Healing music.* The Relaxation Company, CD 3183

Deuter Chaitanya H. *Sea & Silence.* New Earth Records, CD 77159

Deuter Chaitanya H. *Earth Blue.* New Earth Records, CD 77164

Deuter Chaitanya H. *Tibet, Nada Himalaya 2.* New Earth Records, CD 77176

Kamal. *Reiki Whale Song.* New Earth Records, CD 77154

Naegele David. *Temple in the Forest. Valley of the Sun.* New World Music, CD 312

Sayama. *Heart Gems Vol. 2 – Water Miracles.* Koha-Verlag, ISBN 3-936862-41-9

Wiese Klaus/de Jong, Ted, Grassow M. *El-Hadra: The Mystic Dance.* Edition Akasha

Wiese Klaus. *Monsoon,* Aquamarin Verlag CD 6872

Wiese Klaus. *Mudra,* Aquamarin Verlag, CD 6294

Contact address and useful websites

The author is available **internationally** for craniosacral courses, training and continuing professional development (courses can also be arranged in-house or for institutions).

Please address all enquiries to:

SPHINX CRANIOSACRAL INSTITUTE
P.O. Box 629
CH-4003 Basel
Switzerland

e-mail: sphinx@craniosacral.ch
homepage: www.craniosacral.ch

The following details do not constitute a recommendation but are offered solely as a gateway to further information.

Details of craniosacral therapists and practitioners on the Internet:

- **Worldwide:** www.iahp.com
- **UK:** www.cranio-sacral.org.uk
- **Ireland:** www.holisto.com
- **Switzerland:** www.craniosacralflow.ch
- **Germany:** www.craniosacralflow.de

or simply enter details into various search engines.

Craniosacral courses and training on the Internet:

- **Worldwide:** www.upledger.com
- **UK:** www.upledger.co.uk
  www.ccst.co.uk
  www.craniosacral.co.uk
- **Switzerland, Germany and other countries:** www.craniosacral.ch

or simply enter details into various search engines.

Web links:

Energy medicine, Living Matrix and the scientific background, as researched by Dr James L. Oschman: www.energyresearch.bizland.com

Research into fasciae and myofascial release, with Dr Robert Schleip: www.somatics.de

More than 90 studies on touch therapies: www.miami.edu/touch-research/

Phenomenological embryology with Dr med Jaap van der Wal: www.embryo.nl

Polyvagal theory of Prof Dr Stephen W. Porges: www.psych.uic.edu/faculty/porges.htm

Somatic Experiencing®, trauma healing as taught by Dr Peter Levine: www.traumahealing.com

Information on the spread of craniosacral therapy for children requiring care (non-profit organization): www.childrenshelp.ch

Index

References in *italic* indicate pages where a topic can be found only or mainly within a Figure.

D

E

F

L

M

N

O

P

Q

R

S

T

U

V

W

Y

Z

Harmonizing Your Craniosacral System
An Easy and Effective Self-Treatment
by Daniel Agustoni

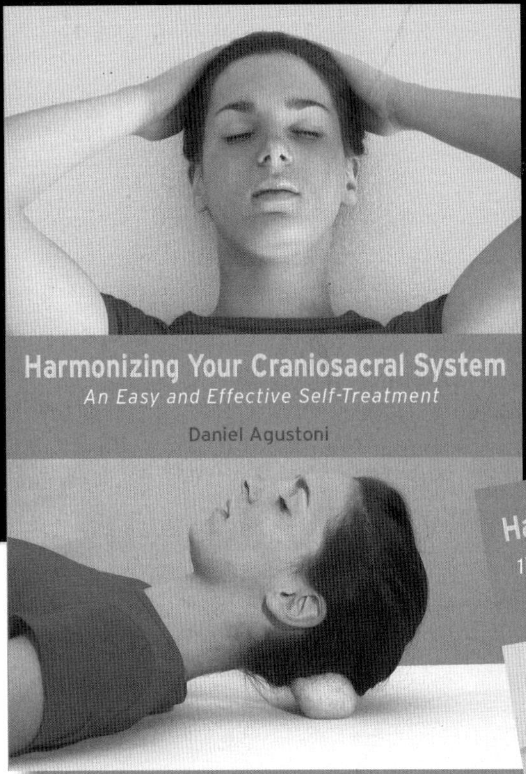

160 pages, full colour,
100 colour photographs & 9 line drawings
ISBN 978 1 844091171
£ 10.99
Publication date: November 2007

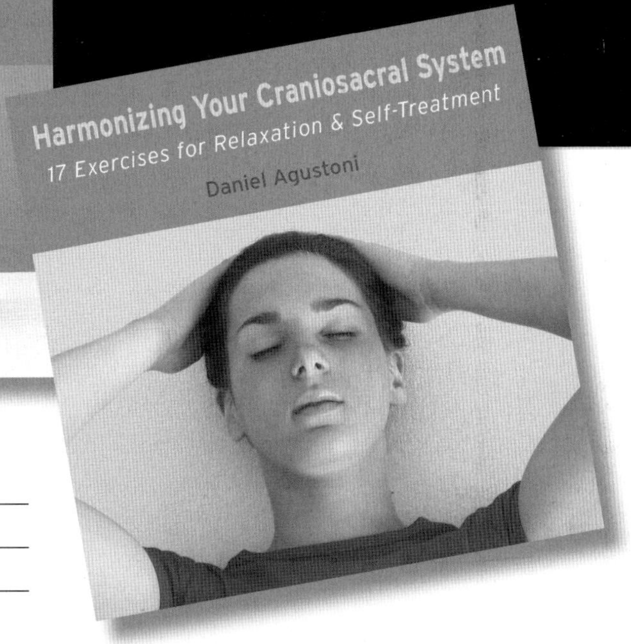

ISBN 978 1 84409 126 3
£ 12.99
Publication date: November 2007

Harmonizing Your Craniosacral System
17 Exercises for Relaxation and Self-Treatment
by Daniel Agustoni

Findhorn Press, 305a The Park, Forres IV36 3TE, Moray, Scotland, Great Britain
Phone: 0044 - 1309 - 690582 • Fax: 0044 - 1309 - 690036
E-mail: sabine@findhornpress.com • www.findhornpress.com